Disability KEY ISSUES AND FUTURE DIRECTIONS

HEALTH AND MEDICINE

The SAGE Reference Series on Disability: Key Issues and Future Directions

Series Editor: Gary L. Albrecht

Disability KEY ISSUES AND FUTURE DIRECTIONS

HEALTH AND
MEDICINE

Ross M. Mullner
University of Illinois at Chicago

SERIES EDITOR
Gary L. Albrecht
University of Illinois at Chicago

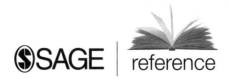

⑤SAGE | reference

Los Angeles | London | New Delhi
Singapore | Washington DC

RENFRO LIBRARY
MARS HILL COLLEGE
MARS HILL, N.C. 28754

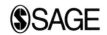

SAGE

Los Angeles | London | New Delhi
Singapore | Washington DC

FOR INFORMATION:

SAGE Publications, Inc.
2455 Teller Road
Thousand Oaks, California 91320
E-mail: order@sagepub.com

SAGE Publications Ltd.
1 Oliver's Yard
55 City Road
London EC1Y 1SP
United Kingdom

SAGE Publications India Pvt. Ltd.
B 1/I 1 Mohan Cooperative Industrial Area
Mathura Road, New Delhi 110 044
India

SAGE Publications Asia-Pacific Pte. Ltd.
33 Pekin Street #02-01
Far East Square
Singapore 048763

Publisher: Rolf A. Janke
Acquisitions Editor: Jim Brace-Thompson
Assistant to the Publisher: Michele Thompson
Project Development, Editing, & Management: Kevin Hillstrom,
    Laurie Collier Hillstrom
Production Editor: Jane Haenel
Reference Systems Manager: Leticia Gutierrez
Reference Systems Coordinator: Laura Notton
Typesetter: C&M Digitals (P) Ltd.
Proofreader: Ellen Howard
Indexer: Terri Corry
Cover Designer: Gail Buschman
Marketing Manager: Kristi Ward

Copyright © 2011 by SAGE Publications, Inc.

All rights reserved. No part of this book may be
reproduced or utilized in any form or by any
means, electronic or mechanical, including
photocopying, recording, or by any information
storage and retrieval system, without
permission in writing from the publisher.

Printed in the United States of America

Library of Congress Cataloging-in-Publication
Data

Mullner, Ross M.

Health and medicine / Ross M. Mullner.

p. cm.—(The Sage reference
series on disability: key issues and
future directions; 1)

Includes bibliographical references
and index.

ISBN 978-1-4129-8110-1 (cloth)

1. People with disabilities—Health
and hygiene. I. Title.

HV1568.M85 2011
617—dc22
2011007693

11 12 13 14 15 10 9 8 7 6 5 4 3 2 1

APR 2 4 2012 R
617
M9599h

Contents

Series Introduction

The SAGE Reference Series on Disability appears at a time when global attention is being focused on disability at all levels of society. Researchers, service providers, and policymakers are concerned with the prevalence, experience, meanings, and costs of disability because of the growing impact of disability on individuals and their families and subsequent increased demand for services (Banta & de Wit, 2008; Martin et al., 2010; Mont, 2007; Whitaker, 2010). For their part, disabled people and their families are keenly interested in taking a more proactive stance in recognizing and dealing with disability in their lives (Charlton, 1998; Iezzoni & O'Day, 2006). As a result, there is burgeoning literature, heightened Web activity, myriad Internet information and discussion groups, and new policy proposals and programs designed to produce evidence and disseminate information so that people with disabilities may be informed and live more independently (see, for example, the World Institute of Disability Web site at http://www.wid.org, the Center for International Rehabilitation Research Information and Exchange Web site at http://cirrie.buffalo.edu, and the Web portal to caregiver support groups at http://www.caregiver.com/regionalresources/index.htm).

Disability is recognized as a critical medical and social problem in current society, central to the discussions of health care and social welfare policies taking place around the world. The prominence of these disability issues is highlighted by the attention given to them by the most respected national and international organizations. The *World Report on Disability* (2011), co-sponsored by the World Health Organization (WHO) and the World Bank and based on an analysis of surveys from over 100 countries, estimates that 17% of the world's population (more than 1 billion people) currently experiences disability. This is the best prevalence estimate available today and indicates a marked increase over previous epidemiological calculations. Based on this work, the British medical journal *Lancet* dedicated an entire issue (November 28, 2009) to disability, focusing attention on the salience of the problem for health care systems worldwide. In addition, the WHO has developed community-based rehabilitation principles and strategies which are applicable to communities of diverse cultures and at all levels of development (WHO, 2010). The World Bank is concerned because of the link between disability and poverty (World Bank, 2004). Disability, in their view, could be a major impediment to economic development, particularly in emerging economies.

Efforts to address the problem of disability also have legal and human rights implications. Being disabled has historically led to discrimination, stigma, and dependency, which diminish an individual's full rights to citizenship and equality (European Disability Forum, 2003). In response to these concerns, the United Nations Convention on the Rights of Persons with Disabilities (2008) and the European Union Disability Strategy embodying the Charter of Fundamental Rights (2000) were passed to affirm that disabled people have the right to acquire and change nationalities, cannot be deprived of their ability to exercise liberty, have freedom of movement, are free to leave any country including their own, are not deprived of the right to enter their own country, and have access to the welfare and benefits afforded to any citizen of their country. As of March 31, 2010, 144 nations—including the United States, China, India, and Russia—had signed the U.N. Convention, and the European Union Disability Strategy had been ratified by all members of the European Community. These international agreements supplement and elaborate disability rights legislation such as the Americans with Disabilities Act of 1990 and its amendments, the U.K. Disability Discrimination Act of 1995, and the Disabled Person's Fundamental Law of Japan, revised in 1993.

In the United States, the Institute of Medicine of the National Academy of Sciences has persistently focused attention on the medical, public health, and social policy aspects of disability in a broad-ranging series of reports: *Disability in America* (1991), *Enabling America* (1997), *The Dynamics of Disability: Measuring and Monitoring Disability for Social Security Programs*, (2002), *The Future of Disability in America* (2007), and *Improving the Presumptive Disability Decision-Making Process for Veterans* (2008). The Centers for Disease Control have a long-standing interest in diabetes and obesity because of their effects on morbidity, mortality, and disability. Current data show that the incidence and prevalence of obesity is rising across all age groups in the United States, that obesity is related to diabetes, which is also on the rise, and that both, taken together, increase the likelihood of experiencing disability (Bleich et al., 2008; Gill et al., 2010). People with diabetes also are likely to have comorbid depression, which increases their chances of functional disability (Egede, 2004).

Depression and other types of mental illness—like anxiety disorders, alcohol and drug dependence, and impulse-control disorders—are more prevalent than previously thought and often result in disability (Kessler & Wang, 2008). The prevalence of mental disorders in the United States is high, with about half of the population meeting criteria (as measured by the *Diagnostic and Statistical Manual of Mental Disorders*, or DSM-IV) for one more disorders in their lifetimes, and more than one-quarter of the population meeting criteria for a disorder in any single year. The more severe mental disorders are strongly associated with high comorbidity, resulting in disability.

Major American foundations with significant health portfolios have also turned their attention to disability. The Bill and Melinda Gates Foundation has directed considerable resources to eliminate disability-causing parasitic and communicable diseases such as malaria, elephantiasis, and river blindness. These efforts are designed to prevent and control disability-causing conditions in the developing world that inhibit personal independence and economic development. The Robert Wood Johnson Foundation has a long-standing program on self-determination for people with developmental disabilities in the United States aimed at increasing their ability to participate fully in society, and the Hogg Foundation is dedicated to improving mental health awareness and services. Taken in concert, these activities underscore the recognized importance of disability in the present world.

Disability Concepts, Models, and Theories

There is an immense literature on disability concepts, models, and theories. An in-depth look at these issues and controversies can be found in the *Handbook of Disability Studies* (Albrecht, Seelman, & Bury, 2001), in the *Encyclopedia of Disability* (Albrecht, 2006), and in "The Sociology of Disability: Historical Foundations and Future Directions" (Albrecht, 2010). For the purposes of this reference series, it is useful to know that the World Health Organization, in the *International Classification of Functioning,*

Disability and Health (ICF), defines disability as "an umbrella term for impairments, activity limitations or participation restrictions" (WHO, 2001, p. 3). ICF also lists environmental factors that interact with all these constructs. Further, the WHO defines impairments as "problems in body function or structure such as significant deviation or loss"; activity limitations as "difficulties an individual may have in executing activities"; participation as "involvement in a life situation"; and environmental factors as those components of "the physical, social and attitudinal environment in which people live and conduct their lives" (WHO, 2001, p. 10). The U.N. Convention on the Rights of Persons with Disabilities, in turn, defines disability as including "those who have long-term physical, mental, intellectual or sensory impairments which in interaction with various barriers may hinder their full and effective participation in society on an equal basis with others." In the introduction to the *Lancet* special issue on disability, Officer and Groce (2009) conclude that "both the ICF and the Convention view disability as the outcome of complex interactions between health conditions and features of an individual's physical, social, and attitudinal environment that hinder their full and effective participation in society" (p. 1795). Hence, disability scholars and activists alike are concerned with breaking down physical, environmental, economic, and social barriers so that disabled people can live independently and participate as fully as possible in society.

Types of Disability

Interest in disability by medical practitioners has traditionally been condition specific (such as spinal cord injury or disabilities due to heart disease), reflecting the medical model approach to training and disease taxonomies. Similarly, disabled people and their families are often most concerned about their particular conditions and how best to deal with them. The SAGE Reference Series on Disability recognizes that there are a broad range of disabilities that can be generally conceived of as falling in the categories of physical, mental, intellectual, and sensory disabilities. In practice, disabled persons may have more than one disability and are often difficult to place in one disability category. For instance, a spinal-cord injured individual might experience depression, and a person with multiple sclerosis may simultaneously deal with physical and sensory disabilities. It is also important to note that disabilities are dynamic. People do experience different rates of onset, progression, remission, and even transition from being disabled at one point in time, to not being disabled at another, to being disabled again. Examples of this change in disability status include disability due to bouts of arthritis, Guillain-Barré Syndrome, and postpartum depression.

Disability Language

The symbols and language used to represent disability have sparked contentious debates over the years. In the *Handbook of Disability Studies* (Albrecht, Seelman, & Bury, 2001) and the *Encyclopedia of Disability* (Albrecht, 2006), authors from different countries were encouraged to use the terms and language of their cultures, but to explain them when necessary. In the present volumes, authors may use "people with disabilities" or "disabled people" to refer to individuals experiencing disability. Scholars in the United States have preferred "people with disabilities" (people-first language), while those in the United Kingdom, Canada, and Australia generally use "disabled people." In languages other than English, scholars typically use some form of the "disabled people" idiom. The U.S. version emphasizes American exceptionalism and the individual, whereas "disabled people" highlights the group and their minority status or state of being different. In my own writing, I have chosen "disabled people" because it stresses human diversity and variation.

In a recent discussion of this issue, DePoy and Gilson (2010) "suggest that maintaining debate and argument on what language is most correct derails a larger and more profound needed change, that of equalizing resources, valuation, and respect. Moreover, . . . locating disability 'with a person' reifies its embodiment and flies in the very face of the social model that person-first language is purported to espouse. . . . We have not heard anyone suggest that beauty, kindness, or even unkindness be located after personhood." While the debate is not likely over, we state why we use the language that we do.

Organization of the Series

These issues were important in conceiving of and organizing the SAGE Reference Series on Disability. Instead of developing the series around specific disabilities resulting from Parkinson's disease or bi-polar disorder, or according to the larger categories of physical, mental, intellectual, and sensory disabilities, we decided to concentrate on the major topics that confront anyone interested in or experiencing disability. Thus, the series consists of eight volumes constructed around the following topics:

- Arts and Humanities
- Assistive Technology and Science
- Disability Through the Life Course
- Education
- Employment and Work
- Ethics, Law, and Policy
- Health and Medicine
- Rehabilitation Interventions

To provide structure, we chose to use a similar organization for each volume. Therefore, each volume contains the following elements:

Series Introduction

Preface

About the Author

About the Series Editor

Chapter 1. Introduction, Background, and History

Chapter 2. Current Issues, Controversies, and Solutions

Chapter 3. Chronology of Critical Events

Chapter 4. Biographies of Key Contributors in the Field

Chapter 5. Annotated Data, Statistics, Tables, and Graphs

Chapter 6. Annotated List of Organizations and Associations

Chapter 7. Selected Print and Electronic Resources

Glossary of Key Terms

Index

The Audience

The eight-volume SAGE Reference Series on Disability targets an audience of undergraduate students and general readers that uses both academic and public libraries. However, the content and depth of the series will also make it attractive to graduate students, researchers, and policymakers. The series has been edited to have a consistent format and accessible style. The focus in each volume is on providing lay-friendly overviews of broad issues and guideposts for further research and exploration.

The series is innovative in that it will be published and marketed worldwide, with each volume available in electronic format soon after it appears in print. The print version consists of eight bound volumes. The electronic version is available through the SAGE Reference Online platform, which hosts 200 handbooks and encyclopedias across the social sciences, including the *Handbook of Disability Studies* and the *Encyclopedia of Disability*. With access to this platform through college, university, and public libraries, students, the lay public, and scholars can search these interrelated disability and social science sources from their computers or handheld and smart phone devices. The movement to an electronic platform presages the cloud computing revolution coming upon us. Cloud computing "refers to 'everything' a user may reach via the Internet, including services, storage, applications and people" (Hoehl & Sieh, 2010). According to Ray Ozzie (2010), recently Microsoft's chief architect, "We're moving toward a world of (1) cloud-based continuous services that connect us all and do our bidding, and (2) appliance-like connected devices enabling us to interact with those cloud-based services." Literally, information will be available at consumers' fingertips. Given the ample links to other resources in emerging databases, they can pursue any topic of interest in detail. This resource builds on the massive efforts to make information available to decision makers in real time, such as computerizing health and hospital records so that the diagnosis and treatment of chronic diseases and disabilities can be better managed (Celler, Lovell, & Basilakis, 2003). The SAGE Reference Series on Disability provides Internet and Web site addresses which lead the user into a world of social networks clustered around disability in general and specific conditions and issues. Entering and engaging with social networks revolving around health and disability promises to help individuals make more informed decisions and provide support in times of need (Smith & Christakis, 2008). The SAGE Reference Online platform will also be configured and updated to make it increasingly accessible to disabled people.

The SAGE Reference Series on Disability provides an extensive index for each volume. Through its placement on the SAGE Reference Online platform, the series will be fully searchable and cross-referenced, will allow keyword searching, and will be connected to the *Handbook of Disability Studies* and the *Encyclopedia of Disability*.

The authors of the volumes have taken considerable effort to vet the references, data, and resources for accuracy and credibility. The multiple Web sites for current data, information, government and United Nations documents, research findings, expert recommendations, self-help, discussion groups, and social policy are particularly useful, as they are being contin-uously updated. Examples of current and forthcoming data are the results and analysis of the findings of the U.S. 2010 Census, the ongoing reports of the Centers for Disease Control on disability, the World Health Organization's *World Report on Disability* and its updates, the World Bank reports on disability, poverty, and development, and reports from major foundations like Robert Wood Johnson, Bill and Melinda Gates, Ford, and Hogg. In terms of clinical outcomes, the evaluation of cost-effective inter-ventions, management of disability, and programs that work, enormous attention is being given to evidence-based outcomes (Brownson, Fielding, & Maylahn, 2009; Marcus et al., 2006; Wolinsky et al., 2007) and compara-tive effectiveness research (Etheredge, 2010; Inglehart, 2010). Such data force a re-examination of policymakers' arguments. For example, there is mounting evidence that demonstrates the beneficial effects of exercise on preventing disability and enhancing function (Marcus et al., 2006). Recent studies also show that some health care reform initiatives may negatively affect disabled people's access to and costs of health care (Burns, Shah, & Smith, 2010). Furthermore, the seemingly inexorable rise in health care spending may not be correlated with desirable health outcomes (Rothberg et al., 2010). In this environment, valid data are the currency of the discus-sion (Andersen, Lollar, & Meyers, 2000). The authors' hopes are that this reference series will encourage students and the lay public to base their discussions and decisions on valid outcome data. Such an approach tem-pers the influence of ideologies surrounding health care and misconcep-tions about disabled people, their lives, and experiences.

SAGE Publications has made considerable effort to make these volumes accessible to disabled people in the printed book version and in the elec-tronic platform format. In turn, SAGE and other publishers and vendors like Amazon are incorporating greater flexibility in the user interface to improve functionality to a broad range of users, such as disabled people. These efforts are important for disabled people as universities, govern-ments, and health service delivery organizations are moving toward a paperless environment.

In the spirit of informed discussion and transparency, may this refer-ence series encourage people from many different walks of life to become knowledgeable and engaged in the disability world. As a consequence, social policies should become better informed and individuals and fami-lies should be able to make better decisions regarding the experience of disability in their lives.

Acknowledgments

I would like to recognize the vision of Rolf Janke in developing SAGE Publications' presence in the disability field, as represented by the *Handbook of Disability Studies* (2001), the five-volume *Encyclopedia of Disability* (2006), and now the eight-volume SAGE Reference Series on Disability. These products have helped advance the field and have made critical work accessible to scholars, students, and the general public through books and now the SAGE Reference Online platform. Jim Brace-Thompson at SAGE handled the signing of contracts and kept this complex project coordinated and moving on time. Kevin Hillstrom and Laurie Collier Hillstrom at Northern Lights Writers Group were intrepid in taking the composite pieces of this project and polishing and editing them into a coherent whole that is approachable, consistent in style and form, and rich in content. The authors of the eight volumes—Linda Barrington, Jerome Bickenbach, Cathy Bodine, Brenda Brueggemann, Susanne Bruyère, Lana Collet-Klingenberg, Cheryl Hanley-Maxwell, Sarah Parker Harris, Tamar Heller, Nancy Mudrick, Ross Mullner, and Peggy Turk—are to be commended for their enthusiasm, creativity, and fortitude in delivering high-quality volumes on a tight deadline. I was fortunate to work with such accomplished scholars.

Discussions with Barbara Altman, Colin Barnes, Catherine Barral, Len Barton, Isabelle Baszanger, Peter Blanck, Mary Boulton, David Braddock, Richard Burkhauser, Mike Bury, Ann Caldwell, Lennard Davis, Patrick Devlieger, Ray Fitzpatrick, Lawrence Frey, Carol Gill, Tamar Heller, Gary Kielhofner, Soewarta Kosen, Jo Lebeer, Mitch Loeb, Don Lollar, Paul Longmore, Ros Madden, Maria Martinho, Dennis Mathews, Sophie Mitra, Daniel Mont, Alana Officer, Randall Parker, David Pfeiffer, Jean-François Raveau, James Rimmer, Ed Roberts, Jean-Marie Robine, Joan Rogers, Richard Scotch, Kate Seelman, Tom Shakespeare, Sandor Sipos, Henri-Jacques Stiker, Edna Szymanski, Jutta Traviranus, Bryan Turner, Greg Vanderheiden, Isabelle Ville, Larry Voss, Ann Waldschmidt, and Irving Kenneth Zola over the years contributed to the content, logic, and structure of the series. They also were a wonderful source of suggestions for authors.

I would also like to acknowledge the hospitality and support of the Belgian Academy of Science and the Arts, the University of Leuven, Nuffield College, the University of Oxford, the Fondation Maison des Sciences de l'Homme, Paris, and the Department of Disability and Human Development at the University of Illinois at Chicago, who provided the time and environments to conceive of and develop the project. While none of these people or institutions is responsible for any deficiencies in the work, they all helped enormously in making it better.

Gary L. Albrecht
University of Illinois at Chicago
University of Leuven
Belgian Academy of Science and Arts

References

Albrecht, G. L. (Ed.). (2006). *Encyclopedia of disability* (5 vols.). Thousand Oaks, CA: Sage.

Albrecht, G. L. (2010). The sociology of disability: Historical foundations and future directions. In C. Bird, A. Fremont, S. Timmermans, & P. Conrad (Eds.), *Handbook of medical sociology* (6th ed., pp. 192–209). Nashville, TN: Vanderbilt University Press.

Albrecht, G. L., Seelman, K. D., & Bury, M. (Eds.). (2001). *Handbook of disability studies*. Thousand Oaks, CA: Sage.

Andersen, E. M., Lollar, D. J., & Meyers, A. R. (2000). Disability outcomes research: Why this supplement, on this topic, at this time? *Archives of Physical Medicine and Rehabilitation, 81*, S1–S4.

Banta, H. D., & de Wit, G. A. (2008). Public health services and cost-effectiveness analysis. *Annual Review of Public Health, 29*, 383–397.

Bleich, S., Cutler, D., Murray, C., & Adams, A. (2008). Why is the developed world obese? *Annual Review of Public Health, 29*, 273–295.

Brownson, R. C., Fielding, J. E., & Maylahn, C. M. (2009). Evidence-based public health: A fundamental concept for public health practice. *Annual Review of Public Health, 30*, 175–201.

Burns, M., Shah, N., & Smith, M. (2010). Why some disabled adults in Medicaid face large out-of-pocket expenses. *Health Affairs, 29*, 1517–1522.

Celler, B. G., Lovell, N. H., & Basilakis, J. (2003). Using information technology to improve the management of chronic disease. *Medical Journal of Australia, 179*, 242–246.

Charlton, J. I. (1998). *Nothing about us without us: Disability, oppression and empowerment*. Berkeley: University of California Press.

DePoy, E., & Gilson, S. F. (2010) *Studying disability: Multiple theories and responses*. Thousand Oaks, CA: Sage.

Egede, L. E. (2004). Diabetes, major depression, and functional disability among U.S. adults. *Diabetes Care, 27*, 421–428.

Etheredge, L. M. (2010). Creating a high-performance system for comparative effectiveness research. *Health Affairs, 29*, 1761–1767.

European Disability Forum. (2003). *Disability and social exclusion in the European Union: Time for change, tools for change.* Athens: Greek National Confederation of Disabled People.

European Union. (2000). *Charter of fundamental rights.* Retrieved from http://www.europarll.europa.eu/charter

Gill, T. M., Gahbauer, E. A., Han, L., & Allore, H. G. (2010). Trajectories of disability in the last year of life. *The New England Journal of Medicine, 362*(13), 1173–1180.

Hoehl, A. A., & Sieh, K. A. (2010). *Cloud computing and disability communities: How can cloud computing support a more accessible information age and society?* Boulder, CO: Coleman Institute.

Iezzoni, L. I., & O'Day, B. L. (2006). *More than ramps.* Oxford, UK: Oxford University Press.

Inglehart, J. K. (2010). The political fight over comparative effectiveness research. *Health Affairs, 29*, 1757–1760.

Institute of Medicine. (1991). *Disability in America.* Washington, DC: National Academies Press.

Institute of Medicine. (1997). *Enabling America.* Washington, DC: National Academies Press.

Institute of Medicine. (2001). *Health and behavior: The interplay of biological, behavioral and societal influences.* Washington, DC: National Academies Press.

Institute of Medicine. (2002). *The dynamics of disability: Measuring and monitoring disability for social security programs.* Washington, DC: National Academies Press.

Institute of Medicine. (2007). *The future of disability in America.* Washington, DC: National Academies Press.

Institute of Medicine. (2008). *Improving the presumptive disability decision-making process for veterans.* Washington, DC: National Academies Press.

Kessler, R. C., & Wang, P. S. (2008). The descriptive epidemiology of commonly occurring mental disorders in the United States. *Annual Review of Public Health, 29*, 115–129.

Marcus, B. H., Williams, D. M., Dubbert, P. M., Sallis, J. F., King, A. C., Yancey, A. K., et al. (2006). Physical activity intervention studies. *Circulation, 114*, 2739–2752.

Martin, L. G., Freedman, V. A., Schoeni, R. F., & Andreski, P. M. (2010). Trends in disability and related chronic conditions among people ages 50 to 64. *Health Affairs, 29*(4), 725–731.

Mont, D. (2007). *Measuring disability prevalence* (World Bank working paper). Washington, DC: The World Bank.

Officer, A., & Groce, N. E. (2009). Key concepts in disability. *The Lancet, 374*, 1795–1796.

Ozzie, R. (2010, October 28). *Dawn of a new day.* Ray Ozzie's Blog. Retrieved from http://ozzie.net/docs/dawn-of-a-new-day

Rothberg, M. B., Cohen, J., Lindenauer, P., Masetti, J., & Auerbach, A. (2010). Little evidence of correlation between growth in health care spending and reduced mortality. *Health Affairs, 29*, 1523–1531.

Smith, K. P., & Christakis, N. A. (2008). Social networks and health. *Annual Review of Sociology, 34*, 405–429.

United Nations. (2008). *Convention on the rights of persons with disabilities.* New York: United Nations. Retrieved from http://un.org/disabilities/convention

Whitaker, R. T. (2010). *Anatomy of an epidemic: Magic bullets, psychiatric drugs, and the astonishing rise of mental illness in America.* New York: Crown.

Wolinsky, F. D., Miller, D. K., Andresen, E. M., Malmstrom, T. K., Miller, J. P., & Miller, T. R. (2007). Effect of subclinical status in functional limitation and disability on adverse health outcomes 3 years later. *The Journals of Gerontology: Series A, 62*, 101–106.

World Bank Disability and Development Team. (2004). *Poverty reduction strategies: Their importance for disability.* Washington, DC: World Bank.

World Health Organization. (2001). *International classification of functioning, disability and health.* Geneva: Author.

World Health Organization. (2010). *Community-based rehabilitation guidelines.* Geneva and Washington, DC: Author.

World Health Organization, & World Bank. (2011). *World report on disability.* Geneva: World Health Organization.

Preface

People with disabilities are a large and growing sector of the world's population that need medical care, healthcare facilities, and public health services. Disabilities are very broad in scope and include such conditions as birth defects, developmental disabilities, behavior/learning problems, substance abuse, injuries, chronic diseases, and mental disorders. Some individuals are born with disabilities, while others acquire them as they age. Over their life spans, the majority of people will experience disabilities or will have friends and family members who do.

Today about 50 million people in the United States—or one in every five Americans—have a disability. However, because of a lack of standard definitions and survey questions, the true number of people with a disability is unknown.

In the future, it is projected that the number of Americans with disabilities will grow significantly with the aging of the large baby boomer generation, many of whom are already experiencing multiple health problems and chronic diseases. Also, the increasing survival rates of premature infants and the successful treatment of cancer and other childhood illnesses often result in disabilities. Additionally, many children and adolescents will likely develop disabilities in the future because of the rising rates of asthma, obesity, diabetes, and other health conditions they are currently experiencing.

To prevent the occurrence of disabilities, better manage the healthcare of those with disabilities, and rehabilitate people with disabilities in the future, new advances as significant and revolutionary as those of the past will need to be accomplished. In the past century, these advances in medicine, healthcare facilities, and public health have greatly lowered population mortality rates, especially infant death rates, and increased overall life expectancy. For example, in 1900 the average life expectancy at birth for Americans was only 48.2 years, while in 2007 it was 77.9 years—an increase of nearly 30 years.

Past advances such as greater sanitation, the chlorination of drinking water, and the discovery and wide use of antibiotics—including sulfa drugs, penicillin, and streptomycin—have resulted in the control of many formerly deadly infectious diseases. Mass public health immunization programs have resulted in the eradication of the deadly disease smallpox, the elimination of the debilitating disease polio, and the control of such diseases as measles, rubella, tetanus, and diphtheria.

The identification of the underlying risk factors of coronary heart disease and stroke, and their modification (such as blood pressure control), early detection, and better treatment, have resulted in a dramatic decline in deaths from those two diseases. The greater public awareness of the deadly health hazards of tobacco, the labeling of cigarette packages identifying the hazards of smoking, the banning of cigarette advertising on television, and the use of antismoking drugs and patches have resulted in the prevention of millions of tobacco-related deaths from lung cancer, heart disease, and other related diseases.

Better hygiene, the availability of antibiotics, greater access to healthcare, and technologic advances in maternal and neonatal medicine have resulted in healthier mothers and babies—with a 90% decrease in infant mortality and a 99% decrease in maternal mortality since 1900 in the United States. Family planning has provided health benefits such as smaller family size and longer intervals between the births of children, which has lowered infant and maternal mortality.

Safer workplaces have resulted in the decrease of severe injuries and deaths related to mining, manufacturing, construction, and transportation. Motor-vehicle safety, including safer vehicles and highways, along with the increased use of safety belts, child safety seats, motorcycle helmets, and behavioral changes such as decreased drinking and driving, have resulted in lower injury and mortality rates. Safer and healthier foods, with decreases in contamination and increases in nutritional content, have resulted in the elimination of major nutritional deficiency diseases such as rickets, goiter, and pellagra. These advances are some of the crowning achievements of the last century, but they also have resulted in tremendous new challenges. The decline of infectious diseases and the aging of the population have given rise to the new burden of chronic diseases, injuries, and other conditions, many of which often result in the limitation of activities and disabilities.

People are now living longer, but many are also living sicker. Specific examples are dramatic: in 1910, children with Down syndrome in the

United States were only expected to survive to age 9. Today, 80% of adults with Down syndrome reach the age of 60, and many live even longer. Prior to World War II, the life expectancy for a person with a spinal cord injury was only a little over one year. Today, many live for decades. In 1973, the average age of survival for a child with cystic fibrosis was 7 years. Today, about one-half of all individuals with the disease are 21 years of age or older. In the 1970s, less than one-third of children with spina bifida reached the age of 20. Today, more than 80% reach adulthood. At the beginning of the HIV/AIDS epidemic in the early 1980s, the disease was a stark death sentence. Today, because of the use of combination antiretroviral drug therapy, a 20 year-old diagnosed with HIV can expect to live 13 years longer than the same person diagnosed with HIV in 1996.

Medicine, healthcare facilities, public health, and indeed all of society must now face a new emerging world. In the near future, for the first time in world history, people age 65 and over will outnumber children under the age 5. Already, the number of people age 85 and over, the oldest-old, are the fastest-growing sector of many national populations. Chronic diseases—such as cardiovascular disease, cancer, dementia and Alzheimer's disease, and diabetes, many of which lead to long-term disabilities—are now the major cause of death among older people in both developed and developing countries.

Realizing that these changes will have an enormous impact on all aspects of society, a number of private organizations and government agencies have called for action. For example, in 1991 the Institute of Medicine (IOM) published the seminal report *Disability in America: Toward a National Agenda for Prevention*, which proclaimed disability to be the nation's largest public health problem. In 2000, the U.S. Department of Health and Human Services' (DHHS) Healthy People 2010 initiative, which is the federal government's ten-year public health agenda for the nation, included a chapter on the health of people with disability for the first time. In 2005, the U.S. Surgeon General published the *Call to Action to Improve the Health and Wellness of Persons With Disability*, the first-ever Surgeon General's Call to Action, which identified equipping healthcare providers with the knowledge and tools to screen, diagnose, and treat persons with a disability with dignity among its four goals. In 2007, the National Institute on Aging and the U.S. Department of State published *Why Population Aging Matters: A Global Perspective*, which identified nine major global aging trends, including the growing burden of chronic diseases. That same year, the Institute of Medicine (IOM) published

The Future of Disability in America, which concluded that American society must do much more to enable people with disabilities to lead full and productive lives. The report also warned that failing to act will lead to individual and societal costs, including avoidable dependency, diminished quality of life, increased stress on individuals and families, and lost productivity. In 2011, the World Health Organization (WHO) and the World Bank published the *World Report on Disability*, which called attention to the global importance of disability for the economies, health, and well-being of the world's population.

Although people with disabilities are no longer the invisible and silent minority they once were, and many federal, state, and local laws have been passed to protect their civil rights, they still often encounter many barriers in daily life and in healthcare environments. These barriers create significant problems for people with disability in receiving timely, safe, and appropriate high-quality healthcare.

People with disabilities often face inaccessible and inadequate public and private transportation systems that can make healthcare appointments difficult to make and keep. People living in rural areas, which often do not have any public transportation systems, have particular difficulty accessing healthcare facilities. Unfortunately, many hospitals, clinics, and other healthcare facilities do not include transportation as part of the regular services they provide.

The health insurance status of people with disabilities also does not guarantee their ability to access healthcare. Those without health insurance are less likely to have a primary physician, and more likely to have trouble finding a physician who understands their disability, and to postpone or to go without needed healthcare. For those with health insurance, their coverage may only provide very limited preventive care and not provide basic technologies that increase safety and functioning. For example, the nation's Medicare program allows only one preventive medical examination to new beneficiaries during the first year they are in the program. Medicare does not pay for routine dental care, eyeglasses or contact lenses, or hearing examinations and hearing aids.

Despite federal regulations and state and local building codes, hospitals and physicians' offices frequently lack buildings, equipment, and services suitable for people with disabilities. For example, individuals with mobility limitations and other impairments often find that medical examination tables, hospital beds, weight scales, imaging devices, and other common medical products are, to some degree, inaccessible. Additionally, many

healthcare facilities do not have adequately trained staff members and technologies to communicate with people who are hearing impaired or have
speech disabilities.

To better serve the needs of people with disabilities, medicine, healthcare facilities, and public health will need to greatly expand their existing
programs as well as create many new, innovative programs and services.
Medical schools will need to change their already crowded curriculums to
better educate students on the healthcare and social needs of those with
disabilities. They must also offer more courses in the medical specialty of
physical medicine and rehabilitation. Physicians will need to increasingly
work in teams to solve complex chronic healthcare problems. They will
also need to train their staff and professional personnel to be more aware
and sensitive on interacting with people with disabilities, and include
those with disabilities in outcome research studies and clinical trials of
new drugs and medical devices. Healthcare facilities such as hospitals,
clinics, and nursing homes will need to provide a wider array of occupational therapy, physical therapy, and rehabilitation services, as well as
provide more social and transportation services. These facilities will also
need to incorporate universal design features to ensure the greatest access
by the disabled. Public health organizations will need to develop more
comprehensive definitions of disability and monitoring systems to track
national and local changes in disability rates. They will also have to work
to prevent secondary health conditions and promote the overall health of
those with disability, and help develop more effective healthcare policies
to better serve them.

This volume of the SAGE Reference Series on Disability will address the
many important health and medical issues concerning people with disabilities. Specifically, Chapter 1, Introduction, Background, and History, dis-
cusses the difficult problem of defining disability, the various widely used
models of disability, the diseases, injuries, and conditions that often lead to
disability, and the role of medicine, healthcare facilities, and public health
in addressing the needs of those with disability. Chapter 2, Current Issues,
Controversies, and Solutions, uses a health services research framework to
discuss access, cost, quality, and the outcomes of healthcare of those with
disabilities. Chapter 3, Chronology of Critical Events, presents a detailed
chronology of the major milestones in the histories of medicine, public
health, and disability from the earliest recorded times to the present.
Chapter 4, Biographies of Key Contributors in the Field, provides the life
stories of selected individuals who have made significant discoveries and

contributions to medicine, public health, and the field of disability. Chapter 5, Annotated Data, Statistics, Tables, and Graphs, presents 14 tables that provide a profile of people with disabilities, healthcare professionals, and facilities. Chapter 6, Annotated List of Organizations and Associations, which is divided into 12 categories, identifies the major academic centers and university programs, government agencies, and national and international organizations and associations involved in the health and medical aspects of disabilities. Lastly, Chapter 7, Selected Print and Electronic Resources, which is divided into nine categories, presents an annotated list of core print and electronic resources for selected topics in health, medicine, and disability.

This book is testament to the efforts of a large number of dedicated and talented people. First, I would like to thank Gary L. Albrecht, the editor of the series, for inviting me to write this volume. Kevin Hillstrom and Laurie Collier Hillstrom of Northern Lights Writers Group provided valuable editorial assistance. I would particularly like to thank Gerard M. Castro, Jessica M. Mazza, Melissa A. Satterlee, and Jacqueline Sieros for writing portions of Chapter 2.

I also appreciate the advice, counsel, and friendship of my colleagues at the University of Illinois at Chicago: Marcia and Gregory Finlayson, Benn Greenspan, Tamar Heller, Kevin Hogan, Anthony LoSasso, Edward Rafalski, Louis Rowitz, and Richard Sewell.

On a personal level, I want to thank my wife, Linda, for her unyielding support, and my two sons, Erik and Jason.

Ross M. Mullner

About the Author

Ross M. Mullner, Ph.D., M.P.H., is a health services researcher and a public health professional. For over 35 years, Dr. Mullner has worked as an academic, healthcare administrator, and consultant. He is currently an associate professor of health policy and administration at the School of Public Health of the University of Illinois at Chicago. He also holds appointments in the University of Illinois's School of Pharmacy, Department of Pharmacy Administration, and the College of Medicine, Department of Psychiatry. Before joining the faculty of the University of Illinois, he was director of research at the American Hospital Association's Healthcare Research and Educational Trust (HRET) and associate director of the Hospital Data Center.

Dr. Mullner has authored or edited eight books and has written more than 90 articles on various areas of healthcare. His work has appeared in the *New England Journal of Medicine, Health Services Research, Medical Care,* and *Social Science and Medicine.* He is the associate editor of the *Journal of Medical Systems* and has served on the editorial boards of *Health Services Research, Inquiry,* and *Quality Management in Health Care.* To keep abreast of the healthcare literature, he has written 45 book reviews for *Library Journal, Choice,* and *Inquiry.*

Dr. Mullner has served on a number of national boards and has been a consultant to a number of healthcare and government organizations, including the national Institute of Medicine (IOM), U.S. Government Accountability Office (GAO), Health Resources and Services Administration (HRSA), Joint Commission, and Cancer Treatment Centers of America. Over the years, Dr. Mullner has received a number of honors for his work, including being elected to *Who's Who in Medicine and Healthcare, Who's Who in America,* and *Who's Who in the World.* He earned a bachelor's degree from Chicago State University, and two master's degrees and a doctoral degree from the University of Illinois.

About the Series Editor

Gary L. Albrecht is a Fellow of the Royal Belgian Academy of Arts and Sciences, Extraordinary Guest Professor of Social Sciences, University of Leuven, Belgium, and Professor Emeritus of Public Health and of Disability and Human Development at the University of Illinois at Chicago. After receiving his Ph.D. from Emory University, he has served on the faculties of Emory University in Sociology and Psychiatry, Northwestern University in Sociology, Rehabilitation Medicine, and the Kellogg School of Management, and the University of Illinois at Chicago (UIC) in the School of Public Health and in the Department of Disability and Human Development. Since retiring from the UIC in 2005, he has divided his time between Europe and the United States, working in Brussels, Belgium, and Boulder, Colorado. He has served as a Scholar in Residence at the Maison des Sciences de l'Homme (MSH) in Paris, a visiting Fellow at Nuffield College, the University of Oxford, and a Fellow in Residence at the Royal Flemish Academy of Science and Arts, Brussels.

His research has focused on how adults acknowledge, interpret, and respond to unanticipated life events, such as disability onset. His work, supported by over $25 million of funding, has resulted in 16 books and over 140 articles and book chapters. He is currently working on a longitudinal study of disabled Iranian, Moroccan, Turkish, Jewish, and Congolese immigrants to Belgium. Another current project involves working with an international team on "Disability: A Global Picture," Chapter 2 of the *World Report on Disability*, co-sponsored by the World Health Organization and the World Bank, to be published in 2011.

He is past Chair of the Medical Sociology Section of the American Sociological Association, a past member of the Executive Committee of the Disability Forum of the American Public Health Association, an early member of the Society for Disability Studies, and an elected member of the Society for Research in Rehabilitation (UK). He has received the Award for the Promotion of Human Welfare and the Eliot Freidson Award for the book *The Disability Business: Rehabilitation in America.* He also has received a Switzer Distinguished Research Fellowship, Schmidt Fellowship, New York State Supreme Court Fellowship, Kellogg Fellowship, National Library of Medicine Fellowship, World Health Organization Fellowship, the Lee Founders Award from the Society for the Study of Social Problems, the Licht Award from the American Congress of Rehabilitation Medicine, the University of Illinois at Chicago Award for Excellence in Teaching, and has been elected Fellow of the American Association for the Advancement of Science (AAAS). He has led scientific delegations in rehabilitation medicine to the Soviet Union and the People's Republic of China and served on study sections, grant review panels, and strategic planning committees on disability in Australia, Canada, the European Community, France, Ireland, Japan, Poland, Sweden, South Africa, the United Kingdom, the United States, and the World Health Organization, Geneva. His most recent books are *The Handbook of Social Studies in Health and Medicine,* edited with Ray Fitzpatrick and Susan Scrimshaw (SAGE, 2000), the *Handbook of Disability Studies,* edited with Katherine D. Seelman and Michael Bury (SAGE, 2001), and the five-volume *Encyclopedia of Disability* (SAGE, 2006).

One

Introduction, Background, and History

Healthcare professionals and healthcare organizations play a vital role in the health and wellness of people with disabilities. They define the nature and extent of disabilities; they work to prevent disabilities from occurring at various levels; they identify and treat the multitude of diseases, injuries, and conditions that cause disabilities; they help patients and clients manage their existing disabilities; and they work to rehabilitate people with disabilities.

Healthcare professionals address disabilities at both the population and individual levels. For example, public health professionals, such as health educators, public health social workers, and public health nurses, work to prevent disabilities from occurring in communities, groups, and populations. They also work to prevent secondary conditions, such as depression, pressure sores, and obesity, from occurring among people with existing disabilities; and they address disaster preparedness and assistance for people with disabilities during natural and man-made disasters, such as floods, hurricanes, and hazardous chemical spills. In contrast, clinical health professionals, such as physicians, nurses, pharmacists, and allied healthcare professionals such as occupational and physical therapists, work with individual patients who are disabled to treat their diseases, injuries, and conditions, help them manage their disabilities by diminishing their pain, and rehabilitate them by restoring their maximum level of functioning.

Healthcare organizations provide a continuum of care across the life span of individuals from before birth (prenatal care) to death (hospice care). For example, community hospitals provide a wide array of acute healthcare services to people with disabilities. And many other organizations, such as rehabilitation facilities, nursing homes, and home healthcare agencies, provide many long-term healthcare services to people with disabilities.

Healthcare professionals and healthcare organizations play an important role in defining the nature, extent, and scope of disability at the conceptual and individual levels. For example, healthcare organizations, such as the World Health Organization (WHO), the National Center for Health Statistics (NCHS), and the National Center for Medical Rehabilitation Research (NCMRR), have attempted to define disability. They have also developed a number of widely used conceptual models of disability. At the individual level, healthcare professionals examine patients who are disabled and certify the existence of a particular disease, injury, or condition and the level of functional impairment it causes. This certification process is required for individuals to receive private and government assistance, such as private insurance payments, and government Social Security Disability Insurance (SSDI), Supplemental Security Income (SSI), state workers' compensation, and Veterans Administration (VA) benefits for service-related disabilities.

First, this introductory chapter will identify how healthcare professionals and healthcare organizations define disability and the various conceptual models they use. Second, it will describe the characteristics of some of the major diseases, injuries, and conditions often associated with a high degree of disability. Third, it will identify the various healthcare professionals who work to prevent, manage, and rehabilitate people with disability. Finally, the chapter will provide an overview of the many healthcare organizations that provide acute and long-term care services to those with disability.

The Difficult Task of Defining Disability

Disability is a complex, multidimensional, and dynamic concept that is very difficult to precisely define. The concept of disability encompasses many different dimensions of health and functioning as well as complex interactions with various dimensions of the environment. As a result, many private and government organizations, public policies, and laws use varying criteria to define disability.

Disability is very difficult to precisely define for numerous reasons. Consider: there are many types of disabilities, such as physical, cognitive, sensory, and mental disabilities, with varying characteristics, and individuals may have multiple disabilities at the same time, such as being both blind and deaf. Disabilities can result from many different causes, such as birth defects, diseases, injuries, and various conditions. Disabilities can occur at every stage of life, with some occurring early in life, such as birth defects, and others often occurring late in life, such as Alzheimer's disease. Disabilities vary in visibility; some disabilities are relatively easy to see, such as in the case of an individual in a wheelchair, while others, such as arthritis, are not. Disabilities vary in their speed of onset, some disabilities have a very sudden and easily identifiable onset, such as having a debilitating stroke, while others occur slowly over many years or decades, such as disabilities caused by chronic progressive multiple sclerosis (MS). Disabilities vary in the length of their duration; some disabilities are permanent, such as a spinal cord injury, while others are temporary, such as a broken leg. Disabilities are also affected by circumstances other than the specific impairment itself. For example, a person who has a college degree and works in an office is less likely than a high school dropout who works in a factory to consider the loss of a leg to be a relevant disability.

Further, societal attitudes and perceptions of disability have significantly changed over time. In the past, society tended to have a much narrower view of disability. Generally, only people with clearly visible and identifiable impairments—the blind, the deaf, and those without limbs—were considered disabled. Today, society recognizes a much larger number of disabilities, such as autism and other learning disabilities, HIV/AIDS, and substance abuse. Even the very words society commonly uses to describe disabilities have changed through time. No longer are people with disabilities referred to as being "crippled," "handicapped" or "retarded."

Accordingly, there is no single, widely accepted definition of disability. However, because disability is such an important issue, a number of healthcare and government organizations have attempted to define it. And many specific, and oftentimes narrow, operational definitions of disability have been developed. These definitions vary greatly across government departments, agencies, and programs. Further, the term disability and its measurement have been applied inconsistently. Disability is often measured in many different ways across surveys and censuses, and this has led to disparate estimates of the prevalence, or occurrence, of disability at the local and national level.

Models and Approaches to Disability

Lacking a single, widely accepted definition, a number of conceptual models of disability, or ways of explaining disability, have been developed. These conceptual models include: the medical model of disability, the functional model of disability, the social model of disability, and integrated models of disability. Each model has a different perspective of disability, and often people view disability through one of these perspectives without thinking about it. The underlying assumptions and the strengths and weaknesses of each model are briefly discussed in this section.

The Medical Model of Disability

The medical model of disability focuses on diseases, injuries, and conditions that impair or disrupt physiological or cognitive functioning of an individual. The medical model conceptualizes disability as a condition or deficit that resides within the individual, which can be cured or ameliorated, or its progression stopped, through a treatment or a particular intervention. The model relies strongly on the notion of the "sick role." The sick role assumes that the sick individual is exempt from certain social obligations, is not responsible for his or her medical condition, should try to get well, and should seek technically competent help and cooperate with healthcare professionals to get well. Under the medical model, disability is generally viewed in categorical terms (e.g., arthritis, cancer, multiple sclerosis) with much less regard for severity (i.e., degree of impairment or symptoms).

The medical model of disability is widely used by healthcare professionals and the general public, but it has been strongly criticized by many disability activists and scholars.

One of the medical model's main strengths is its ability to consistently and efficiently determine the eligibility of people with disabilities, a necessary step if they are to receive private or government assistance and services. Physicians are arduously trained for years to use standardized medical tests (i.e., x-rays, CT scans, MRI scans, and ultrasound) and pathological studies (biopsies) to confirm their diagnoses. Each year, physicians examine and certify millions of patients with disabilities and assist them in applying for private or government assistance. Some of the model's weaknesses include: it tends to exclusively emphasize the physiological basis of disability; it creates an assumption that disability is a non-normative or abnormal state; it is oriented toward "curing" or "fixing" the disabled individual and decreasing his or her care needs; and it tends to ignore the larger role society plays in impacting health status and creating disability through prejudice or other negative attitudes (Committee on Disability in America, 2007).

The Functional Model of Disability

The functional model of disability acknowledges an individual's medical conditions or impairments, but focuses primarily on the expression of disability, such as the inability to perform a number of functional activities. For example, an individual has a disability under the functional model if, due to an underlying condition or impairment, he or she is unable to perform vital physical or mental activities. The model stresses the adoption of treatment regimens, strategies, and services that improve functional capacity, such as prosthetics, portable oxygen units, and other assistive technologies, rather than exclusively addressing the underlying condition or impairment. Under the functional model, disability is generally viewed as being dichotomous—individuals with major functional limitations are classified as being disabled, while those without major functional limitations are not classified as being disabled and are therefore considered able-bodied.

The functional model of disability is used by several government agencies, such as the Social Security Administration (SSA), to determine disability status. For example, the Social Security Act, Section 223(d)(1), defines disability as the "inability to engage in any substantial gainful activity by reason of any medically determinable physical or mental impairment which can be expected to result in death or which has lasted or can be expected to last for a continuous period of not less than 12 months" (U.S. Social Security Administration, 2009, p. 2).

One of the functional model's main strengths is its pragmatic approach to measuring disability. The model takes thousands of potentially disabling diseases, injuries, and conditions and ultimately classifies people into a much smaller, more manageable group. In the case of the Social Security Administration, the classification is based on whether an individual can work (non-disabled) or not (disabled). Some of the model's weaknesses include: It is overly simplistic in its view of disability, ignoring the fact that disabilities occur along a continuum from very mild to severe; and it overlooks the important role physical, cultural, environmental, and political factors play in creating disability status.

The Social Model of Disability

The social model of disability shifts the concept of disability from an individual's diseases or impairments and inability to perform functional activities to the barriers an individual with disabilities faces when interacting with the environment. The model takes the view that many problems lie not within the individuals with disabilities, but in the environment that fails to accommodate their disabilities and in the negative attitudes of people without disabilities. For example, proponents of the model argue that a wheelchair user is "disabled" by a public transportation system that lacks wheelchair lifts and by buildings and facilities that do not have ramps or elevators.

The social model broadly defines the environment, which includes social, physical, economic, and political dimensions. Social dimensions include such things as discriminatory policies, stereotyping, and the oppression of individuals with disabilities. Physical dimensions include the built environment, such as commercial buildings, housing, and public transportation systems. Economic dimensions include excluding individuals with disabilities from educational and occupational opportunities. Finally, the political dimension includes such things as elected officials failing to involve people with disabilities in public policies and not addressing the needs of the disabled.

The landmark Americans with Disabilities Act of 1990 (ADA) incorporates the social model of disability. The ADA is the most comprehensive federal civil rights statute that creates broad legal protection for people with disabilities. Its goal is to provide equal participation of individuals with disabilities in the "mainstream" of society. The ADA affects access to employment; state and local government programs and services; places of public accommodation, such as businesses; transportation; and telecommunications.

One of the social model's main strengths is that it places a much greater emphasis on society to provide greater access for people with disability. One of the model's weaknesses is that it tends to overemphasize barrier removal and other social changes. An entirely barrier-free world is a utopian dream because the natural environment cannot be made accessible; it is impractical to make many existing buildings or systems accessible; and different impairments necessitate different accommodations, many of which are mutually contradictory. The model also is difficult to understand, particularly by health-care professionals and others. It tends to ignore the complexity of various diseases and impairments and the potential of public health and medicine to cure and care for people with disabilities (Drum, Krahn, & Bersani, 2009).

Integrated Models of Disability

Several models of disability have attempted to integrate various components of the medical, functional, and social models of disability. One integrated model of disability is the World Health Organization's International Classification of Functioning, Disability, and Health (ICF). Released in 2001, the ICF integrates the medical and social models to form what it calls a "biopsychosocial" model of disability.

In the ICF model (Figure 1), disability and functioning are viewed as the outcomes of the interactions between health conditions and contextual factors. Health conditions include a wide array of acute and chronic diseases, injuries, and various conditions, while contextual factors include environmental factors (e.g., products and technology, support and relationships, social attitudes, and the natural and human-made environment) and personal factors (e.g., age, gender, education, and health conditions). The ICF identifies three dimensions of human functioning: body function and structure, activity, and participation. The term disability is used to denote decrements, or decreases, of functioning on a continuum at each level: impairment, activity limitation, and participation restriction.

Thus, in the ICF, disability is used as an umbrella term, covering impairments, activity limitations, and participation restrictions. Specifically, the ICF defines impairments as "problems in body function or structure such as significant deviations or losses"; activity limitations as "difficulties an individual may have on executing activities"; and participation restrictions as "problems an individual may experience in involvement in life situations."

The ICF has been widely adopted around the world, both as an organizational model of disability and as a classification platform for assessment and measurement tools and data management and analysis.

The ICF's main strength is that it provides a standard language and framework of disability, enabling health professionals, researchers, and policy analysts to identify local trends in disabilities as well as compare disabilities across regions and countries. Its weaknesses include: it does not address what causes or is responsible for disabilities; it does not incorporate "quality of life" in its framework of health and disability; it needs to more fully develop personal and environmental factors that influence the outcome of potentially disabling health conditions; and it needs to better depict functioning and disability as a dynamic process.

Figure 1   The ICF Model of Functioning, Disability, and Health

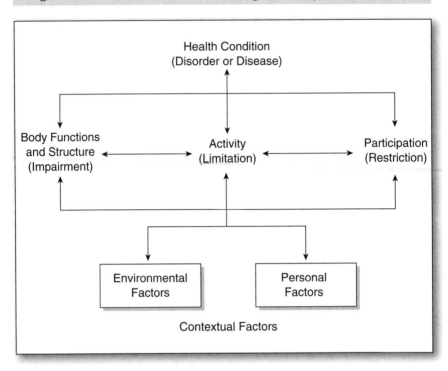

Although the ICF is not perfect, it is a significant step forward in describing the full spectrum of human functioning, and it provides a better understanding of the complex processes that create disabilities. Because of its standardized language and definitions, the ICF is increasingly becoming an important tool in the systematic collection and analysis of disability data by healthcare professionals, researchers, and policy analysts (World Health Organization, 2001).

Diseases, Injuries, and Conditions

As described in the ICF, health conditions, such as acute and chronic diseases, injuries, and various conditions, play an important role in disability. This section presents a general overview of diseases associated with disability, and it also describes the causes and occurrences of some of the major disabling diseases.

General Overview of Diseases

Many diseases associated with disability are chronic versus acute in nature. Chronic diseases are generally of long duration, progressive, and not cured once they are acquired. Examples of chronic diseases include arthritis, diabetes, and heart disease. In contrast, acute diseases are generally of short duration, sometimes curable, and are oftentimes self-limiting. Examples of acute diseases are the common cold, the flu (influenza), and sore throat (Falvo, 2009).

It should be noted that individuals may respond differently to the same disease, injury, or condition. There is a biological as well as a psychological gradient of response. Biologically, a particular disease may have little impact on some individuals (a sub-clinical response), while other individuals may be very severely impacted (death). Psychologically, some individuals may consider themselves severely disabled by a disease, while others may not consider themselves disabled at all. For example, some blind individuals consider themselves disabled, while others do not.

Major Disabling Diseases, Injuries, and Conditions

Some of the major diseases, injuries, and conditions associated with a high degree of disability are briefly summarized below. They are grouped into four very broad and overlapping categories: physical diseases and conditions; injury and trauma conditions; mental diseases and conditions; and other diseases and conditions. Within each category, the specific diseases, injuries, and conditions are presented in alphabetical order.

The physical diseases and conditions category includes: amyotrophic lateral sclerosis (ALS) or Lou Gehrig's disease; arthritis; back pain; cancer; chronic obstructive pulmonary disease (COPD); diabetes; epilepsy; fibromyalgia; hearing disorders; heart disease; HIV/AIDS; multiple sclerosis (MS); muscular dystrophy (MD); osteoporosis; Parkinson's disease; stroke; and vision impairment.

The injury and trauma conditions category includes: amputation; hip fracture; spinal cord injury; and traumatic brain injury (TBI).

The mental diseases and conditions category includes: Alzheimer's disease; depression; and mental disorders.

Finally, the other diseases and conditions category includes: attention deficit hyperactivity disorder (ADHD); autism; development disabilities (DD); obesity; and substance abuse.

Physical Diseases and Conditions

Amyotrophic Lateral Sclerosis (ALS). Often referred to as Lou Gehrig's disease, after the world-famous baseball player for the New York Yankees who died from it in 1941, Amyotrophic Lateral Sclerosis (ALS) is a degenerative disease of the nerve cells in the brain and spinal cord. As the disease progresses, weakness may appear in the legs, arms, or in the muscles used for speech, swallowing, or breathing. Risk factors for ALS include heredity (having a parent with the disease), increasing age, gender (the disease is more common in men than women by a ratio of 3:2), geography, and military service. It is estimated that about two out of every 100,000 people in the United States have ALS. There are about 30,000 Americans living with the disease at any given time (Vincent & Williams, 2010).

Arthritis. Arthritis is one of the most common causes of disability among American adults. Arthritis comprises more than 100 different rheumatic diseases and conditions, the most common of which is osteoarthritis. Other frequently occurring forms of arthritis include rheumatoid arthritis, lupus, and gout. Common symptoms include pain, aching, stiffness, and swelling in or around the joints. Some forms of arthritis, such as rheumatoid arthritis and lupus, can affect multiple organs and cause widespread symptoms. Risk factors for arthritis include gender (women are more likely to develop arthritis than men), increasing age, having a family history of the disease, and smoking. Over 46 million Americans—about one in every five adults—had arthritis as of 2006 (Lorig & Fries, 2000).

Back Pain. Back pain is a common health problem that can range from a dull, constant ache to a sudden, sharp pain that can leave a person incapacitated. It can come on suddenly—from an accident, a fall, or lifting something too heavy—or it can develop slowly as the result of age-related changes to the spine. Risk factors associated with back pain include: age, fitness level, diet, heredity, race and ethnicity, the presence of other diseases, and occupation. Back pain affects an estimated eight out of every ten Americans at some point in their lifetime (Kostuik, Jan de Beur, & Margolis, 2003).

Cancer. Cancer is not a single disease but many diseases. Cancer is a term used for diseases in which abnormal cells divide without control and are able to invade other tissues. Cancer can spread to other parts of the body through the blood and lymph system. There are more than 100 different types of cancer, which can be grouped into five broad categories: carcinomas, which are cancers that begin in the skin or in tissues that line or cover internal organs; sarcomas, which are cancers that begin in bone, cartilage, fat, muscle, blood vessels, or other connective or supportive tissue; leukemia, which are cancers that start in blood-forming tissues such as bone marrow and cause large numbers of abnormal blood cells to be produced and enter the blood; lymphoma and myeloma, which are cancers that begin in the cells of the immune system; and central nervous system cancers, which are cancers that begin in the tissues of the brain and spinal cord. Many cancers are named for the organ or type of cell in which they start (e.g., breast cancer, lung cancer, and prostate cancer). Common risk factors for cancer include: increasing age; tobacco use; sunlight; ionizing radiation such as x-rays; certain chemicals and other substances; some viruses and bacteria; certain hormones; having a family history of cancer; alcohol use; and poor diet, lack of physical activity, or being overweight. The most common type of cancer is nonmelanoma skin cancer, with more than 1 million new cases of the disease occurring annually in the United States. Skin cancer represents about half of all cancers diagnosed in the country. Excluding skin cancer, about 1.5 million Americans will be annually diagnosed with cancer, and over 500,000 people will die from the disease (Tobias, Hochhauser, & Souhami, 2010).

Chronic Obstructive Pulmonary Disease (COPD). Chronic obstructive pulmonary disease (COPD) is a leading cause of illness, disability, and death in the United States. COPD refers to a group of diseases, including emphysema, chronic bronchitis, and in some cases asthma, that cause airflow blockage and breathing-related problems. COPD can cause coughing, wheezing, shortness of breath, chest tightness, and other symptoms. Cigarette smoking is a key factor in the development and progression of COPD. Other risk factors include: exposure to air pollution in the home and workplace, genetic factors, and respiratory infections. About 12 million Americans have been diagnosed with COPD, and another 12 million Americans are considered likely to have the disease, but it is undiagnosed (MacNee & Rennard, 2009).

Diabetes. Diabetes is a group of diseases marked by high levels of blood glucose (sugar) resulting from problems in insulin production, insulin action, or both. There are two main types of diabetes: type 1 diabetes and type 2 diabetes. Type 1 diabetes, which usually occurs in children and young adults, develops when the body's immune system destroys pancreatic cells that make insulin, a hormone that regulates blood glucose. People with type 1 diabetes must take insulin by injection or pump. Type 1 diabetes accounts for 5 to 10% of all diagnosed cases of diabetes. Type 2 diabetes, which usually occurs in adults, often begins as insulin resistance, a disorder in which the body's cells do not use insulin properly. As the need for insulin rises, the pancreas gradually loses its ability to produce it. Untreated diabetes can lead to very serious health complications, such as blindness, kidney problems, nerve damage, lower-limb amputation, and premature death. An estimated 23.6 million Americans, or about 7.8% of the country's population, have diabetes, including both those who are diagnosed and undiagnosed with the disease (Holt & Kumar, 2010).

Epilepsy. Epilepsy is a chronic neurological condition characterized by recurrent seizures. Epilepsy can be caused by: stroke, head trauma, complications during childbirth, infections, and certain genetic disorders. Children younger than two years of age and adults older than 65 years of age are most likely to be affected by the condition. In addition, people of low socioeconomic status, those who live in urban areas, and members of some minority populations are at increased risk for epilepsy. Epilepsy affects an estimated 2.5 million Americans (Fisch, 2010).

Fibromyalgia. Fibromyalgia is a chronic condition characterized by fatigue, muscle pain, and "tender points." Tender points are places on the neck, shoulders, back, hips, arms, or legs that hurt when touched. People with fibromyalgia may also have other symptoms, such as trouble sleeping, morning stiffness, headaches, and problems with thinking and memory. The cause of the disorder is unknown. However, people with rheumatoid arthritis and other autoimmune diseases are at higher risk of developing fibromyalgia. The disorder is most common in middle-aged women. Fibromyalgia affects an estimated 5 million Americans 18 years of age or older, about 2% of the country's population (Jones & Hoffman, 2009).

Hearing Disorders. Hearing disorders can lead to disability. People with hearing loss may have difficulty conversing with friends and family. They may also have trouble understanding healthcare professionals and responding to warnings and alarms. Hearing loss can be caused by a number of factors, including: heredity, diseases such as ear infections and meningitis, trauma, certain medicines, long-term exposure to loud noise, and aging. Hearing loss is one of the most common conditions affecting older adults. About one-third of Americans 65 to 74 years of age, and one-half of those 75 and older, have hearing loss. An estimated 1 million Americans are functionally deaf, and about 8 million Americans are hard of hearing (that is, they have some difficulty hearing normal conversation even with the use of a hearing aid; Fiedler & Krause, 2009).

Heart Disease. Heart disease is the leading cause of death in the United States, and it is a major cause of disability. There are many different forms of heart disease. The most common form is coronary artery disease (CAD). CAD, the major reason people have heart attacks, is caused by the narrowing or blockage of coronary arteries, the blood vessels that supply blood to the heart. Other forms of heart disease involve problems with the valves in the heart, or the inability of the heart to pump enough blood throughout the body, which may cause heart failure. Some heart conditions are congenital, with the heart not fully developing. Symptoms of heart disease include: dizziness or lightheadedness, chest pain, numbness in the arms, sweating, irregular heartbeat or pulse, shortness of breath, and nausea. The risk factors of CAD include: hypertension or high blood pressure, being overweight or obese, having high amounts of certain fats and cholesterol in the blood, smoking, having high amounts of sugar in the blood due to insulin resistance or diabetes, and lack of exercise. About 26.6 million non-institutionalized American adults have diagnosed heart disease, or about 12% of the non-institutionalized population of the country. Annually, there are about 16 million visits to physicians' offices by patients with heart disease as a primary diagnosis. There are about 4.2 million hospital discharges with heart disease as the first-listed diagnosis. And there are about 635,000 nursing home residents in the country, about 43% of all residents, with heart disease (Dunn, Everitt, & Simon, 2007).

HIV/AIDS. HIV/AIDS was first recognized as a disease in 1981. HIV (human immunodeficiency virus) is the virus that causes AIDS (acquired immunodeficiency syndrome). HIV attacks the body's immune system by destroying a type of white blood cell (T cells or CD4 cells) that the immune system must have to fight disease. AIDS is the final stage of HIV infection. It can take years for a person infected with HIV to reach this stage. Having AIDS means that the virus has weakened a person's immune system to the point at which the body has a difficult time fighting infection. When a person has one or more specific infections, certain cancers, or a very low number of T cells, they are considered to have AIDS. In 2006, an estimated 1.1 million Americans had HIV/AIDS (Stolley & Glass, 2009).

Multiple Sclerosis (MS). Multiple sclerosis (MS) is a progressive neurodegenerative disease characterized by inflammation, destruction, and scarring of cells that protect the neurons in the central nervous system. MS is one of the most common disabling neurological diseases in young people, with typical onset of the disease being 30 to 40 years of age. The disease is about twice as common in women than men. Most people with MS are mildly affected, but in the worst cases MS can render a person unable to write, speak, or walk. The cause of MS is unknown. Some scientists believe MS is an autoimmune disease—one in which the body, through its immune system, launches a defensive attack against its own tissues. About 350,000 Americans have been diagnosed with MS (Coyle & Halper, 2001).

Muscular Dystrophy (MD). Muscular Dystrophy (MD) is a group of more than 30 inherited diseases that causes slow, progressive muscle weakness. Some forms of MD appear in infancy or childhood, while others may appear in middle age or later. The different types of MD vary in symptoms. Some people with MD have mild cases that worsen slowly, while other cases are disabling and severe. The main types of MD include: Duchenne, Becker, limb-girdle, faciosapulohumeral, oculopharyngeal, and myotonic dystrophy. Most types of MD are rare. The most common type is Duchenne MD, which occurs in about one in 3,000 males (Abramovitz, 2008).

Osteoporosis. Osteoporosis is a disease that makes a person's bones weak and more likely to break. It is often called the "silent disease" because calcium is lost from the bones with no symptoms. People with osteoporosis often break bones in the hip, spine, and wrist. Risk factors for developing osteoporosis include: getting older, being small and thin, having a family history of osteoporosis, taking certain medicines, being a white or Asian woman, and having osteopenia, which is low bone mass. Nearly 34 million Americans have low bone mass that puts them at increased risk of developing the disease, and about 10 million Americans over the age of 50 have osteoporosis (Mattingly & Pillare, 2009).

Parkinson's Disease. Named after the English physician James Parkinson, who first described the disease in 1817, Parkinson's disease is one of a group of conditions called motor system disorders, which are the result of the loss of dopamine-producing brain cells. According to the National Institutes of Health, the primary symptoms of Parkinson's disease include: tremor, or trembling in the hands, arms, legs, jaw, and face; rigidity, or stiffness of the limbs and trunk; bradykinesia, or slowness of movement; and postural instability, or impaired balance and coordination. As these symptoms become more pronounced, individuals with Parkinson's disease may have difficulty walking, talking, or completing other simple tasks. Parkinson's disease usually affects people over the age of 50. Risk factors for developing Parkinson's disease include: increasing age; heredity; gender, as males are more likely to develop the disease than females; and exposure to environmental toxins such as herbicides and pesticides. About 500,000 Americans have Parkinson's disease (Sharma, 2008).

Stroke. Stroke is one of the leading causes of serious, long-term disability. A stroke occurs when blood flow to the brain is interrupted. When this happens, brain cells in the immediate area begin to die because they stop getting the oxygen and nutrients they need. There are two types of stroke: ischemic stroke and hemorrhagic stroke. Ischemic stroke is caused by a blood clot that blocks or plugs a blood vessel or artery leading to or in the brain. About 80% of all strokes are ischemic. Hemorrhagic stroke occurs when a blood vessel breaks and bleeds into the brain. About 20% of strokes are hemorrhagic. The symptoms of stroke are sudden: numbness or weakness of the face, arm, or leg (especially on one side of the body); confusion, trouble speaking or understanding speech; trouble seeing in one or both eyes; trouble walking, dizziness, loss of balance or coordination; and severe headache with no known cause. Risk factors for developing a stroke include various individual and behavioral characteristics, as well as medical conditions. Specifically, individual characteristics include: increasing age; having a family history of stroke; gender, as men are at greater risk of stroke than women; and race and ethnicity, as American Indians/Alaska Natives have a greater risk of stroke than do non-Hispanic whites or Asians. Behavioral characteristics include: tobacco use, alcohol use, and physical inactivity. Medical conditions include: having high blood pressure, high blood cholesterol, heart disease, or diabetes; and being overweight or obese. The effects of a stroke can range from mild to severe. About 50 to 70% of stroke survivors regain some functional independence, but 15 to 30% are seriously disabled. Each year about 780,000 Americans suffer a stroke (Brainin & Heiss, 2010).

Vision Impairment. Vision impairment can range from mild to severe. Normal vision is referred to as 20/20 vision, which means that an individual can see clearly at 20 feet what should be normally be seen at that distance. In contrast, 20/40 vision means that an individual must be as close as 20 feet to see what a person with normal vision can see from 40 feet. Vision impairment is defined as having 20/40 or worse vision in the better eye, even with corrective eyeglasses. Blindness is severe vision impairment, not correctable by standard glasses, contact lenses, medicine, or surgery. "Legal blindness" is defined as visual acuity in the better eye worse than or equal to 20/200 with correction, or a visual field of less than 20 degrees in diameter. Legal blindness is significant in determining eligibility for disability benefits from the federal government. The leading causes of vision impairment and blindness are: cataracts, age-related macular degeneration, diabetic retinopathy, and glaucoma. Eye injuries and birth defects can also cause vision loss. More than 1 million Americans are legally blind, and 12 million are visually impaired (McLannahan, 2008).

Injury and Trauma Conditions

Amputation. Amputation, or limb loss, is often the result of illness or injury. The most frequent cause of amputation is peripheral vascular disease, which is often associated with diabetes mellitus. Other causes of amputation include trauma, cancer, and congenital-related problems. It is estimated that about one out of every 200 people in the United States have had an amputation. Approximately 1.7 million Americans live with limb loss (Kirkup, 2006).

Hip Fracture. Hip fracture is a break in the upper quarter of the femur (thigh) bone. Hip fracture, which is the most common major injury among elderly Americans, can cause severe health problems and lead to a reduced quality of life and premature death. About half of the people who have a hip fracture never regain their previous level of functioning, and 15 to 20% of them die within one year of the fracture. More than 90% of hip fractures are caused by falling, most often sideways onto the hip. Risk factors of having a hip fracture include: increasing age; being a woman, because women lose bone density at a faster rate than men do; having chronic medical conditions such as osteoporosis; taking certain medications; nutritional problems, such as having a diet lacking in calcium and vitamin D; and lack of physical activity. About 300,000 Americans have hip fractures each year (Onslow, 2005).

Spinal Cord Injury. Spinal cord injury is any injury or disease that damages the spinal cord or spinal column. The spinal cord is the largest nerve in the body. It is the pathway that messages use to travel between the brain and the other parts of the body. The spinal column or backbone consists of vertebrae. It provides the main support for the body. Spinal cord injury may be traumatic or non-traumatic. Traumatic spinal cord injury may be caused by motor vehicle crashes, falls, acts of violence, or sports and recreation injuries. Non-traumatic spinal cord injury may be caused by arthritis, cancer, infections, or disk degeneration of the spine. After a spinal cord injury, all the nerves above the level of injury keep working as they did before the injury. However, from the point of injury and below, the spinal cord nerves cannot send messages between the brain and parts of the body. Several terms are used to describe the level of spinal cord injury. Tetraplegia (formerly called quadriplegia) generally describes the condition where the individual experiences a loss of feeling and/or movement in their head, neck, shoulder, arms and/or upper chest, while paraplegia generally describes the condition where the individual experiences a loss of feeling in the chest, stomach, hips, legs and feet. Every year, about 10,000 Americans sustain a spinal cord injury. An estimated 200,000 Americans live with a disability related to a spinal cord injury (Mayo Clinic, 2009).

Traumatic Brain Injury (TBI). Traumatic brain injury (TBI) is caused by a blow or jolt to the head or a penetrating head injury that disrupts the normal function of the brain. The severity of a TBI may range from mild (a brief change in mental status or consciousness) to severe (unconsciousness or death). The leading causes of TBI in the United States are: falls, motor vehicle crashes, blows to the head, and assaults. TBI can cause a wide range of functional changes affecting thinking, sensation, language, and/or emotions. It can also cause epilepsy and increase the risk for conditions such as Alzheimer's disease, Parkinson's disease, and other brain disorders that become more prevalent with age. Each year about 1.4 million Americans sustain a TBI, resulting in 50,000 deaths, 235,000 hospitalizations, and 1.1 million individuals treated and released from the nation's hospital emergency departments. It is also estimated that at least 5.3 million Americans, about 2% of the population, currently have a long-term or lifelong need for help to perform activities of daily living (ADLs) such as feeding, bathing, dressing, and grooming as a result of a TBI (Ashley, 2010).

Mental Diseases and Conditions

Alzheimer's Disease. Named after the German physician Alois Alzheimer, who first described the disease in 1906, Alzheimer's disease is a neurodegenerative disease that leads to progressive intellectual decline, confusion, and disorientation. Increasing age is the greatest known risk factor for Alzheimer's disease. One in ten individuals over 65 years of age and nearly half of those over 85 are affected. It is the most common cause of dementia among people 65 years of age and older. Alzheimer's disease affects an estimated 4.5 million Americans (National Institute on Aging, 2008).

Depression. Depression, or major depressive disorder, is the leading cause of disability in the United States for individuals between the ages of 15 and 44. Depression is a potentially life-threatening disorder. It can contribute to a higher morbidity and mortality of other medical conditions. A variety of biochemical, genetic, and environmental factors may cause depression. The risk factors for developing or triggering depression include: having other biological relatives with depression; having family members who have taken their own life; stressful life events, such as the death of a loved one;

having a depressed mood as a youngster; having an illness, such as cancer, heart disease, or HIV/AIDS; the long-term use of certain medications, such as sleeping pills and some drugs used to control high blood pressure; having certain personality traits, such as low self-esteem and being overly dependent, self-critical, or pessimistic; alcohol, nicotine, and drug use; having recently given birth; and being in a lower socioeconomic group. Depression can also co-occur with anxiety disorders and substance abuse. While depression can develop at any age, the median age at onset is 32. Depression tends to be more prevalent in women than in men. Depression affects about 14.8 million American adults, or about 6.7% of the population age 18 or older in a given year (Manderscheid & Berry, 2006).

Mental Disorders. Mental disorders, such as anxiety disorders, mood disorders, personality disorders, and schizophrenia, are major causes of disability. The causes of mental disorders are complex, and vary according to the particular disorder and individual. Possible causes of mental disorders include: heredity, infections, brain injury, poor nutrition, exposure to toxins, severe psychological trauma, and substance abuse. About one-quarter of Americans 18 years of age and older—about one in four adults—suffer from a diagnosable mental disorder in a given year. Although mental disorders are widespread in the population, the main burden of illness is concentrated in a much smaller proportion—about 6% or one in 17—that suffers from a serious mental illness. Many people suffer from more than one mental disorder at a given time. Nearly half of those with any mental disorder meet criteria for two or more disorders, with severity strongly related to multiple illnesses (Manderscheid & Berry, 2006).

Other Diseases and Conditions

Attention Deficit Hyperactivity Disorder (ADHD). Attention deficit hyperactivity disorder (ADHD) is one of the most common behavioral disorders in children and adolescents. The main characteristics of ADHD are inattention, hyperactivity, and impulsiveness. ADHD usually becomes evident in preschool or early elementary years and is about three times more common in boys than girls. Although the cause of ADHD is not known, the disorder may be the result of a combination of genetic, social, and environmental factors. Possible risk factors include: alcohol and tobacco use during pregnancy, premature delivery, very low birth weight, and brain injuries. About 5 million American children 3 to 17 years of age have been diagnosed with ADHD—about 8% of children in this age category (Stahl, Mignon, & Muntner, 2010).

Autism. Autism is part of a group of disorders called autism spectrum disorders (ASDs). Symptoms of ASDs include: significant language delays, social and communication problems, and unusual behaviors and interests. ASDs symptoms range in severity, with autism being the most debilitating form, while other disorders, such as Asperger syndrome, produce milder symptoms. Autism and other ASDs develop in childhood and generally are diagnosed by age three. Autism is about four times more common in boys than girls. However, girls with the disorder tend to have more severe symptoms and greater cognitive impairment. The cause or causes of ASDs are not known, but they may be due to environmental, biological, and genetic factors. It is estimated that about one in 110 American children have ASDs (Chez, 2010).

Developmental Disabilities (DD). Developmental disabilities (DD) are a diverse group of severe chronic conditions. DD originate at birth or during childhood, and they usually last throughout a person's lifetime. DD can be divided into various categories that include: nervous system disabilities, sensory-related disabilities, metabolic disorders, and degenerative disorders. Specific conditions commonly included under the DD term are autism, cerebral palsy, epilepsy, hearing and visual impairments, and intellectual disability, among others. Individuals with DD have substantial limitations in major life activities, such as language, mobility, learning, self-help, and independent living. Although estimates vary, over 6 million Americans have DD (Dryden-Edwards & Combrinck-Graham 2010).

Obesity. Obesity refers to having an abnormally high proportion of body fat, which is defined as having a body mass index (BMI) of 30 or more, calculated from a person's weight and height. A person can be overweight without being obese. However, many people who are overweight are also obese. Obesity is a major risk factor for heart disease, certain types of cancer (breast, colorectal, endometrial, and kidney), and type 2 diabetes. The prevalence of obesity has steadily increased in America over the years among all age groups, ethnic and racial groups, and educational levels. The increase in obesity is due to environments that encourage increased food intake, the promotion and greater use of non-healthful foods, and lack of physical activity. Nearly one-third of all American adults and nearly one-fifth of all American children are obese (Bouchard & Katzmarzyk, 2010).

Substance Abuse. Substance abuse includes two areas: alcohol and drug abuse. Alcohol is the most commonly abused substance in the United States. Many people who abuse alcohol are alcoholics. Alcoholism is a serious disease that has four main features: craving, or a strong need to drink; loss of control, or not being able to stop drinking once started; physical dependence, or having withdrawal symptoms, such as nausea, sweating, or shakiness, after stopping drinking; and tolerance, or the need to drink greater amounts of alcohol in order to get "high." Alcoholism can lead to many health problems, including increased risk of developing various cancers and liver and brain disease. Excessive alcohol consumption among pregnant women can cause birth defects. And it increases the risk of death from motor vehicle crashes and other injuries as well as the risk of homicide and suicide.

Drug abuse includes the use of amphetamines, anabolic steroids, club drugs, cocaine, heroin, inhalants, marijuana, and prescription drugs. Drug abuse plays a major role in many social problems, such as violence, stress, and child abuse. It can lead to homelessness, crime, missed work, or problems with keeping a job. Risk factors for substance abuse are complex and include such factors as: early aggressive behavior, lack of parental supervision, substance abuse among peers, the availability of alcohol and drugs, and poverty. About 17.6 million American adults are alcoholics or have alcohol problems. Each year drug abuse results in about 40 million serious illnesses or injuries among Americans (Scheier, 2010).

Healthcare Professionals

To address the multitude of diseases, injuries, and conditions associated with disability, healthcare professionals differ in their perspectives and the approaches they take. This section presents the two fundamental approaches of healthcare professionals, that of public health professionals and that of clinical health professionals. Although they differ, the two professional groups complement each other. Each group is discussed below.

Public Health Professionals

Public health can be broadly defined as the practice of preventing disease and promoting health within groups of people, from small communities to entire countries. To protect the public's health, public health professionals implement educational programs, develop public policies, administer services, and conduct research to understand and address issues such as infant mortality, chronic diseases, and disability in particular populations.

Public health includes professionals from many different fields (e.g., biology, economics, medicine, nursing, and nutrition) with the common purpose of protecting the public's health. Public health professionals include: scientists and researchers, health educators, public policymakers, public health physicians, public health nurses, occupational health and safety professionals, social workers, sanitarians, nutritionists, and others.

Many public health professionals receive their academic training at Schools of Public Health, which are often university colleges (e.g., the School of Public Health at the University of Illinois at Chicago). Although Schools of Public Health differ in the number and types of courses they offer, they all address certain core areas. These core areas include: biostatistics, a field of study that applies statistical procedures, techniques, and methods to medical and public health problems; epidemiology, which identifies the causes and risk factors of diseases in order to prevent them from occurring; maternal and child health, which works to improve the health of women, children, and their families, nutrition, which examines how food and nutrients affect the wellness and lifestyle of populations; behavioral science/health education, which identifies ways of helping people make healthier choices and develops educational programs; environmental health, which determines environmental risk factors that cause diseases such as asthma, cancer, and food poisoning; public health laboratory practice, which trains people to test biological and environmental samples in order to diagnose and control diseases; health services administration/management, which teaches various skills needed to manage clinics, hospitals, and other healthcare institutions; health policy, which works to improve the public's health through legislative action at the federal, state, and local levels; international/global health, which addresses and compares the levels of health among different countries; and public health practice, which trains physicians, dentists, nurses, and pharmacists to apply public health principles to improve their practices.

A large number of government agencies conduct public health activities. For example, at the federal level they include such agencies as the Centers for Disease Control and Prevention (CDC), the Food and Drug Administration (FDA), and the Health Resources and Services Administration (HRSA). At the state level, each state in the United States has a public health department, such as the Illinois Department of Public Health. And at the local level, counties and cities have public health departments, such as the Cook County Department of Public Health and the Chicago Department of Public Health. There are about 500,000 public health professionals employed by federal, state, and local public health agencies (Turnock, 2009).

Many private organizations also conduct public health activities, including: academic centers and university programs (e.g., Coleman Institute for Cognitive Disabilities, University of Colorado); disease, injury, and condition associations (e.g., Alzheimer's Association); group/population associations (e.g., American Association of People with Disabilities); professional and trade associations (e.g., American Academy of Physical Medicine and Rehabilitation); contract-research and policy organizations (e.g., Center for Studying Disability Policy [CSDP], Mathematical Policy Research, Inc.); healthcare accrediting organizations (e.g., Commission on Accreditation of Rehabilitation Facilities); and various foundations and philanthropies (e.g., American Foundation for the Blind).

At the core of public health is the concept of prevention. Prevention aims to stop or minimize the occurrence of disease and its consequences. Specifically, public health attempts to prevent diseases, injuries, and various conditions at three different levels: primary prevention, secondary prevention, and tertiary prevention.

Primary prevention seeks to stop a disease, injury, or condition from occurring by decreasing or eliminating its risk factors and by promoting healthy lifestyles. Examples of primary prevention activities that decrease risk factors include: obtaining recommended immunizations; women taking daily doses of folic acid before conception through the first trimester of pregnancy to reduce the risk of certain birth defects (spina bifida, anencephaly, and some heart defects); using a condom to prevent the spread of sexually transmitted diseases; taking blood-pressure and cholesterol medications to prevent heart disease and stroke; and wearing a safety helmet while skateboarding, or riding a bicycle or motorcycle, to prevent head injuries. Examples of primary prevention activities to promote healthy lifestyles include: avoiding tobacco use; not abusing alcohol and other drugs; maintaining a healthy diet; getting adequate exercise and rest; successfully managing stress; and maintaining a positive outlook on life.

Secondary prevention, or screening, seeks to identify and control diseases in their early stages, before signs and symptoms develop. Examples of secondary prevention activities include: taking mammograms to detect early-stage breast cancer; blood pressure checks to reveal hypertension; eye screening for glaucoma and cataracts; pap smears to check for cervical cancer; prostate exams for prostate cancer; blood screening for diabetes and high cholesterol; EKGs to reveal problems with the heart; skin checks to identify possible skin cancer; and colonoscopy to detect colorectal cancer.

Tertiary prevention seeks to prevent long-term impairments and disabilities by restoring individuals to their optimal level of functioning after a disease or injury has occurred. Examples of tertiary prevention activities include: providing insulin to diabetes patients; preventing the reoccurrence of heart attacks with anticlotting medications; and providing occupational therapy for individuals with a recent stroke (Holland & Stewart, 2005).

Emerging Areas of Public Health and Disability

An emerging area of public health concerns the prevention of secondary conditions among people with disabilities. Secondary conditions are any conditions to which a person is more susceptible by virtue of having a primary disabling condition. They include such conditions as depression, substance abuse, hip fracture, obesity, decubitus ulcers (pressure sores), lost muscle tone, and gait instability. To prevent and reduce secondary conditions, public health professionals are promoting healthy habits and lifestyles of people with disabilities, changing the environmental factors that undermine their health and well-being, and routinely including people with disabilities in policy, planning, reporting, and legislation practices, and other areas of society.

Another emerging area of public health concerns disaster preparedness and assistance for people with disabilities. People with disabilities often have special, unique needs during natural and man-made disasters. During disasters, they are often at greater risk than others. For example, a disaster may force people with disabilities to leave behind their wheelchairs, service dogs, medications, and other adaptive aids and medical supplies necessary for daily living. They may find that elevators in hospitals, nursing homes, and other facilities are not working and streets are flooded or filled with debris, making it difficult to evacuate or move about. People in need of personal assistance services may be separated from their attendants. And medical records may be lost or destroyed.

To help address these needs at the federal level, President George W. Bush signed Executive Order 13347 on July 22, 2004. The Executive Order, *Individuals with Disabilities in Emergency Preparedness*, called for the federal government to support the safety and security of individuals with disabilities in all types of emergency situations through a coordinated effort among federal agencies. It also established the Interagency Coordinating Council on Emergency Preparedness and Individuals with Disabilities (ICC), which is composed of 23 federal departments and agencies.

The vital importance of disaster preparedness and emergency response was starkly shown in late August 2005, when Hurricane Katrina struck the Gulf coasts of Louisiana, Alabama, and Mississippi. Hurricane Katrina, one of the greatest single natural disasters in the country's history, blew down and washed away entire neighborhoods, broke down protective levees, and flooded much of the City of New Orleans. Although the exact numbers will never be known, the hurricane displaced 1 million people, and killed over 1,300 people. People with disabilities were particularly hard hit by the devastating storm. Dozens died in nursing homes and medical centers, and more died in their own homes or in the streets.

Learning from the failures in planning and response to Hurricane Katrina, federal, state, and local government agencies (i.e., Centers for Disease Control and Prevention [CDC], U.S, Department of Homeland Security [USDHS], and the Federal Emergency Management Agency [FEMA]), as well as many private organizations (i.e., American Association on Health and Disability [AAHD], American Red Cross, and the National Organization on Disability [NOD]), are working to ensure that the public health needs of persons with disabilities are met before, during, and after a disaster (Drum, Krahn, & Bersani, 2009).

Clinical Health Professionals

Clinical health professionals examine and treat individual patients or clients. To a varying degree, all clinical health professionals provide services to and treat people with disabilities. There are many types of clinical health professionals, including: physicians, nurses, pharmacists, allied health professionals, and other professionals and paraprofessionals. Each type is briefly discussed below.

Physicians

Although physicians constitute a small part of the entire clinical health professional workforce, they control the greatest amount of resources and make the critical decisions with regard to admitting and discharging hospital patients, diagnosing a patient's illness, and conceptualizing the overall medical treatment plan. Physicians play a vital role in providing services to and treating people with disabilities. They also evaluate and certify the degree of physical or mental impairment(s) of individuals to determine their eligibility to receive disability assistance. In 2007, there were an estimated 816,727 active physicians in the United States (U.S. Census Bureau, 2009).

Being a physician is one of the most demanding of all occupations. To practice medicine, physicians must undergo many years of formal education and training. After receiving their undergraduate degrees, they must go to medical school for four years, and then go on to receive internship and residency training for an additional three to eight years.

The vast majority of physicians in the United States (about 95%) are trained in allopathic medicine, with a small minority of physicians (about 5%) being trained in osteopathic medicine. Allopathic medicine is a therapeutic system in which diseases are treated by using drugs, radiation, or surgery to produce effects different from those caused by the disease. In contrast, osteopathic medicine tends to take a holistic perspective, treating the "whole person" (mind-body-spirit), and it emphasizes the role of the musculoskeletal system in health and the use of manipulation in treatment. Over the years, the training of allopathic and osteopathic physicians has become increasingly similar, and today there is little difference between the two.

In order for physicians to practice medicine, all states, the District of Columbia, and U.S. territories require licensing. The specific licensure requirements include graduation from an accredited allopathic medical school that awards a Doctor of Medicine (MD) degree or a osteopathic medical school that awards a Doctor of Osteopathic Medicine (DO) degree, successful completion of a licensing examination governed by either the National Board of Medical Examiners or the National Board of Osteopathic Medical Examiners, and completion of a supervised internship/ residency program.

Most practicing physicians in the United States received their medical school training in the United States or Canada. However, about one-quarter of all physicians practicing medicine in the country received their medical school education somewhere other than in an approved North American medical school. These physicians are known as International Medical Graduates (IMGs), and formerly they were referred to as Foreign Medical Graduates (FMGs). For IMGs to practice medicine in the United States they must pass an English proficiency examination as well as a national medical licensing examination.

Only about 30% of all practicing physicians in United States are generalist versus specialist physicians. Generalist physicians, or primary care physicians, include physicians in the areas of family medicine, general internal medicine, and general pediatrics. Primary care physicians are often the first point of contact for patients in the healthcare system with undiagnosed diseases, signs, symptoms, or other health concerns. They also take responsibility for coordinating the overall care of the patient's health problems, referring patients to appropriate medical specialists when necessary. Primary care physicians diagnose and treat many common acute and chronic diseases, and they also provide health promotion, disease prevention, health maintenance, counseling, and patient education. Most osteopathic physicians are primary care physicians.

The majority of practicing physicians (about 70%) in the country are specialists. Specialist physicians focus their practices on a particular area of medicine or patient care, concentrating on certain body systems (e.g., cardiology), specific age groups (e.g., pediatrics), or scientific techniques to diagnose or treat particular medical conditions (e.g., radiology). The American Board of Medical Specialties (ABMS) recognizes and accredits more than 145 medical specialties and subspecialties. Medical specialties include such areas as anesthesiology, oncology, surgery, and urology. Most allopathic physicians are specialists (Bujak, 2008).

The number, type, and geographic distribution of physicians have important implications regarding the access to, and the quality of, healthcare for people with disabilities. Some healthcare researchers and public policy analysts believe there are too many specialist physicians and too few primary care physicians practicing medicine in the United States. They argue that specialist physicians focus too narrowly on a particular disease, condition, or treatment method and tend to ignore the patient's other important medical conditions and not treat the whole person. Some believe there is a problem with the overall geographic distribution of physicians, often referred to as a maldistribution of physicians, with too few physicians practicing in rural and poor inner city areas and too many physicians practicing in affluent urban and suburban areas. And many believe there is a growing national shortage of physicians, which is expected to intensify in the future as the generation known as the baby boomers ages and the need for healthcare grows (Association of American Medical Colleges, 2009).

Physical Medicine and Rehabilitation

One medical specialty that treats a relatively large proportion of people with disabilities is physical medicine and rehabilitation (PM&R). Physical medicine and rehabilitation, which is also referred to as rehabilitation medicine, is concerned with evaluating, diagnosing, and treating patients with physical disabilities. The specialty of PM&R is also divided into six subspecialties: hospice and palliative medicine, neuromuscular medicine, pain medicine, pediatric rehabilitation medicine, spinal cord injury medicine, and sports medicine.

Physicians who specialize in PM&R are known as physiatrists. The term physiatrist was coined by Frank Krusen, an American physician who established the country's first Department of Physical Medicine at the Mayo Clinic. It is derived from the Greek words "physis," pertaining to physical phenomena, and "iatreia," referring to healer or physician. Physiatrists treat a wide range of diseases, injuries, and conditions, from back pain to spinal cord injuries. The role of the physiatrist is to manage a patient's medical issues as the patient participates in the rehabilitation process. There are about 10,000 physiatrists practicing in the United States. Most physiatrists work in community hospitals, rehabilitation facilities, and private offices (Weiss, Weiss, & Pobre, 2010).

Nurses

Nurses are the largest single group of clinical health professionals in the United States. There are two major types of nurses: registered nurses (RNs) and licensed practical nurses (LPNs).

RNs are responsible for overseeing the nature and quality of all nursing care patients receive, supervising licensed practical nurses and other health personnel involved in providing patient care, and following the instructions of physicians regarding patients. Specifically, RNs treat patients by recording their medical histories and symptoms, help perform diagnostic tests and analyze results, operate medical machinery, administer treatments and medications, and help with patient follow-up and rehabilitation.

All states in the country require RNs to be licensed. To obtain a license, individuals must obtain a bachelor's degree, an associate's degree, or a diploma from an approved nursing program. They must then pass a national licensing examination, known as the National Council Licensure Examination, or NCLEX-RN. Other eligibility requirements for licensure vary by state.

Some RNs obtain more formal education and go on to become advanced degree nurses, including advanced practical nurses (APN), nurse anesthetists (CRNA), nurse practitioners (NP), and doctors of nursing (DPN).

About 60% of all RNs in the country work in hospitals, while others work in the offices of physicians, in home health care, in nursing homes, and for employment services. In 2007, there were over 2.4 million licensed RNs in the United States (U.S. Census Bureau, 2009).

Licensed practical nurses (LPNs), called licensed vocational nurses (LVNs) in some states, often provide basic bedside care to patients. Working under the supervision of an RN or physician, LPNs measure and record patients' vital signs, prepare and give injections, monitor catheters, dress wounds, give rubs and massages, and assist patients in eating, dressing, and walking. LPNs may also supervise nursing assistants and aides.

Most LPNs receive their nursing training by taking one year of course work at a vocational or technical school or community college. To practice, an individual must complete a state-approved training program and pass the National Council Licensure Examination, or NCLEX-PN. Eligibility for licensure may vary by state. LPNs also may become credentialed in specialties such as IV therapy, gerontology, long-term care, and pharmacology. Some LPNs also choose to become registered nurses through LPN-to-RN training programs. LPNs work in a variety of settings, including hospitals, nursing homes, home health care, and the offices of physicians. In 2007, there were 719,240 LPNs in the United States (U.S. Census Bureau, 2009).

As of 2010, there is a growing shortage of nurses, particularly RNs, in the United States. Over 100,000 RN positions in the country's hospitals are vacant. These vacancies are the result of the aging of the nursing workforce, the declining number of students seeking careers in nursing, insufficient numbers of nursing faculty, and competition from non-hospital employers. The shortage of nurses is expected to worsen in the future, with the nation's hospitals facing an estimated 1 million nursing vacancies by 2020 (American Hospital Association, 2009).

Pharmacists

Pharmacists are generally the most accessible of all clinical health professionals, as they practice in a wide range of settings, including community retail pharmacies, hospitals, and clinics, and they also provide mail and telephone services. In 2007, there were 253,110 pharmacists in the United States (National Center for Health Statistics, 2009).

Pharmacists are the most knowledgeable clinical health professionals concerning medications and their use. Although pharmacists cannot dispense prescription drugs without authorization from a licensed physician or other legally sanctioned practitioner, they explain the effects of medications and recommend levels or doses—primarily to patients and at times to practitioners—as well as provide instructions for their use.

Some pharmacists specialize in specific drug therapy areas, such as intravenous nutrition support, which provides nutrients to patients who are unable to ingest or tolerate various foods; oncology, which provides anticancer drugs; nuclear pharmacy, which provides chemotherapy; geriatric pharmacy, which provides drugs to elderly patients; and psychiatric pharmacy, which provides drugs to treat patients with various mental conditions.

All states and the District of Columbia require pharmacists to be licensed in order to practice. To obtain a license, individuals must earn a Doctor of Pharmacy (Pharm. D.) degree from an accredited college or school of pharmacy and pass several examinations.

The demand for pharmacists is expected to increase in the future as prescription drugs increase in number and become more complex, and the number of people taking multiple medications increases.

Allied Health Professionals

Allied health professionals are clinical health professionals who are not physicians, nurses, or pharmacists. Allied health professionals include a very large number of professionals, encompassing more than 100 occupational titles. They include, to name a few, dental hygienists, diagnostic medical sonographers, dietitians, medical technologists, respiratory therapists, and speech language pathologists. There are about 3 million allied health professionals employed in the United States. As a group, they comprise more than 20% of all healthcare workers.

Some allied health professionals practice independently, while others work as part of a healthcare team. Allied health professionals often provide continual evaluation and assessment of patients needs. They also play a major role in informing the attending clinician of the patient's progress and response to treatment. The training and licensure of allied health professionals varies greatly by occupation. To practice, most allied health professionals must receive one or more years of formal education, and most must pass one or more examinations.

Two examples of allied health professionals who work with a relatively large proportion of people with disabilities are occupational therapists and physical therapists. Both occupational and physical therapists are concerned with improving the health and quality of life of their clients through treatments that allow them to perform everyday activities. Their approaches are different, but their treatments are complementary.

Occupational Therapists

Occupational therapists, sometimes referred to as simply OTs, focus on evaluating and improving their clients' functional abilities. Although they do not directly treat a client's disease, injury, or condition, occupational therapists help their clients optimize their independence and ability to accomplish their daily activities, from using a computer to caring for daily needs such as dressing, cooking, and eating. For clients with permanent disabilities, such as spinal cord injuries, cerebral palsy, or muscular dystrophy, occupational therapists often demonstrate the use of adaptive equipment, such as wheelchairs, orthoses, and dressing and eating aides. They also may design or build customized equipment for their clients to help them improve their communication and better control their environment at home or work.

Although many clients of occupational therapists have a medical condition, some do not. For example, occupational therapists may work with clients who are making life transitions, such as retirement, homelessness, or displacement because of a disaster, or who are just struggling with everyday activities, such as a child who is having difficulty with handwriting in school.

To practice, all states require that occupational therapists be licensed. To obtain a license, individuals must obtain a master's degree or higher in occupational therapy, and then they must pass a national examination. Occupational therapists work in hospitals, offices of other health practitioners, schools, and nursing homes. In 2007, there were 91,920 occupational therapists in the United States (National Center for Health Statistics, 2009).

Physical Therapists

Physical therapists, or PTs, focus on assessing, diagnosing, and treating musculoskeletal and neuromuscular problems that affect how people move and perform physical functions, such as standing up, walking, and lifting. Typical clients of physical therapists include individuals with back pain, elderly persons with arthritis or balance problems, injured athletes, infants with developmental disabilities, and persons who have had severe burns, strokes, or spinal cord injuries. Physical therapists treat clients with therapeutic exercise, functional training, manual therapy techniques, assistive and adaptive devices and equipment, and physical agents and electrotherapeutic modalities.

All states regulate the practice of physical therapists. Although eligibility requirements vary by state, the typical requirements include graduating from an accredited physical therapy education program and passing a national and state examination. A number of states also require physical therapists to take continuing education courses as a condition of maintaining their licensure.

Physical therapists practice in a variety of settings, including private practices, hospitals, rehabilitation centers, nursing homes, schools, and home health agencies. In 2007, there were 161,853 physical therapists in the United States (National Center for Health Statistics, 2009).

Other Professionals and Paraprofessionals

Some people with disabilities seek care from other clinical health professionals as well as paraprofessionals. These professionals often include chiropractors, and acupuncturists, while paraprofessionals include home health aides and personal and home care aides.

Chiropractors and acupuncturists practice complementary and alternative medicine (CAM). CAM is difficult to precisely define because it is such a broad field that is constantly changing. Generally speaking, though, the term covers a group of diverse medical and healthcare systems and products that are not usually considered part of conventional medicine, as practiced by physicians, nurses, pharmacists, and allied health professionals. It should be noted, however, that the boundaries between CAM and conventional medicine are not absolute and change over time, with some CAM practices and products becoming part of conventional "mainstream" medicine (Zollman, Richardson, & Vickers, 2008).

Chiropractors

Chiropractors, also known as doctors of chiropractic or chiropractic physicians, are the largest and most widely recognized group of CAM practitioners. In 2007, there were 89,161 licensed chiropractors in the United States. Chiropractors focus on disorders of the musculoskeletal and nervous systems and the effects of these disorders on general health. They often treat back pain, neck pain, pain in the joints of the arms and legs, and headaches by manipulating the patient's spine.

To practice, chiropractors must be licensed, which requires an undergraduate education, the completion of four years of chiropractic college courses, and passing scores on national and state examinations. Each state in the country and the District of Columbia licenses chiropractors.

Most chiropractors work in a solo practice, although some are in group practice or work for other chiropractors. Unlike many other CAM practitioners, chiropractors are authorized to receive federal Medicare payments for the treatments they provide, as well as payments from major private health insurance carriers. Many people go to chiropractors rather than physicians to receive care because chiropractors usually charge less than physicians, spend more time with patients, and tend to explain medical problems in easily understandable terms (Haldeman, 2005).

Acupuncturists

Another type of CAM practitioner that often treats people with disabilities is an acupuncturist. Acupuncture, which has been practiced for thousands of years in China and other Asian countries, uses needles, herbs, and other devices to treat disorders such as headaches, back problems, and foot pain. By inserting fine needles into the body at various sites, acupuncture appears to stimulate the nervous system, releasing various chemicals, such as endorphins, in the muscles, spinal cord, and brain. This process may influence bodily systems and improve healing. Acupuncture appears to be effective in some cases and is moving into mainstream medicine.

The training of acupuncturists varies greatly. Some acupuncturists are formally trained at various schools, while others have no formal educational training in the practice, learning acupuncture from a family member or friend. The licensing of acupuncturists also varies greatly. In some states, only licensed physicians and chiropractors are permitted to practice acupuncture. In other states, acupuncturists must pass an examination to be licensed, while in still other states, there are no laws governing the practice of acupuncture at all. In 2007, there were about 28,000 licensed acupuncturists in the United States, in addition to an unknown number of acupuncturists who are not licensed. During that same year, about 3.1 million adults and 150,000 children in the country used acupuncture (Barnes, Bloom, & Nahin, 2008).

Home Health Aides and Personal and Home Care Aides

Home health aides and personal and home care aides (also called caregivers, companions, homemakers, and personal attendants) are paraprofessionals who provide medical and personal care to the elderly or disabled living in their own home or a residential care facility. Aides may provide light housekeeping and homemaking tasks as well as helping their clients get out of bed, bathe, dress, and groom. Some may also accompany their clients to medical or other appointments. Although home health aides and personal and home care aides have similar job duties, there are some differences. Home health aides are typically employed by home health or hospice agencies, where they work under the direct supervision of a nurse or other medical professional. Home health aides often provide some basic health-related services, such as checking the patients' pulse rate, temperature, respiration rate, changing dressings, and administrating medications, while some experienced aides assist their clients with medical equipment such as ventilators. Personal and home care aides tend to work for various public and private agencies that provide home care services. A nurse, social worker, or other non-medical manager may supervise these aides. However, some aides are hired directly by the client or the client's family. Some personal and home care aides, often called direct-support professionals, work with individuals with development disabilities (DD), assisting them in implementing behavior plans, teaching self-care skills, providing employment support, and a range of other personal assistance services. In terms of education, training, and licensure, home health aides are often required to complete a training program and successfully pass a competency evaluation or state certification program. In contrast, personal and home care aides are not required to be certified. Most aides work part-time and weekends or evenings to suit the needs of their clients. Some aides may work for a short amount of time with many clients, while others may work for many years with one client. In 2008, home health aides and personal and home care aides held about 1.7 million jobs in the United States (National Association for Home Care and Hospice, 2008).

Healthcare Organizations

Hospitals, nursing homes, and various long-term care organizations play a vital role in providing a continuum of medical care and social services to people with disabilities. A brief overview and a description of the importance of each type of healthcare organization are presented below.

Hospitals

Hospitals are the cornerstone of the clinical healthcare system. Hospitals are multipurpose institutions that bring together a vast array of clinical health professionals, medical technology, and other resources. Specifically, hospitals provide inpatient and outpatient diagnostic and therapeutic medical services, conduct medical research, train healthcare practitioners, provide laboratory and other medical facilities, and sponsor health education and preventive healthcare programs.

The importance of hospitals to patients and the communities they serve is enormous. In 2007, the 4,915 community hospitals in the United States provided care to 35 million inpatients, performed 27 million surgeries, responded to 121 million patients in their emergency departments, and delivered more than 4 million babies. Hospitals are also very important to the national and local economies, providing 5.3 million jobs (American Hospital Association, 2009).

Hospitals are defined by the various organizations that license, regulate, and accredit them. As a result, the definition of a hospital varies widely across countries, states, and programs. The World Health Organization (WHO) defines a hospital broadly as an organization that is permanently staffed by at least one physician, can offer inpatient accommodations, and can provide active medical and nursing care. In contrast, the American Hospital Association (AHA) more narrowly defines a hospital as an organization that has at least six inpatient beds that are continuously available for care; is constructed to ensure patient safety; has an identifiable governing authority responsible for running it, a chief executive who reports to the authority, a medical staff with licensed physicians, and at least one registered nurse supervisor and continuous nursing services; admits patients only by the authority of a member of the organization's medical staff; maintains medical records; and provides pharmacy services and patient food services, including special diets.

Hospitals are very complex organizations. They can be classified and compared in many different ways, such as by their size or number of beds, ownership status, teaching status, the type of services they provide to patients, whether they are a community hospital, and whether they are a member of a multihospital healthcare system.

Hospitals can be classified by bed size, the number of beds they have that are licensed, or the number of beds they have that are set up and staffed. Small hospitals have 25 beds or less, while large hospitals have 500 or more beds. The average bed size of hospitals in United States is about 175 beds.

By ownership status, hospitals can be classified as being non-government not-for-profit institutions (i.e., church operated, or other), government-owned institutions (i.e., federal, state, or local), or investor-owned (for-profit) institutions. Most hospitals in the United States are non-government not-for-profit institutions, followed by government-owned institutions, and investor-owned institutions.

By teaching status, hospitals can be classified as being either a teaching or non-teaching hospital. Teaching hospitals are affiliated with a medical school, have at least one medical residency program, and are members of the Association of American Medical Colleges' Council of Teaching Hospitals and Health Systems (COTH).

By the services they provide, hospitals can be classified as being general hospitals, special hospitals, rehabilitation and chronic disease hospitals, or psychiatric hospitals. General hospitals provide a wide array of patient services, diagnostic and therapeutic, for a variety of medical conditions. Special hospitals provide services to patients with specific medical conditions, both surgical and nonsurgical. Psychiatric hospitals provide diagnostic and treatment services for patients who have psychiatric-related illnesses. Rehabilitation and chronic disease hospitals provide diagnostic and treatment services to patients with disabilities requiring restorative and adjustive services.

By community status, hospitals can be classified as being either a community or non-community hospital. The American Hospital Association (AHA) defines community hospitals as all nonfederal, short-term (having an average length of inpatient stay of less than 30 days), general and other special hospitals (e.g., children's hospitals, obstetrics and gynecology, rehabilitation hospitals) whose facilities and services are available to the public. Examples of well-known community hospitals in the United States include: Bellevue Hospital Center, New York City (America's oldest public hospital); John H. Stroger Jr. Hospital of Cook Country (formerly Cook County Hospital, Chicago); and Los Angeles County-USC Medical Center. In contrast, U.S. Department of Veterans Affairs (VA) hospitals are not community hospitals because they are federal hospitals and they are not available to the general public, only to U.S. veterans.

Lastly, hospitals can also be classified as being either a member of a multihospital healthcare system or a single, stand-alone institution. A multihospital healthcare system is defined as two or more hospitals owned, leased, sponsored, or contract managed by a central organization. Examples of multihospital systems include: the Mayo Clinic, which has hospitals in Rochester, Minnesota, Jacksonville, Florida, and Phoenix and Scottsdale, Arizona; Baylor Healthcare System, which has 15 hospitals in the Dallas, Texas, area; and Advocate Health Care, which owns 12 hospitals in the Chicago area.

Rehabilitation Facilities

Although all hospitals provide some medical care and services to people with disabilities, rehabilitation inpatient and outpatient units within community hospitals and rehabilitation hospitals treat a high proportion of people with disabilities.

Treatment for a disability often begins in a community hospital. After an illness, injury, or surgery, many patients receive additional treatment and services in the hospital's rehabilitation inpatient and/or outpatient units. In 2007, a total of 1,480 community hospitals in the United States had a physical rehabilitation inpatient unit, and 3,636 community hospitals had physical rehabilitation outpatient units (American Hospital Association, 2009).

Rehabilitation hospitals are specialty facilities, often single, stand-alone institutions, which provide treatment programs to patients to enhance their functional ability. These hospitals provide coordinated multidisciplinary care using treatment teams that often consist of physiatrists, nurses, physical and occupational therapists, and other allied health professionals. They typically treat patients with spinal cord injuries, brain injuries, stroke, amputation, neurological disorders, and musculoskeletal and orthopedic conditions. Some of the major rehabilitation hospitals in the United States include the Rehabilitation Institute of Chicago (RIC), the Kessler Institute of Rehabilitation in West Orange, New Jersey, and the Spaulding Rehabilitation Hospital in Boston.

Veterans Health Administration Hospitals

The Veterans Health Administration (VHA), the medical component of the U.S. Department of Veterans Affairs (VA), is an important source of medical care and services for U.S. veterans with disabilities. Specifically, one of the VHA's major strategic goals is to "restore the capability of veterans with disabilities to the greatest extent possible, and improve the quality of their lives and that of their families" (U.S. Department of Veterans Affairs, 2010).

The VHA provides a broad spectrum of medical, surgical, prescriptive, and rehabilitation care for veterans through its giant national healthcare system. The VHA's integrated healthcare system—the largest in the world—employs a staff of 255,000 individuals and consists of a nationwide network of 153 hospitals, 956 outpatient clinics, 134 nursing homes, 90 domiciliary residential rehabilitation treatment programs, and 232 readjustment counseling centers. The system provides care to nearly 6 million veterans each year.

An important feature of the VHA is its pioneering integrated clinical database and electronic patient medical records system. The VHA's electronic medical records system stores all of a VHA patient's inpatient and outpatient medical records and makes all of the information available at any of its facilities. The system increases access to care, lowers costs, and improves the quality of care. It enables veterans who move, travel, or go on vacation to easily access their medical records and receive medical care at any VHA facility in the country.

The VHA also plays a major role in both health education and research. It is the nation's largest provider of education and training for medical residents and other trainees. Each year nearly 34,000 medical residents and 19,000 medical students receive training at the VHA. And more than 65% of all practicing physicians in the United States have at some point in their careers trained at VHA facilities. In terms of research, the VHA is one of the 10 largest research and development agencies in the federal government. Its major areas of research and development include biomedical laboratory science, clinical science, health services research, and rehabilitation research.

To address the special needs of disabled veterans with post-traumatic stress disorders, visual impairment, and polytrauma (multiple traumatic injuries), the VHA has established a number of programs and centers. For example, the VHA provides polytrauma care through a system of four dedicated rehabilitation centers and 21 network sites to veterans and returning service members with multiple injuries, one of which is considered life threatening. Polytrauma includes such conditions as traumatic brain injury (TBI), hearing loss, amputation, fractures, burns, and visual impairment.

Although telemedicine accounts for only a small part of its total medical services, the VHA is increasingly using interactive audiovisual media to provide in-home medical care via computer and other special devices to increase accessibility for rural and disabled veterans (U.S. Department of Veterans Affairs, 2010).

Nursing Homes

Nursing homes, also called nursing facilities, play a vital role in providing medical care and social services to many people with disabilities as well as elderly people. These facilities provide different levels of medical care designed to meet the wide range of the needs of their residents. They may specialize in short-term or acute nursing care, intermediate care, or long-term, custodial nursing care.

Nursing homes are state-licensed residential facilities with professional staff that provide continuous nursing care and health-related services for individuals who do not require hospitalization but cannot be cared for at home. They provide 24-hour care for residents who are not in the acute phase of illness, but who have significant functional deficiencies, such as the inability to independently dress, eat, bathe, get around, and use the toilet themselves. Nursing home residents may need care for a short period of time, such as for rehabilitation or recovery after an injury or illness, or they may require long-term or permanent care for chronic or progressive physical or mental illness or infirmity.

There are three major types of nursing homes: skilled nursing facilities, intermediate care facilities, and custodial care facilities. Although each type of nursing facility provides a different level of care, many nursing homes in the United States provide more than one level of care. For example, they may have one unit that provides skilled nursing care and another separate unit that provides intermediate care within the same building. And each unit is individually licensed by the State.

Skilled Nursing Facilities

Skilled nursing facilities (SNFs) often provide short-term nursing and rehabilitation care, generally to assist individuals during their recovery following hospitalization for acute medical conditions. For individuals with short-term care needs, SNFs play a transitional role in facilitating care that is less intensive than that provided in hospitals and more intensive than that provided at home. For individuals with long-term care needs, SNFs provide services that may be rendered until the end of their lives. SNFs are staffed by registered nurses (RNs), licensed practical nurses (LPNs), and other clinical health professionals, such as therapists, social workers, and dietitians, all of whom work under the supervision of a physician.

There are about 15,000 SNFs in the United States. Their average size is about 100 beds. SNFs can be hospital-based units or freestanding facilities. Some hospitals, typically small, rural hospitals and critical-access hospitals, also provide skilled nursing care through swing beds, which are hospital beds that are used for either acute care inpatients or skilled nursing care, depending upon the need. Both the Medicare and Medicaid programs certify most SNFs, although a small number of them are only certified by Medicare. Smaller facilities and those only certified by Medicare are often designated units within hospitals.

The majority of SNFs in the country are investor-owned (for-profit) facilities, followed by not-for-profit facilities, with the smallest number of facilities being government owned. Regardless of ownership, most SNFs are affiliated with a corporate chain, while a much smaller number are independent facilities. Some of the largest corporate nursing home chains in the country are HCR Manor Care, Kindred Healthcare, and Genesis Healthcare (Pratt, 2010).

Intermediate Care Facilities

Intermediate care facilities (ICFs) often provide care for individuals who are recovering from acute medical conditions but who do not need continuous care or daily therapeutic services. At ICFs, medical care services are provided to residents by registered nurses (RNs), licensed practical nurses (LPNs), therapists, and other health professionals, under the supervision of a physician.

Many ICFs also provide care for people with intellectual and developmental disabilities. Known as Intermediate Care Facilities for the Developmentally Disabled or ICFs/DD, these residential facilities are certified by the Federal Centers for Medicare and Medicaid Services (CMS) and individual state Medicaid programs. The health services and/or rehabilitation care provided at these facilities is an optional benefit for Medicaid recipients who qualify.

To be eligible for benefits, residents in an ICF/DD must require and receive "active treatment," which consists of aggressive, consistent implementation of a program of specialized and generic training, treatments, and health and related services directed toward helping the individuals acquire the behaviors necessary to function with as much self-determination and independence as possible.

ICFs/DD provide a wide variety of services for the complex needs of intellectual and developmentally disabled individuals who also have significant physical impairments and need 24-hour nursing care. Residents of ICFs/DD are often non-ambulatory and may have seizure disorders, behavior problems, mental illness, visual or hearing impairments, or a combination of these conditions. Many residents of ICFs/DD remain in these facilities from youth until old age. For some residents, the ICF/DD becomes their home and the staff becomes like a family.

There are about 7,000 ICFs/DDs in the United States. The number and size of ICFs/DDs vary widely by state. All 50 states have at least one ICF/DD (Braddock, Hemp, & Rizzolo, 2008).

Custodial Care Facilities

Custodial care facilities provide assistance to residents in activities of daily living (ADL), such as bathing, dressing, eating, and toileting. Individuals who are recovering from a disabling injury or illness may temporarily need custodial care. For other individuals, who are losing their ability to function independently due to chronic or progressive disease or frailty due to advanced age, custodial care may be a long-term need. For some, ongoing professional nursing and other services may be required along with custodial care. If custodial care residents become ill or injured, they may spend time in skilled care and then return to custodial care.

Examples of the types of custodial care services provided at these facilities include: assistance in dressing, eating, and toileting; periodic turning and positioning of residents in bed to prevent bed sores; routine care of incontinent residents, including the use of diapers and protective sheets; changing dressings for chronic conditions; routine care in connection with braces and other devices; and the administration of medications.

The number of custodial care facilities in the United States is unknown (Shi & Singh, 2008).

Other Long-Term Care Organizations

In the past, people with disabilities and elderly people had very few alternatives where they could receive long-term care other than state institutions or nursing homes. Over time, however, there has been a major shift in thinking and public policy encouraging them to live in their own homes, control their own lives, and be an integral part of their community.

To help people remain at home, a number of long-term care organizations are now available. They include such organizations as adult day service centers, home healthcare agencies, assisted living facilities, and continuing care retirement communities.

Adult Day Service Centers

Adult day service centers provide a coordinated program of services for adults in a community-based group setting. Services are designed to provide social and a limited number of health services to adults who need supervised care outside their homes during the day. Most centers operate during normal business hours, five days a week, but some offer services in the evening and on weekends.

There are three major types of adult day service centers: social, medical/ health, and specialized centers. Social adult day service centers provide meals, recreation, and some health-related services. Medical/health adult day service centers provide social activities as well as more intensive health and therapeutic services. Specialized adult day service centers provide services only to specific care recipients, such as those with dementias or intellectual and developmental disabilities (DD).

In 2007, there were 4,601 adult day service centers in the United States. These centers provided care to about 150,000 recipients each day. Most of the centers are not-for-profit organizations, and they are affiliated with other organizations, such as skilled nursing facilities (SNF), hospitals, and senior organizations. The average capacity of adult day centers is 40 recipients. The average age of adult day care recipients is 72. About half of all recipients have some cognitive impairment (MetLife Mature Market Institute, 2009).

Home Healthcare Agencies

Home healthcare agencies provide healthcare and homemaker services in an individual client's residence on a part-time basis for those who are chronically ill, recovering from surgery, or are disabled. These agencies promote, maintain, and restore health as well as maximize the level of independence of the client while minimizing the effects of illness and disability, including terminal illness. Accordingly, home healthcare agencies provide a wide range of healthcare services, including skilled nursing services and occupational, physical, and speech therapy. They also provide help with basic activities of daily living, such as getting in and out of bed, dressing, bathing, eating, and toileting, as well as help with light housekeeping, laundry, shopping, and cooking.

Home healthcare agencies provide and help coordinate the care that the client's physician orders. In support of the physician, home healthcare agency staff develop written care plans describing what services the client will receive in order to reach and maintain his or her best physical, mental, and social well-being. The staff also keeps the physician up-to-date on how the client is doing and amends the care plan as needed.

Specific examples of what the home healthcare staff provide during a typical home visit include: checking what the client is eating and drinking; checking their blood pressure, temperature, heart rate, and breathing; checking the safety of the client's residence; teaching the client about their care so, if possible, they can take care of themselves; and coordinating the client's care by communicating with them, their physician, and others who provide care to them.

In 2007, there were 9,284 Medicare-certified home healthcare agencies in the United States. The number of non-certified agencies that provide home healthcare services is unknown (National Association for Home Care and Hospice, 2008).

Assisted Living Facilities

Assisted living facilities are group living facilities that provide or coordinate personal services, 24-hour supervision and assistance, activities, and health-related services. These facilities are for individuals who are mobile but may need assistance with one or two activities of daily living. Residents of assisted living facilities often live in their own room or apartment within a building, but they have some or all of their meals together.

Assisted living facilities typically provide a range of services, including: personal care services, such as help with eating, bathing, dressing, and toileting; various health services; medication management; social services; transportation services; laundry and linen services; and housekeeping and maintenance services.

The typical assisted living resident is a woman in her mid-80s who is mobile but needs assistance with two activities of daily living, often preparing meals and managing medications. The average length of stay in an assisted living facility is a little over two years.

In 2007, there were about 38,000 assisted living facilities in the United States housing about 975,000 people. The average assisted living facility has 54 units. However, facilities can vary greatly in size (Assisted Living Federation of America, 2009).

Continuing Care Retirement Communities

Continuing care retirement communities (CCRCs), sometimes referred to as life-care communities, are residential facilities that provide their residents access to three levels of housing and care in one location: independent living, assisted living, and skilled nursing home care. Residents who are healthy and self-sufficient live in independent homes or apartments. Residents requiring assisted living are provided help with the daily tasks of living. And residents with greater healthcare needs are provided with skilled nursing home care. Depending upon their health, residents move in and out of these settings, but always remain in the CCRC.

CCRCs are unique compared to other healthcare organizations because they offer prospective residents a contract that says they will provide the individuals with housing and services for life. Most CCRCs require a substantial one-time entrance fee and then monthly payments thereafter.

These fees vary by community and depend on the type of housing and services they provide. However, other CCRCs operate on a rental basis and do not require an entrance fee.

Often established in a campus-like setting, CCRCs offer independent living units such as apartments, cottages, town homes, or small, single-family homes for incoming residents who are healthy and self-sufficient. They provide residents the option of purchasing their meals, housekeeping, and laundry services. They also frequently provide their residents various amenities, such as fitness centers, libraries, health clinics, and emergency services.

CCRCs vary greatly in size and ownership. Some CCRCs are owned and operated by religious orders or fraternal organizations, some are not-for-profit, and others are for-profit entities. In 2009, there were 1,861 CCRCs in the United States with over 745,000 residents (U.S. Government Accountability Office, 2010).

Conclusion

The concept of disability is difficult to precisely define. However, because disability is such an important concept, many narrow, programmatic definitions of disability have been developed by various government agencies and other organizations. All of the definitions of disability have a medical component within them, which may be either explicitly or impliedly stated. Including the medical component in the definitions is important and appropriate, because a large number of diseases, injuries, and conditions have a high degree of disability associated with them. To prevent disabilities from occurring, to manage the disabilities, and to rehabilitate people with disabilities, healthcare professionals use either a public health or a clinical approach. Public health works to prevent disabilities from occurring in groups of people at various levels, while clinical health professionals work directly with individual patients/clients to relieve pain and restore their function. Healthcare organizations, such as hospitals, rehabilitation facilities, and nursing homes, provide a continuum of care to people with disabilities. Although there are many healthcare resources available to them, people with disabilities often face a fragmented and uncoordinated healthcare system, as well as complex healthcare financing systems. People with disabilities, and indeed the general public, face many problems in the access, cost, quality, and outcomes of their healthcare.

References

Abramovitz, M. (2008). *Muscular dystrophy*. San Diego, CA: Lucent Books.

American Hospital Association. (2009). *AHA hospital statistics*. Chicago: Author.

Ashley, M. J. (Ed.). (2010). *Traumatic brain injury: Rehabilitation, treatment, and case management* (3rd ed.). Boca Raton, FL: CRC Press.

Assisted Living Federation of America. (2009). *2009 overview of assisted living*. Alexandria, VA: Author.

Association of American Medical Colleges. (2009). *Recent studies and reports on physician shortages in the U.S.* Washington, DC: Author.

Barnes, P. M., Bloom, B., & Nahin, R. L. (2008, December 10). *Complementary and alternative medicine use among adults and children: United States, 2007*. National Health Statistics Reports, 12. Hyattsville, MD: U.S. Dept. of Health & Human Services.

Bouchard, C., & Katzmarzyk, P. T. (Eds.). (2010). *Physical activity and obesity* (2nd ed.). Champaign, IL: Human Kinetics.

Braddock, D., Hemp, R., & Rizzolo, M. C. (2008). *The state of the states in developmental disabilities 2008* (7th ed.). Washington, DC: American Association on Intellectual and Developmental Disabilities.

Brainin, M., & Heiss, W.-D. (Eds.). (2010). *Textbook of stroke medicine*. New York: Cambridge University Press.

Bujak, J. S. (2008). *Inside the physician mind: Finding common ground with doctors*. Chicago: Health Administration Press.

Chez, M. G. (2010). *Autism and its medical management: A guide for parents and professionals*. Philadelphia, PA: Jessica Kingsley.

Committee on Disability in America, Board on Health Policy, Field, M. J., & Jette, A. M. (Eds.). (2007). *The future of disability in America*. Washington, DC: National Academies Press.

Coyle, P. K., & Halper, J. (2001). *Meeting the challenge of progressive multiple sclerosis*. New York: Demos.

Drum, C. E., Krahn, G. L., & Bersani, H. (Eds.). (2009). *Disability and public health*. Washington, DC: American Public Health Association/American Association on Intellectual and Developmental Disabilities.

Dryden-Edwards, R., & Combrinck-Graham, L. (Eds.). (2010). *Developmental disabilities from childhood to adulthood: What works for psychiatrists in community and institutional settings*. Baltimore, MD: Johns Hopkins University Press.

Dunn, N., Everitt, H., & Simon, C. (2007). *Cardiovascular problems*. New York: Oxford University Press.

Falvo, D. R. (2009). *Medical and psychosocial aspects of chronic illness and disability* (4th ed.). Sudbury, MA: Jones and Bartlett.

Fiedler, D., & Krause, R. (Eds.). (2009). *Deafness, hearing loss, and the auditory system*. Hauppauge, NY: Nova Science.

Fisch, B. J. (Ed.). (2010). *Epilepsy and intensive care monitoring: Principles and practice.* New York: Demos Medical.

Haldeman, S. (Ed.). (2005). *Principles and practice of chiropractic* (3rd ed.). New York: McGraw-Hill.

Holland, W. W., & Stewart, S. (2005). *Screening in disease prevention: What works?* Seattle, WA: Nuffield Trust/European Observatory.

Holt, T. A., & Kumar, S. (2010). *ABC of diabetes* (6th ed.). Hoboken, NJ: Wiley-Blackwell/BMJ.

Jones, K. D., & Hoffman, J. H. (2009). *Fibromyalgia.* Santa Barbara, CA: Greenwood Press/ABC-CLIO.

Kirkup, J. (2006). *A history of limb amputation.* New York: Springer.

Kostuik, J. P., Jan de Beur, S. M., & Margolis, S. (2003). *Back pain and osteoporosis.* Baltimore, MD: Johns Hopkins Medical Institution.

Lorig, K., & Fries, J. F. (2000). *The arthritis helpbook: A tested self-management program for coping with arthritis and fibromyalgia.* New York: Perseus Books.

MacNee, W., & Rennard, S. I. (2009). *Fast facts: Chronic obstructive pulmonary disease* (2nd ed.). Oxford, UK: Health Press.

Manderscheid, R. W., & Berry, J. T. (Eds.). (2006). *Mental health, United States, 2004.* Rockville, MD: Substance Abuse and Mental Health Services Administration.

Mattingly, B. E., & Pillare, A. C. (Eds.). (2009). *Osteoporosis: Etiology, diagnosis, and treatment.* Hauppauge, NY: Nova Science.

Mayo Clinic. (2009). *Mayo Clinic guide to living with a spinal cord injury: Moving ahead with your life.* New York: Demos Medical.

McLannahan, H. (Ed.). (2008). *Visual impairment: A global view.* New York: Oxford University Press.

MetLife Mature Market Institute. (2009). *Market survey of long-term care costs: The 2009 MetLife market survey of nursing home, assisted living, adult day services, and home care costs.* New York: Metropolitan Life Insurance Company.

National Association for Home Care and Hospice. (2008). *Basic statistics about home care.* Washington, DC: Author.

National Center for Health Statistics. (2009). *Health, United States, 2008 with chartbook.* Hyattsville, MD: Author.

National Institute on Aging. (2008). *Alzheimer's disease: Unraveling the mystery.* Bethesda, MD: Author.

Onslow, L. (2005). *Prevention and management of hip fracture.* Philadelphia, PA: Whurr.

Pratt, J. R. (2010). *Long-term care: Managing across the continuum* (3rd ed.). Sudbury, MA: Jones and Bartlett.

Scheier, L. M. (Ed.). (2010). *Handbook of drug use etiology: Theory, methods, and empirical findings.* Washington, DC: American Psychological Association.

Sharma, N. (2008). *Parkinson's disease.* Westport, CT: Greenwood Press.

Shi, L., & Singh, D. A. (2008). *Delivering health care in America: A systems approach* (4th ed.). Sudbury, MA: Jones and Bartlett.

Stahl, S. M., Mignon, L., & Muntner, N. (2010). *Attention deficit hyperactivity disorder*. New York: Cambridge University Press.

Stolley, K. S., & Glass, J. E. (2009). *HIV/AIDS*. Santa Barbara, CA: Greenwood Press.

Tobias, J. S., Hochhauser, D., & Souhami, R. L. (2010). *Cancer and its management*. Hoboken, NJ: Wiley-Blackwell.

Turnock, B. J. (2009). *Public health: What it is and how it works* (4th ed.). Sudbury, MA: Jones and Barlett.

U.S. Census Bureau. (2009). *The 2010 statistical abstract: The national data book*. Washington, DC: U.S. Government Printing Office.

U.S. Department of Veterans Affairs, Office of Human Resources and Administration. (2010). *2010 organizational briefing book*. Washington, DC: Author.

U.S. Government Accountability Office. (2010). *Older Americans: Continuing care retirement communities can provide benefits, but not without some risk*. GAO-10-611. Washington, DC: Author.

U.S. Social Security Administration. (2009). *Annual statistical report on the Social Security Disability Insurance Program, 2008*. SSA Pub. No. 13-11826. Washington, DC: Author.

Vincent, N., & Williams, B. J. (2010). *Principles of ALS care*. Sudbury, MA: Jones and Bartlett.

Weiss, L., Weiss, J., & Pobre, T. (Eds.). (2010). *Oxford American handbook of physical medicine and rehabilitation*. New York: Oxford University Press.

World Health Organization. (2001). *International classification of functioning, disability and health: ICF*. Geneva: Author.

Zollman, C., Richardson, J., & Vickers, A. (2008). *ABC of complementary medicine* (2nd ed.). Malden, MA: Blackwell.

Two

Current Issues, Controversies, and Solutions

People with disabilities often face a multitude of problems seeking and receiving needed healthcare services. To systematically address some of these problems, this chapter uses the conceptual framework of health services research. Health services research is a multidisciplinary field that focuses on the study of the access, costs, quality, and outcomes of healthcare services. Access to healthcare consists of everything that facilitates or impedes (i.e., geographic barriers, and not having health insurance coverage) the use of healthcare services. Costs of healthcare include provider costs and charges and the payments made by insurers and individuals for healthcare services. Quality of healthcare encompasses the elements of structure, process, and the outcomes of healthcare. Outcomes of healthcare generally include such measures as changes in mortality (deaths), life expectancy, morbidity (diseases, injuries, and conditions), disability, degree of pain or discomfort, and patient satisfaction with the care they receive. Ideally, all health professionals and healthcare organizations should strive to provide their patients and the communities they serve with the greatest possible access to care, at the lowest possible costs, and with the highest possible level of quality, and to achieve the best possible outcomes of care.

Health services researchers work to improve the effectiveness, efficiency, and equity of healthcare, mainly by influencing, developing, and evaluating public policies. Effectiveness may be broadly defined as meeting the stated goals and objectives of a program or organization, efficiency as the ratio of inputs to outputs, and equity as fairness or justice (Mullner, 2009).

First, this chapter will identify some of the major problems people with disabilities often face when accessing healthcare. Second, it will describe the different government programs in the United States and the unique problems people with disabilities have with them. Third, it will discuss the complex task of measuring the quality of healthcare. Fourth, it will describe some of the summary and condition-specific outcome measures of care. Finally, the chapter will provide an overview of the recently passed federal healthcare reform legislation and its likely impact upon people with disabilities.

Access to Healthcare

Access to healthcare by people with disabilities is influenced by a multitude of factors, many of which can interact to reduce access. For example, a disabled person may have difficulty getting or keeping appointments with a physician because of a lack of public transportation. The public transportation system they must depend on may be inadequate or unreliable, making the disabled person repeatedly late for their appointments. At the physician's office, because they are late, the physician may not see them until the end of all of his or her appointments. And a disabled person may also have to wait for a long time for appropriate medical equipment (i.e., wheelchair, oxygen unit) or personnel (i.e., interpreter) before they can receive care.

Facing such difficulties can be enormously frustrating for both the individual with a disability as well as their loved ones. The entire process of arranging transportation, arriving, and following through with a medical procedure can be so complex and taxing, both physically and emotionally, that some disabled individuals simply give up needed care. For the disabled person who does access care, relationships with family members and friends can be strained by difficulties in making needed physician visits, having to cancel appointments, sitting through long wait times, and struggling to use medical equipment. Lack of access to healthcare can also lower social participation for the disabled who rely on their medical equipment and care to maintain independence. Additionally, any physical deterioration in health or mobility can cause an extra economic hardship on a patient and his or her family.

This section will provide an overview of some of the main barriers to access to healthcare people with disability face. Specifically, it will discuss transportation, architectural, medical equipment, and patient-provider communication barriers. It will conclude with a brief discussion of the promising concept of universal design.

Transportation Barriers

Of the various barriers to access of healthcare, transportation is one of the most visible and obvious challenges for all individuals. For people with disability, there are even more complications around planning transportation to and from medical appointments and other required services. Because of physical, sensory, and cognitive impairments, many people with disability cannot drive a vehicle. Additionally, very few medical offices, clinics, or hospitals include transportation as part of the regular service delivery system.

Private Transportation

Some individuals with disability rely on family members, friends, or personal assistants to provide transportation to medical appointments, but this option can be taxing on all persons involved. For one, an individual with a disability may have friends and family who are willing to help out with transportation, but work schedules and availability make it difficult to continually rely on this type of support. Paid personal assistants may only be available a few hours a week, making coordination of care difficult. Further, because arranging transportation with family and friends must often be handled in advance, it makes responding to urgent care situations difficult.

Public Transportation

Public transportation systems offer fixed routes, meaning that an individual can take a planned bus, train, or subway route from one location to another. However, access to public transportation systems varies greatly across the country, and is contingent upon many factors. Primarily, many people with disabilities do not live in communities with a viable public transportation system. Available public transportation is quite often both inaccessible and unreliable. For those individuals who live in regions with a public transit system, not all fixed-route vehicles and stops are compliant with the federal Americans with Disability Act (ADA) of 1990.

For example, buses may not have wheelchair ramps, and some subway or train stops are only accessible via a set of staircases. Further, patients' ability to use a fixed route can also depend on how close their home is to a nearby route, and how close the same route is to their destination.

Paratransit

The ADA requires public transportation systems to provide complimentary paratransit for those individuals whose disabilities make it unfeasible for them to use the fixed routes within the transit system. Paratransit, or "dial-a-ride," provides individualized rides without fixed routes or schedules. They are typically provided by vans or mini-buses. However, operation and utilization of paratransit is not without its challenges. For one, paratransit services are expensive. It can cost up to ten times more to operate than a fixed route within the same system. Also, not all persons with disabilities are considered eligible for paratransit services, and most people must go through an eligibility assessment before being granted access to transportation. That is, disability is required to receive paratransit benefits, but is not sufficient. As public transit systems across the country struggle to maintain their costs, more individuals with disabilities must demonstrate that they meet the requirements for paratransit use.

Some individuals must reserve transportation with a private paratransit agency, if public paratransit services are not generally available where they live. The quality of both public and private paratransit varies greatly. Persons with disabilities often state that it can be challenging to even arrange a reservation with a paratransit agency, to reserve a pick-up early enough to make sure that they arrive on time for their appointments, and to coordinate pick-up or drop-off with other necessary services. Many individuals complain that paratransit drivers sometimes do not show up, arrive late, or are unable to provide adequate assistance in the transportation process (Sanchez & Brenmen, 2008).

Rural Considerations

About 54 million Americans live in rural areas of the country, where access to healthcare services is often very difficult to obtain. Many rural areas suffer from chronic shortages of physicians, specialty care practices, and other needed healthcare and social services.

People with disabilities living in rural areas frequently have more problems receiving healthcare than their non-disabled counterparts. For example, disabled persons often have difficulty finding physicians who are knowledgeable about their disabilities, and they also frequently have to educate physicians about their specific disabilities. Many people with disabilities believe that physicians in urban areas, unlike those in rural areas, are both more physically accessible and more knowledgeable about various disabilities and their associated restrictions. Frequently, disabled persons who live in rural areas have to travel to distant, large urban medical centers to receive any specialized care, and the transportation to these centers is often very difficult to coordinate. Again, difficulty in arranging transportation for medical services is one of the greatest barriers to accessing healthcare by people with disabilities, and this is further compounded for those persons living in rural areas (Glasgow, Morton, & Johnson, 2004)

Architectural Barriers

Just as public transit systems often do not comply with federal disability standards, people with disabilities often find that the healthcare facilities they use are also non-compliant. Recognizing this important problem, the U.S. Surgeon General in 2005 released the first *Call to Action to Improve the Health and Wellness of Persons With Disability*, encouraging all of the nation's healthcare facilities to give more attention to providing sufficient physical access for people with disabilities (Carmona, 2005).

Unfortunately, many patients with disabilities still encounter significant physical barriers while entering and navigating physicians' offices, clinics, and hospitals. Patients often encounter healthcare facilities that do not have accessible doorbells, doors, toilets, or rooms. Other barriers that patients encounter when accessing care include office/hospital parking (the condition and location of the parking lot in relation to an accessible entrance), stairs without an elevator or wheelchair lift device, or an architectural layout that is difficult or impossible to navigate independently (Fischer & Meuser, 2009).

Barriers to Medical Equipment

Another important challenge to providing patient care to people with disabilities is the availability of appropriate assistive medical equipment. Such equipment as wheelchairs, walkers, and oxygen tanks is imperative for maintaining the functional ability and independence of the disabled. However, many health insurance policies do not cover or pay for maintaining such equipment. For example, it is estimated that nearly one-half of mobility devices such as wheelchairs and scooters are purchased without the assistance of insurance. Sometimes, patients can only gain access to less-expensive models, or equipment replacement is not covered. Further, repairs and other parts required for equipment, such as batteries, are not always covered by insurance.

Medical office equipment accessibility also poses challenges to providing quality care to persons with disabilities. This includes such equipment as non-adjustable medical examination tables and mammography machines that cannot be used by non-standing patients. Also relevant to accessible medical equipment is the availability of staff members to safely transfer a patient onto an examination table or into an imaging machine (Reis, Breslin, Iezzoni, et al., 2004).

Barriers to Patient-Provider Communication

Patient-provider communication also poses a threat to access for people with disabilities. Although appropriate patient-provider communication is mandated by an array of regulatory guidelines and accreditation standards, patients with communication impairments are at an increased risk of having ineffective means of communicating with healthcare providers. If a patient is unable to adequately convey his or her symptoms to a provider, there is a threat to access of care, which can also impact the quality of care and patient satisfaction. There are many factors that can impede patient-provider communication for people with disabilities, including a lack of systematic assessment, evaluation, and monitoring of patient-provider communication, along with the unavailability of medical equipment, personnel, and a set of standardized procedures for communication-impaired patients.

Patients' rights grant individuals the ability to be more informed about their care, make informed decisions about medical procedures, and have providers understand their concerns and complaints. However, for patients with disabilities, this right may be threatened by an unavailability of appropriate accommodations or services, or standardized procedures that are infrequently used.

One example of poorly executed communication is when "ad hoc" interpreters are used in the patient setting, meaning healthcare providers rely on family, friends, or other administrative staff to facilitate communication with patients. Reliance on such techniques has been shown to lead to patient-provider miscommunication. For those patients who are non-speaking, many providers have tended to rely on nonverbal gestures, such as head nodding and pointing, which has been shown to be both ineffective for communication and frustrating to both the patient and the provider.

Some common forms of communication support are through teletypewriter (TTY), a device that allows users to type back and forth using regular telephone lines, and American Sign Language (ASL) interpretation for those with hearing impairments, and large-print material and Braille for those with visual impairments. However, not all healthcare providers are required to have these types of communication support available, and the range of communication impairment for people with disabilities varies widely.

Although accommodating all disabilities can be difficult, communication resources should be made readily available for all healthcare providers, and those who are involved in facilitating patient-provider communication. These communication resources include writing instruments (pen and paper), communication boards, language/ASL interpreters, hearing aids, and electronic communication devices. Further, patient-provider communication should be assessed and evaluated, and subsequent standardization of best practices should be developed to ensure that providers are adequately providing accommodations for their patients who need extra assistance with communication needs. It is also important to allow extra time for these patients, so that providers are able to fully communicate any information about medical conditions, patients can receive information and ask medical questions, and providers can acquire any consent needed for medical procedures (Iezzoni, 2006).

The Universal Design Concept

To address some of the barriers faced by people with disabilities, the promising new concept of universal design has emerged. Universal design is the concept of designing all products and environments to be usable to the greatest extent possible by everyone, regardless of their age, ability, or status in life. Architects and medical equipment designers are increasingly incorporating the concepts of universal design to improve both the physical environment as well as the personal interactions of patients with disability. Examples of some recommended universal design features include power door operators at interior and exterior entrances; chairs for use by people who cannot stand while transacting business; scales that allow people to be weighed while sitting in a wheelchair; motorized, adjustable-height treatment and examining tables and chairs; portable, amplified communication systems or devices with volume control at service desks and treatment spaces for people who are hard of hearing; and awareness and sensitivity training for all staff and professional personnel on interacting with people with disabilities (Mace, 1998).

Costs of Healthcare

Although the healthcare needs of people with disabilities vary by type and severity, their healthcare costs are greater than that of the general population. The disabled often have poorer health status and more chronic medical conditions, and they face greater access-to-care barriers. Their disabilities result in a greater number of medical visits to address and manage their healthcare needs. Often, their disabilities take precedence over preventative care, such as immunizations and health screening tests. In addition, people with disabilities tend to visit medical specialists more frequently than the general population, resulting in a greater number of expensive healthcare bills.

As a result of their increased usage and need, costs associated with healthcare for people with disabilities are expensive. In 2006, an estimated total of $397.9 billion was spent on healthcare services for the disabled, representing 26.7% of all healthcare costs for the United States (Anderson, Armour, Finkelstein, et al., 2010). Although these numbers are substantial, they underestimate the true cost because they do not take into consideration the economic costs of assistance from family members and friends—a major source of support for the daily physical care needs of the disabled.

The economic costs of disability are great for both people with disability as well as society. Often, people with disabilities who are unable to work rely on government programs, such as Social Security Disability Insurance (SSDI) and Supplemental Security Income (SSI) for economic security and Medicare and/or Medicaid for their health insurance needs. However, the disabled who cannot work and who are also ineligible for government programs often face the enormous problem of paying their healthcare costs themselves.

The SSDI and SSI Programs

The federal Social Security Disability Insurance (SSDI) program provides wage replacement income for individuals who have worked and paid Social Security taxes who become disabled according to Social Security criteria. The SSDI program is financed with Social Security taxes paid by workers, employers, and self-employed workers. Its benefits are paid to disabled workers, their widows, widowers, and children, and eligible adults disabled since childhood.

In 2008, disabled workers accounted for the largest share of SSDI beneficiaries (87%); the average age of beneficiaries was over 52; men represented slightly more than half (53%) of individuals in the program; and people with mental disorders account for about a third of the beneficiaries. That same year, the SSDI program paid over 8.5 million beneficiaries in the country approximately $100 billion—an average monthly payment of $1,063 (O'Brien, 2009).

In contrast, Supplemental Security Income (SSI) is a federal income supplement program funded by general tax revenues (not Social Security taxes). The SSI program is designed to help low-income people who are elderly, blind, or disabled. It provides cash to meet people's basic needs for food, clothing, and shelter.

In 2008, most SSI recipients (84%) were eligible on the basis of disability; most (58%) were aged 18 to 64; 6 out of 10 recipients under age 65 were diagnosed with a mental disorder; and more than half (56%) had no income other than their SSI payment. That same year, the SSI program paid 7.5 million recipients in the country $43 billion—an average monthly payment of $478 (Social Security Administration, 2009).

Some people receive income from both the SSDI and SSI programs. About 1 out of 7 SSDI disabled beneficiaries also receive SSI payments.

The process of obtaining SSDI and SSI is often lengthy and cumbersome. Applicants must prove their level of disability by having physicians certify their degree of functional impairment. Based on interviews and client reports, officials then make a decision on whether or not the person should be given funds. Often people with disabilities who apply for the programs are initially denied, and they must reapply in order to receive benefits. And completion of forms and medical visits to prove disability are costly. To further complicate the process, people in this transitional stage are often uninsured and unable to access healthcare.

Employment Problems and Policies

In addition to healthcare costs, the economic impact of disability is manifested in missed work, unemployment, and underemployment. People with disabilities often miss workdays for reasons related to their disability. They also face discrimination from employers as well as the inability to perform job-related tasks as a result of their disability status. Often people with disabilities are employed in lower wage or part-time employment. They often have lower incomes than their non-disabled counterparts, and the disabled report higher rates of poverty. For disabled individuals, underemployment results in lost wages and lower socioeconomic status. People with disabilities often face a lack of employer-based health insurance and a poorer quality of life. And many are unable to work and must face the reality of unemployment.

Missed Work and Loss of Productivity

Missed work and loss of productivity are frequent occurrences for people with disabilities. Missed work occurs when disabled persons cannot work because of their disability. Alternatively, the loss of productivity occurs when disabled persons are at work but are unable to perform their task to the fullest capacity due to their disability. Both missed work and loss of productivity are hidden costs of disability and significantly decrease earning power for individuals with disability. For the disabled person, lost days translates to lost wages and decreased job security, while for industry, lost productivity increases the cost of goods and services that are produced.

Employment Discrimination

Discrimination and stigma are commonplace for many people with disabilities. Stigma can be defined as having an attribute, behavior, or reputation that is socially discrediting. Stigma, which devalues and taints the individual or group within a particular social context, can limit the ability to obtain and keep a job, earnings, as well as social interactions, housing, health, and life itself.

There are many categories of stigma, which may overlap, including: physical deformities (e.g., individuals with extremes in height or weight, those lacking limbs, those who are badly burned); weakness or defects of individual character (e.g., individuals who have a criminal record, addiction, mental illness); and tribal stigma, which refers to a person's membership in an ethnic, racial, religious, or gender that is thought to disqualify all members of the group (e.g., being an member of an ethnic minority group, being an immigrant, being a women who does not live up to gender expectations). Stigma can also be categorized as public stigma (the ways the public reacts to the individual or group that is stigmatized) and self-stigma (the ways the individual turns against him or herself because they are a member of a stigmatized group) (Goffman, 1963).

Stigma may lead to workplace or employment discrimination. Employment-related discrimination occurs when employees suffer unfavorable or unfair treatment due to their race, religion, national origin, disability status, or other legally protected characteristics (Switzer, 2003).

Employment-related discrimination is an obstacle that many disabled people face. Such discrimination can occur at all junctions of the employment process. During job interviews, people with obvious disabilities must convince their prospective employers of their abilities. Once a person with disability is hired, many employers perceive disability to impact that person's ability to work, even in cases where ability to work is not hindered. Often people with disabilities must prove their ability to perform tasks throughout the duration of their employment. For a disabled person, this translates to a daily struggle to obtain or maintain employment status. Employment discrimination of people with disabilities leads to greater unemployment and higher reliance on government programs.

Unemployment

Unemployment is another reality that people with disabilities frequently face. In 2008, the American Community Survey (ACS), a large national survey conducted by the U.S. Census Bureau, identified the employment rate of working-age (ages 21 to 64) people with disabilities as 39.5%, while the employment rate of working-age people without disabilities was 79.9%—a gap of 40.4 percentage points. Among the six types of disabilities identified in the ACS, the highest employment rate was for people with a "hearing disability," 56.0%. In contrast, the lowest employment rate was for people with a "self-care disability," 18.7%. In the face of chronic unemployment, people with disabilities must rely on government programs such as SSI and SSDI for their primary sources of income. For a disabled person, this translates to reliance on government programs for economic security and health insurance. For society, low employment of people with disabilities translates to healthcare costs being borne by government programs (Erickson, Lee, & von Schrader, 2010).

Public Policies

A number of public policies have been developed to address the employment and general barriers that people with disabilities face. In order to end discrimination in the workplace, the federal Americans with Disabilities Act of 1990 (ADA) and the Ticket to Work and Work Incentives Improvement Act of 1999 (TWWIIA) were implemented to help pave avenues to employment for people with disabilities. These policies reflect an increase in federal government support to address the needs of the disabled. The landmark ADA highlighted a broad range of issues for people with disabilities. It focused on areas of daily living, while the TWWIIA focused more specifically on employment for people with disabilities. The passage of the TWWIIA allows people with disabilities to maintain Medicare eligibility for four additional years (Roessler, 2002).

Many policymakers anticipated that the passage of the ADA and the TWWIIA would allow people with disabilities to participate more fully in life and enter the workforce in greater numbers. Instead, however, people with disabilities continue to have lower rates of employment than their non-disabled counterparts, which indicates that current policies are insufficient to fully address their needs.

Health Insurance

People with disabilities often do not have employer-sponsored health insurance coverage due to their underemployment or unemployment. And they are often unable to purchase individual health insurance policies because of economic reasons and their disability/pre-existing health conditions. As a result, many of the disabled rely on the government's Medicare and Medicaid programs for their health insurance.

Employer-Sponsored Health Insurance

Most working Americans obtain their health insurance through their employers. Health insurance is generally part of the worker's employment benefits package. Employers offer health insurance through the workplace because of the tax advantage of doing so, because of the increase in worker productivity that results from improved access to healthcare, and because providing health benefits allows them to recruit and retain high-quality workers. Large employers are most likely to offer their workers health insurance. In contrast, employers least likely to offer health insurance are medium- and small-size firms, those with low-wage workers, high turnover, no unions, and many part-time employees (Morrisey, 2007).

People with disabilities are less likely than their non-disabled counterparts to have access to employer-sponsored health insurance. Those who are underemployed or employed part-time are often not offered health insurance as part of their employment benefits package. Given their higher rate of unemployment, people with disabilities are often excluded from the opportunity to have employer-based health insurance.

Individually Purchased Health Insurance

Individually purchased health insurance is often very costly. Because employer-sponsored health insurance spreads the risk of loss over a large group of people, it is generally less expensive than individually purchased health insurance. Further, individually purchased health insurance tends to provide a smaller set of benefits than employer-sponsored health insurance.

Medicare

Medicare (Title XVIII of the Social Security Act) is a federal healthcare program that covers almost everyone in the United States age 65 years or older, individuals under age 65 with certain disabilities, and individuals of all ages with permanent kidney failure requiring dialysis or a kidney transplant. Medicare consists of four parts: Part A (hospital insurance), Part B (medical insurance), Part C (managed-care plans, also called Medicare Advantage), and Part D (prescription drug coverage).

Although the Medicare program covers many of the health services of people with disabilities, it has a number of important limitations. For example, Medicare allows only one preventive medical examination to new beneficiaries during the first year they are in the program. It does not pay for routine dental care, eyeglasses or contact lenses, or hearing examinations and hearing aids. And most importantly, Medicare generally does not cover long-term care services such as custodial nursing home care (Kaiser, 2010c).

Medicaid

Medicaid (Title XIX of the Social Security Act) is a federal-state health insurance program for individuals and families with low incomes and limited resources. Medicaid covers children, the elderly, blind, and/or the disabled, and people who are eligible to receive federally assisted income maintenance payments. The program generally pays for physicians' services, inpatient and outpatient hospital care, prescription drugs, dental care, physical therapy, rehabilitation services, and hospice care. Medicaid is the largest payer of long-term care services in the nation, paying about 50% of the care being provided in nursing homes.

The Medicaid program also has a number of important limitations. Although the federal government establishes broad guidelines for the program, each state establishes its own eligibility standards, benefit packages, payment rates, and program administration. Thus, a disabled person may be eligible for Medicaid in one state, but may not be eligible in another (Kaiser, 2010b).

Dual Eligibility

Some low-income people with disabilities are dual eligible, meaning that they are covered by both the Medicare and Medicaid programs. Medicare covers their acute care services, while Medicaid covers their Medicare premiums and cost sharing and, for those below certain income and asset thresholds, long-term care services. Dual eligibility may seem ideal, but in reality it has limitations. Medicare and Medicaid are separate programs with different benefits and payment policies. This can lead to confusion for the individual about which services are covered, and individuals may use services that are not covered by either program. As a result, people who are dual eligible often report high out-of-pocket expenses (Medicare Payment Advisory Commission, 2010).

In summary, people with disabilities have increased needs for healthcare services, which often result in higher costs. The disabled often face employment discrimination and unemployment in greater numbers than their non-disabled counterparts, and public policies and laws such as the ADA and TWWIIA have not resulted in higher rates of employment. As a result of unemployment and underemployment, people with disabilities rely on government programs such as SSDI and SSI for economic support and Medicare and/or Medicaid for their health insurance needs. Because of this reliance on government programs, the healthcare and societal costs for people with disabilities are high.

Quality of Healthcare

Despite the passage of the landmark federal Americans with Disabilities Act (ADA) of 1990, which was intended to decrease discrimination, promote integration, and improve accommodation/programmatic access, patients with disabilities continue to receive disproportionately poor quality healthcare. People with disabilities receive fewer preventive medical, dental, and psychiatric services; report less satisfaction with their healthcare; experience more medical errors; and have more barriers to accessing care, equipment, and medications than their non-disabled counter parts. This decrease in quality healthcare is present for both children and adults with disabilities and whether the disability is congenital or acquired. As the population of the United States ages and technology improvements allow more people to live with disabilities, the number of the disabled will greatly increase in the future. A top priority should be closing the gap in healthcare quality for people with disabilities by providing appropriate, efficient, effective, and coordinated care that meets the unique needs of each person with a disability (Carmona, 2005).

Defining Quality of Healthcare

The definition of quality healthcare is complex, multidimensional, and dependent on the perspective of the definer or stakeholder. Whereas physicians place more emphasis on technical performance (e.g., number and type of medical tests and procedures given), patients tend to define quality of healthcare by their ease of access to services (e.g., waiting times for medical tests), amenities provided (e.g., tastiness of hospital food), and their satisfaction with the interpersonal communication between themselves and their provider (e.g., friendly bedside manner).

A widely used definition, which encompasses many perspectives, is that of the Institute of Medicine (IOM) (Lohr, 1990), which defines quality of care as "the degree to which health services for individuals and populations increase the likelihood of desired health outcomes and are consistent with current professional knowledge" (p. 21). By including "desired" health outcomes, the IOM definition emphasizes patient preferences as well as a patient's desire for broad health status and quality of life outcomes. By including patient experience, the definition of quality moves beyond the medical definition, which is primarily concerned with diagnosis, treatment, and clinical outcome, to include these psychosocial aspects of medical care. This expansion of the definition of quality is particularly important in the population of disabled patients, whose medical care interacts with other essential social and vocational needs, such as community reintegration and returning to work. Besides clinical technical performance by providers and responsiveness to patient preferences, other elements of quality healthcare also include access and management of the interpersonal relationships between provider and client, including shared decision making and equity of care.

Measuring Quality Healthcare

Health services researchers often use the framework of structure, process, and outcome to analyze the quality of healthcare. Developed by Avedis Donabedian, a physician and professor of public health at the University of Michigan, this framework is often referred to as the Donabedian model. Each component of this framework is an aspect of healthcare that is measurable. Standardized and rigorous measures allow researchers to better identify and address problems in all areas of healthcare (Donabedian, 2002).

Structure Measures

Structure measures of healthcare include the static components of individuals who provide care, such as the licensing of physicians and nurses, as well as the physical components of facilities where the care is provided, such as number of hospital beds and ownership status (private not-for-profit, for-profit, or state and local government). But Donabedian's broader definition of structure also includes the human, physical, and financial resources that are needed to provide medical care. Thus, structure measures can include access to services, an aspect of care that is particularly challenging to disabled patients due specifically to these physical and organizational barriers. As discussed earlier, disabled patients are more susceptible to being affected by poor transportation infrastructure, lack of community health systems, and office limitations such as medical examination tables. Many studies indicate that rural residents with disabilities face even more substantial barriers to obtaining healthcare than most disabled patients due to lower incomes and increased distance to tertiary care centers. Access to technology, equipment, and medications that could ease the burden of their disability is often not available to people with disabilities because of financial and bureaucratic barriers, with a profound effect. The functional status of disabled patients who do not receive appropriate equipment and assistive technology often declines. Studies also show that children with special needs and adults with mobility-related disabilities experience the most difficulty in accessing medical specialists and advanced care. Organizational barriers include difficulties in attaining timely appointments and poor processes in information sharing between shifts and specialists, which is especially seen in persons with disabilities who have multiple healthcare providers.

Process Measures

Process measures can be defined as what takes place during the delivery of care. Two aspects of process measures can be examined: the appropriateness of care, and the skill of care. A number of process measures have an impact on the quality of care for patients with disabilities. One particularly important measure is the use of appropriate preventive healthcare. A number of studies have found that persons with disabilities were less likely to receive preventive testing. A review of Medicare data confirms that the disabled were 57% less likely to receive pap smears or mammograms than their non-disabled counterparts. Possible reasons for this underuse of preventive services include physical obstacles (such as difficult-to-use medical examination tables), multiple acute problems taking priority over preventive services, and poor coordination among clinicians (Chan, Doctor, MacLehose, et al., 1999).

Other process quality-related issues include the undertreatment of co-morbid conditions, poor provider knowledge of disabling conditions, and the existence of barriers to effective provider-patient communication. For example, patients with mental impairment are most at risk for undertreatment of co-morbidities. Data from the Cooperative Cardiovascular Project, a large national study of a cohort of Medicare patients, found that individuals with co-morbid mental disorders were substantially less likely to undergo coronary revascularization procedures than those patients without mental disorders. Finally, people with disabilities often suffer from decreased patient safety. Many times, the disabled have more than one medical condition that contributes to their disability. Also, since they experience more contact with the healthcare system and take multiple medications, they are often at a higher risk for medical errors and adverse drug interactions (Druss, Bradford, Rosenheck, et al., 2000).

Outcome Measures

Outcome measures are the desired states resulting from healthcare structure and processes. While originally outcome measures included only clinical or technical outcomes, patient satisfaction with care has increasingly been included. A clinical outcome typically encompasses the physical aspects of care, such as mortality and complications from procedures, but sometimes includes functional improvement. Patient satisfaction with care is a measure of the IOM's aim to make healthcare patient centered. It includes the goal of achieving the patient's desired quality of life. There is often a disconnect between what the provider considers a positive outcome of therapy and what the patient with a disability considers a positive quality-of-life outcome. Patient-centered care also depends on shared decision making between the provider and the disabled patient, adequate information provision, and absence of stigmatization. Persons with more visible disabilities, such as cerebral palsy, often experience a greater degree of bias than those with less visible disabilities, such as mental disabilities. Both situations have resulted in decreased access to preventive measures and provision of quality care.

General Problems in Measurement

While structure, process, and outcome measures provide a useful framework or model of the healthcare encounter, their link to each other and to quality healthcare is not robust. Good structure measures, such as licensing, high level of medical equipment, or adequate access to care, are necessary for quality healthcare, but do not guarantee it. Once the patient is in the healthcare system, there is no guarantee that a good process encounter or a good outcome will ensue. Evidence of poor structure is actually more meaningful, since a quality healthcare experience cannot occur in that situation. Similar to structure measures, process measures do not always link well to outcome measures. If the right things are done and done well by the provider, good outcomes may occur. And sometimes, process measures are poor and good outcomes still occur. Since process measures are directly related to medical care, they do have several advantages. They are sensitive to quality differences across providers and over time, and they are often easier to interpret and place accountability. Process measures are also easy to obtain, since data can be compared to guidelines. Clinical practice guidelines and standards are consensus opinions derived from strong, valid, scientific evidence—often described as evidence-based medicine. Therefore, process measures, when compared to these guidelines, can indicate areas where improvement is needed. For example, yearly mammograms are recommended for women after the age of 50. Indicators of poor process measures will be observed when providers fail to order mammograms for these women. Interventions can be directed to improve the quality of patient encounters for this parameter.

Clinical outcome measurements, such as mortality, readmission, and medical complications, are advantageous because they are easy to measure, concrete, and well defined. They can be used to determine which processes may need further evaluation to improve healthcare quality. But outcome measures have several limitations. Certain sets of clinical processes do improve the likelihood of better health outcomes, but many factors besides these process measures of technical skill and appropriate use of treatment affect clinical outcomes. These factors include patient genetics and their environment, both of which cannot be measured and providers often have no control over. Patient compliance also will affect outcomes and is very difficult to quantify and measure.

A second limitation to outcome measures is that broad measures might not adequately depict the variance of these measures among geographical areas and among hospitals, even in the same region. Those healthcare regions where social and financial barriers prevent patient compliance and access to healthcare and equipment will have decreased health outcomes when measured. If outcome measures do not take into account these differences and are used for comparison between healthcare organizations, inequities and diminished care for certain populations, such as people with disabilities, may increase.

A third limitation to clinical outcome measures is that they are a measure of aggregate population data, not individual cases. Each patient will have his or her own desired quality health outcome as set forth in the IOM definition of quality healthcare, which can also be quite different from that of the clinician's optimal outcome goal. Providers are increasingly attempting to incorporate this concept of patient-centered care by improving provider-client communication. Outcome measures often now include patient satisfaction, attempting to quantify this emotion and desired outcome, although still not adequately (Kane & Radosevich, 2011).

Problems in Measurement for People With Disability

Using the structure, process, and outcome framework poses three important problems to measuring the quality of healthcare for the population of people with disabilities. First, defining disability is difficult and varied. No single definition works for all purposes. Potentially impairing conditions differ in their causes, nature, timing, and societal implications. Disability can be defined medically, as well as socially, with the social model often recognizing the influence of prejudices, discrimination, and an inaccessible environment. The World Health Organization (WHO) calls disability an "umbrella term for impairments, activity limitations or participation restrictions," underscoring the dynamic interaction between health conditions and contextual factors, such as environmental and personal attributes (World Health Organization, 2001). What is a disability for one person may not be considered a disability by another. For this reason, it is often difficult to define the disabled population when determining quality measurements.

Second, the causes of disability are varied. Some are congenital, whereas others are acquired. Some forms of disability may be caused by visible physical impairments such as limb amputations, others by sensory deficits such as hearing loss or blindness, and still others by mental impairments such as depression. Although clinical guidelines do exist for preventive measures for people with disabilities, and for treating some of the individual disease symptoms that cause the disability, there are not any guidelines for how to treat "disability," the functional impairment. Guidelines for treating disability may not even be in the best interest of the person with a disability, since healthcare should be patient centered and since adaptation to a disability will be different for each patient, depending on the cause and the situation. Measuring the process of healthcare is more difficult when guidelines do not exist, and outcome measures cannot be uniform when desired health outcomes may be different for each category of disability and for each patient within those categories. These issues increase the difficulty in measuring quality in disabled populations.

Third, persons with disabilities often have many providers besides the ones taking care of the disability itself. They also interact with many healthcare organizations that provide services, medications, equipment, and social and vocational counseling. Process and outcome measures cannot delineate accurately which provider or organization holds the responsibility for the measure. Some health services researchers are expanding the traditional framework of structure, process, and outcome to accommodate the broader complexity of the healthcare experience for persons with disabilities. For example, some researchers are now including the coordination of services in their models. Coordination of care allows smooth and consistent communication between providers and institutions and prevents delays between various services. The essential components of coordination include identifying patients' needs that may increase their risk of adverse health events, providing patient self-care education, and monitoring individuals for potential problems. These components can be combined into one of two programs, case management or disease management, and can be incorporated into process measures to better determine the quality of care for the disabled. Better definitions of coordination and how to measure it are also necessary before it can be fully implemented into quality measures for persons with disabilities.

In summary, persons with disabilities can have decreased quality of healthcare as measured by structure, process, and outcome measures. This is demonstrated as decreased access, physical building limitations, and lack of preventive treatment. To improve health outcomes of this population, coordination of care measures needs to be added to the traditional framework so that interventions can be implemented to help people meet essential medical, social, and vocational needs.

Outcomes of Healthcare

Health services for people with disabilities focus on helping those individuals reach and maintain optimal physical, sensory, intellectual, psychiatric, and/or social functional levels, or restore or compensate for the loss of function. In this model, outcomes are a function of access to care, cost, and quality. The study of outcomes in the context of the health services research model is defined as investigations of the end result of medical care, or the effect of healthcare on the health and well-being of patients and populations. Outcomes of healthcare are typically measured in terms of changes in mortality, life expectancy, morbidity, and satisfaction with care. In the case of disability, outcome measurement considers assessment of disability, health status of individuals with a disability, and quality of life given the individual's capabilities. Assessment of these outcomes is essential for determining service needs, predicting hospital lengths of stay, or improving level of functioning in the patient's home or community.

Summary Outcome Measures

Summary measures of population health offer a broader representation of overall health. Summary measures combine mortality, morbidity, and other social and personal attributes using several different methods to represent overall population health in a single number. Usually optimal health is assigned the value of 1.0 and death is assigned a value of 0.0. This number is then linked to life expectancy to form an overall measure of health.

Disability-adjusted life years (DALY), quality-adjusted life years (QALY), and healthy life expectancy (HLE) are examples of summary measures of population health.

Disability-Adjusted Life Years

The disability-adjusted life years measure was created by the World Health Organization (WHO) to represent the burden of disease in terms of years of life lost due to either disability or premature death. The DALY is constructed using weight for the additional years of life remaining at each age and weights for health deficits resulting from different diseases and injuries. One DALY is equivalent to one lost year of "healthy" life. The sum of DALYs across a population can be thought of as a relative measure of the burden of disease for that population compared to an ideal health situation, where the entire population lives to an advanced age, free of disease and disability.

Quality-Adjusted Life Years

Quality-adjusted life years is a measure of disease burden that includes both the quality and quantity of life. A year in perfect health is considered equal to 1.0 QALY, whereas a year in poor health is less than 1.0 QALY. For example, a year confined to bed might have a value equal to 0.5 QALY.

Healthy Life Expectancy

Healthy life expectancy (HLE) is the expected number of remaining years of life spent in good health from a particular age, assuming current rates of mortality and morbidity. HLE is a summary measure composed of two sets of partial measures. The first partial measure is composed of age-specific death rates and accounts for the mortality component of the measure. Age-specific rates of population morbidity, disability, or health-related quality of life compose the second partial measure.

Summary measures of health can be used in many different ways. They can be used in health comparisons between one population and another, or within the same population over different points in time. Better comparisons can be made between fatal and chronic diseases, because summary measures combine information on morbidity and mortality to form a single scale for comparison. Summary measures also can be used to identify and quantify health inequities within and among populations, which can inform priorities for health services, planning, and research. Finally, they can be used for analyzing the effectiveness and benefits of health interventions.

With increasing use of summary measures to inform decision making, it is important to recognize and consider their technical limitations. An understanding of what is being assessed and current measurement strategies is necessary to determine appropriateness for different purposes. Partial measures or weights developed using a segment of a population or a particular data set may not apply to a local community population, for example, leading to misinterpretation or misleading information. In addition, the methodology of summary measure development continues to evolve as researchers seek to improve weaknesses in different measures and resolve differences in methods. These decisions involve value judgments in measure construction and application. Value judgments come into play when summary measures are used to make resource allocation decisions. In measure construction, value judgments are used in determining what partial measures will compose the summary measure and how weights will be assigned to different health states. Partial measures may not adequately capture important dimensions characterizing a particular disease, and relying on expert consensus to assign weights to health states is subject to the biases of the expert panel. Coming to agreement on standards for summary measures to help alleviate measurement weaknesses and biases is an ongoing effort (McDowell, 2006).

Condition-Specific Outcome Measures

For some purposes and individual patient care decisions, diagnostic, physiologic, cognitive, and functional assessments and evaluations of quality of life can inform clinical decisions and the provision of services at organizational or local levels. Most of these types of outcome measures focus on specific conditions and can be assessed using a self-administered questionnaire or an assessment administered by a clinician. Some examples of condition-specific outcome measures are presented below.

Arthritis Impact Measurement Scales (AIMS/AIMS2)

Developed by the Boston University Arthritis Center, the Arthritis Impact Measurement Scales (AIMS/AIMS2) is used to assess the physical, social, and emotional well-being of patients with rheumatic diseases. The AIMS contains nine scales (mobility, physical activity, dexterity, house activities, social activities, activities of daily living, pain, depression, and anxiety) to assess a person's health and functioning over the previous month. There are many variations of AIMS, including the original version, a shortened version, an expanded version (AIMS2), a short form of the AIMS2 (AIMS2-SF), a child version, and a version for the elderly (Geri-AIMS) (Meenan, Mason, Anderson, et al., 1992).

Disabilities of the Arm, Shoulder, and Hand (DASH) Outcome Measure

Developed by the American Academy of Orthopedic Surgeons (AAOS) and the Institute for Work and Health (IHW), the Disabilities of the Arm, Shoulder, and Hand (DASH) Outcome Measure is a self-administered questionnaire that assesses the physical function and symptoms for several musculoskeletal disorders of the upper limbs. Questionnaire responses are ranked from 0, indicating the least disability, to 100, indicating the most disability (Dixon, Johnston, McQueen, et al., 2008).

Kurtzke Expanded Disability Status Scale (EDSS)

Developed by John Kurtzke, a physician at the Veterans Administration (VA), the Kurtzke Expanded Disability Status Scale (EDSS) is a widely used outcome measure of multiple sclerosis (MS). The EDSS allows neurologists to quantify disability in eight physiological functional systems (pyramidal [motor function]; cerebellar; brainstem; sensory; bowel and blander; visual; cerebral or mental; and other). Each functional system is assigned a score ranging from 0 to 10, with 0 being "normal neurological examination," 5 being "disability severe enough to impair full daily activities," and 10 being "death due to multiple sclerosis" (Kurtzke, 2008).

In summary, improving outcome measures will require much more work on methodological, clinical, and ethical levels. In addition, appropriate use of measures will require informed decisions on which measures to use and better understanding of the interpretation and limitations of those measures. These elements are essential to help inform policymakers to make decisions and set priorities for public health, research, and distribution of health services.

Recent Healthcare Reform Legislation

As mentioned earlier, the overall aim of health services research is to improve the effectiveness, efficiency, and equity of healthcare, mainly by influencing, developing, and evaluating public policies. In 2010, after much acrimonious debate, the U.S. Congress passed sweeping new healthcare reform legislation. The new legislation, the Patient Protection and Affordable Care Act (PPACA; P.L. 111-148) and the Health Care and

Education Reconciliation Act (HCERA; P.L. 111-152), which made modifications to the PPACA, was signed into law by President Barack Obama. This legislation constitutes the largest change to America's healthcare system since the creation of the Medicare and Medicaid programs in 1965.

The new healthcare reform legislation greatly increases the role of the federal government in all aspects of the nation's healthcare system. It fundamentally overhauls how health insurance is regulated and purchased; it changes the way healthcare is delivered and paid for; and it finances changes through many new taxes, fees, fines, and cost reductions.

The healthcare reform legislation is both comprehensive and incremental in scope. The complex legislation will be implemented in stages over a 10-year time period. Many new regulations will have to be promulgated to determine the exact details. Dozens of new federal and state agencies, commissions, committees, and offices will need to be created to administer the regulations. Many pilot and demonstration programs and new research on treatments and systems of care will have to be conducted. And the nation's healthcare delivery system will need to be reorganized, which will require many changes in existing laws.

A brief overview of the legislation and its likely impact upon people with disabilities is presented below.

Overview of the Healthcare Reform Legislation

The new healthcare reform legislation will provide greater access to health insurance coverage for the uninsured. To increase access, the legislation regulates the nation's health insurance industry; it creates new state-run health insurance exchanges for individuals to purchase coverage; it changes Medicare coverage and premiums; it expands Medicaid eligibility; and it requires most U.S. citizens and legal residents to have health insurance coverage or pay a penalty tax.

Under the new legislation, health insurance companies can no longer deny children coverage because of a preexisting medical condition. And as of 2014, they cannot deny coverage to anyone with a preexisting medical condition. Insurance companies are now required to extend dependent coverage to adult children up to age 26. They are prohibited from rescissions of coverage (the cancellation of a policy because a policyholder withheld or concealed vital information, such as failing to disclose a preexisting condition) and from having waiting periods for coverage of greater than 90 days. The new law also requires group insurance plans to eliminate lifetime limits on coverage and, by 2014, to eliminate annual limits on coverage (Kaiser, 2010d).

The new legislation also requires each state to establish and manage a health insurance exchange where individuals and small employers can purchase coverage. Most of the exchanges will operate as online market-places where individuals can review and compare a variety of private health insurance plans. Consumers will be able to compare what services are covered, the premiums they will pay, the extent of their co-payments and deductibles, as well as their out-of-pocket limits on expenses. It is hoped that these exchanges, with their competing private plans written in easy-to-understand language, will enable consumers to purchase health insurance with lower premiums and better coverage (Kaiser, 2010a).

The legislation changes Medicare coverage and premiums. It expands prevention services for Medicare beneficiaries by covering, with no co-payment or deductible, an annual wellness visit and creation of a personalized prevention assessment and plan. Prevention services include referrals to education and preventive counseling or community-based interventions to address various health risk factors. It increases the premiums for Medicare Part B (medical insurance) and Part D (prescription drug coverage), and it applies a Medicare tax on net investment income for individuals making $200,000 and over and couples making $250,000 and over. Government payments to Medicare Part C (privately run managed-care plans, also called Medicare Advantage) will be frozen in 2011 and decline in subsequent years. The legislation also gradually eliminates the Medicare Part D "doughnut hole" (when Medicare temporarily stops paying for prescriptions and the beneficiary has to pay the entire cost of prescriptions until reaching a certain level before Medicare will start paying again) by 2020 (Davis, Hahn, Morgan, et al., 2010)

To provide health insurance coverage to more people, state Medicaid programs will expand eligibility to non-Medicare individuals age 64 and under with incomes up to 133% of the federal poverty level. The legislation also increases federal Medicaid matching funds to all states (Stone, Baumrucker, Binder, et al., 2010).

One of the most controversial parts of the new legislation is its requirement that most U.S. citizens and legal residents have health insurance coverage by 2014 or pay a penalty tax. Specifically, those without coverage will pay a penalty tax of $95.00 in 2014, gradually rising to $695.00 by

2016, or up to 2.5% of their income. Large employers will also be required to provide health insurance coverage to their workers, or pay a fine of $2,000 per worker. However, small employers, those with fewer than 50 workers, are exempt from this rule (Chaikind & Peterson, 2010).

The Likely Impact of Healthcare Reform for People With Disabilities

All Americans will feel the impact of the new healthcare reform legislation, but it will likely have the greatest impact upon people with disabilities. The legislation will make the once-common insurance practice of denying health insurance coverage because of a preexisting medical condition a thing of the past, which is a particular benefit to people with disabilities who have long struggled against this obstacle. The legislation, however, goes much further in helping people with disabilities. Some of the major new innovative programs, insurance plans, and regulations the legislation will create are briefly discussed below.

New Long-Term Care Insurance: The CLASS Program

The new legislation creates the Community Living Assistance Services and Supports or CLASS program, a new voluntary national long-term care insurance program that provides individuals with a cash benefit if they have functional limitations or disability. The intent of CLASS is to provide additional options for individuals with disabilities to help them purchase community living assistance services and supports, enabling them to remain independent, employed, and participate in their communities. CLASS is designed to be self-supporting and prohibits any use of taxpayer money to fund benefit payments.

Although the details of the CLASS program still need to be defined by the federal government, to be eligible for the program individuals will need to be active workers, 18 years of age or older, and receive income subject to Social Security tax. The voluntary program will be offered by employers and paid for by employees, and CLASS premiums will be withheld from the employees' paychecks, similar to Social Security and Medicare payroll deductions. To receive CLASS benefits, individuals must be unable to perform a specific number of activities of daily living, or have an equivalent cognitive impairment, for a continuous period of more than 90 days. CLASS benefits will be paid on a daily or weekly basis, based on a scale of functional ability. The benefits will average no less than $50 per day (adjusted annually for inflation). To be eligible for benefits, individuals must pay CLASS premiums for at least five years, and earn wages for at least three of those years (Watts, 2009).

Greater Nursing Home Transparency and Quality Assurance

The legislation will create more transparency and quality assurance efforts in the nation's nursing homes. The law specifically requires all nursing homes to disclose their finances, owners, operators, suppliers, and others with whom they do business so they can be held accountable for the care their residents receive. It also requires the federal government to implement a system to collect and report information about how well nursing homes are staffed, including information about the hours of nursing care residents receive, staff turnover rates, and how much the facilities spend on wages and benefits. It also establishes a Quality Assurance and Performance Improvement Program to improve quality assurance standards. It implements a pilot program to improve the federal government's oversight of nursing home chains that have quality of care problems. And it provides funds for the training of workers who care for nursing home residents with dementia, and for the prevention of abuse (Williams & Redhead, 2010).

New Accessibility Standards for Medical Equipment

The legislation contains a provision that will significantly affect many types of medical equipment used by people with disabilities. Section 4203 of the PPACA amends Title V of the Rehabilitation Act of 1973 requiring the independent federal U.S. Access Board (formerly known as the Architectural and Transportation Barriers Compliance Board) to work with the U.S. Food and Drug Administration (FDA) to develop and implement technical regulatory standards for medical equipment. These new standards will ensure that the medical equipment used in physicians' offices, clinics, hospitals, and other medical settings are accessible by individuals with disabilities, allowing them to independently enter and exit from the equipment to the maximum extent possible. The medical equipment covered under this section includes examination tables, examination chairs (including chairs used for eye and dental examinations), weight scales, mammography equipment, x-ray machines, and other radiological equipment used for diagnostic purposes (Williams & Redhead, 2010).

Independence at Home Demonstration Program and Accountable Care Organizations

One provision of the new healthcare reform legislation with perhaps the greatest potential to transform the nation's healthcare system is the creation of the Independence at Home Demonstration Program. This new demonstration program will utilize Accountable Care Organizations to provide high-need Medicare beneficiaries with multiple chronic conditions primary care services in their homes.

Accountable Care Organizations, or ACOs, are new emerging models of healthcare that attempt to improve patient outcomes and save money by better coordinating all of the care patients receive. A number of well-known healthcare systems are already experimenting with ACOs, including: Montefiore Medical Center in New York City; Kaiser Permanente in Oakland, California; Intermountain Healthcare in Salt Lake City, Utah; Mayo Clinic in Rochester, Minnesota; and a handful of other healthcare systems (Arnst, 2010).

Although a precise definition of ACOs does not exist, these organizations may be broadly defined as healthcare networks that provide and help patients better coordinate and manage their care, along a continuum that includes primary care, inpatient and outpatient care, home care, pharmacy, and other services. ACOs, which may consist of a hospital, a large physician group practice, or a combination of the two, are held accountable for the overall health of a community or group of patients, many of whom often reside in a geographic area surrounding the healthcare facility. ACOs are generally funded through a flat fee per year from each patient's insurer or employer, based on his or her health and age. Health professionals, mainly primary care physicians and nurse practitioners, within the ACOs provide care and work with their patients to keep them as healthy as possible. To lower costs and improve the quality of care provided to their patients, ACOs rely heavily on home visits, electronic patient records, and sophisticated home monitoring systems. They also try to prevent their patients from using unnecessary and expensive hospital services, such as the use of emergency departments for non-emergency care (Devers & Berenson, 2009).

The new healthcare reform legislation requires the secretary of the U.S. Department of Health and Human Services (HHS) to establish an Independence at Home Demonstration Program by January 1, 2012. The demonstration program will likely fund some existing ACOs as well as lead to the creation of many new ones. To receive government funding, the ACOs will have to bring primary care services to the homes of at least 200 high-need Medicare beneficiaries—those with two or more chronic conditions, such as Alzheimer's disease, chronic obstructive pulmonary disease, ischemic heart disease, stroke, and other diseases. The ACOs will be eligible for shared savings if they achieve high-quality outcomes, high patient satisfaction, and cost savings. The specific goals of the demonstration program are to reduce preventable hospitalizations, prevent hospital readmissions, reduce emergency room visits, and improve health outcomes commensurate with the individuals' stage of chronic illness (Shortell, Casalino, & Fisher, 2010).

Although there is no guarantee that ACOs will succeed in both lowering the costs and increasing the quality of healthcare patients receive, these organizations do offer a novel approach to care that appears to be promising.

Conclusion

Using the conceptual framework of health services research, this chapter addressed some of the multitude of problems people with disabilities face in seeking and receiving needed healthcare services. They often face difficulties and disparities in access, costs, quality, and outcomes of care. The recent passage of national healthcare reform legislation will likely help eliminate some of these problems. The new legislation has an enormous potential for improving the nation's healthcare system and the daily lives of people with disabilities. Access to healthcare will be greatly increased by removing the insurance barrier of preexisting medical conditions, establishing state-run health insurance exchanges with competitive health insurance plans, expanding the number of people eligible for the Medicaid program, and establishing long-term care insurance through the CLASS program. The quality of healthcare should be greatly improved by making the operations of the nation's nursing homes more transparent and holding them more accountable for the quality of care they provide to their residents. And the outcomes of care should also be improved by paying for more preventive health-care services and wellness programs.

Although the new legislation is a very important step forward, it still has a number of problems. Many of the details of the legislation still have to be developed, which will take many years to complete. Even without the details, the legislation is enormously large and complex (the PPACA is over 2,000 pages in length), adding a new layer of complexity to an already cumbersome national healthcare system. Perhaps most importantly, the new legislation—despite what many politicians say—will likely increase the overall cost of healthcare, which is already enormously expensive. Arguably, the new complexity and increasing cost of healthcare is the price that each of us will have to pay to live in a healthier, organized modern society (Monheit, 2010).

References

Anderson, W. L., Armour, B. S., Finkelstein, E. A., et al. (2010, January/February). Estimates of state-level health-care expenditures associated with disability. *Public Health Reports, 125*(1), 44–51.

Arnst, C. (2010, August). The hospital, your care coordinator: Some centers now take charge of keeping people healthy and at home. *U.S. News and World Report, 147*(7), 12–18.

Carmona, R. M. (2005). *The Surgeon General's call to action to improve the health and wellness of people with disabilities*. Rockville, MD: Office of the Surgeon General, Public Health Service, U.S. Department of Health and Human Services. Retrieved from http://www.surgeongeneral.gov

Chaikind, H., & Peterson, C. L. (2010). *Summary of potential employer penalties under the Patient Protection and Affordable Care Act (PPACA)* (R41159). Washington, DC: Congressional Research Service. Retrieved from http://www.crs.gov

Chan, L., Doctor, J. N., MacLehose, R. F., et al. (1999, June). Do Medicare patients with disabilities receive preventive services? A population-based study. *Archives of Physical Medicine and Rehabilitation, 80*(6), 642–646.

Davis, P. A., Hahn, J., Morgan, P. C., et al. (2010). *Medicare provisions in PPACA (P.L. 111-148)* (R41196). Washington, DC: Congressional Research Service. Retrieved from http://www.crs.gov

Devers, K. J., & Berenson, R. A. (2009). *Can accountable care organizations improve the value of health care by solving the cost and quality quandaries?* Washington, DC: Urban Institute. Retrieved from http://www.rwjf.org/files/research/acobrieffinal.pdf

Dixon, D., Johnston, M., McQueen, M., et al. (2008). The Disabilities of the Arm, Shoulder and Hand Questionnaire (DASH) can measure the impairment, activity limitations and participation restriction constructs from the International Classification of Functioning, Disability and Health (ICF). *BMC Musculoskeletal Disorders, 9*, 114–120.

Donabedian, A. (2002). *An introduction to quality assurance in health care.* New York: Oxford University Press.

Druss, B. G., Bradford, D. W., Rosenheck, R. A., et al. (2000, January 26). Mental disorders and use of cardiovascular procedures after myocardial infarction. *Journal of the American Medical Association, 283*(4), 506–511.

Erickson, W. A., Lee, C. G., & von Schrader, S. (2010s). *2008 disability status report: The United States.* Ithaca, NY: Cornell University Rehabilitation Research and Training Center on Disability Demographics and Statistics. Retrieved from http://www.ilr.cornell.edu/edi/disabilitystatistics

Fischer, J., & Meuser, P. (Eds.). (2009). *Accessible architecture: Age and disability-friendly planning and building in the 21st century.* Berlin, Germany: Dom Publishers.

Glasgow, N., Morton, L. W., & Johnson, N. E. (Eds.). (2004). *Critical issues in rural health.* Ames, IA: Blackwell.

Goffman, E. (1963). *Stigma: Notes on the management of a spoiled identity.* Englewood Cliffs, NJ: Prentice Hall.

Iezzoni, L. I. (2006, Fall). Make no assumptions: Communication between persons with disabilities and clinicians. *Assistive Technology, 18*(2), 212–229.

Kaiser Family Foundation. (2010a). *Explaining health care reform: Questions about health insurance exchanges* (Pub. #7908-02). Menlo Park, CA: Author. Retrieved from http://kff.org/healthreform/upload/7908-02.pdf

Kaiser Family Foundation. (2010b). *Medicaid: A primer 2010* (Pub. #7334). Menlo Park, CA: Author. Retrieved from http://www.kff.org/medicaid/7334.cfm

Kaiser Family Foundation. (2010c). *Medicare: A primer 2010* (Pub. #7615). Menlo Park, CA: Author. Retrieved from http://www.kff.org/medicare/7615.cfm

Kaiser Family Foundation. (2010d). *Summary of new health reform law* (Pub. #8061). Menlo Park, CA: Author. Retrieved from http://www.kff.org/healthreform/8061.cfm

Kane, R. L., & Radosevich, D. M. (2011). *Conducting health outcomes research.* Sudbury, MA: Jones and Bartlett.

Kurtzke, J. F. (2008). Historical and clinical perspectives of the Expanded Disability Status Scale. *Neuroepidemiology, 31*(1), 1–9. Retrieved from http://content.karger.com/produktedb/produkte.asp?typ=fulltext&file=000136645

Lohr, K. N. (Ed.). (1990). *Medicare: A strategy for quality assurance*. Washington, DC: National Academy Press.

Mace, R. L. (1998). *Removing barriers to health care: A guide for health professionals*. Raleigh: Center for Universal Design, College of Design, North Carolina State University. Retrieved from http://www.fpg.unc.edu/~ncodh/rbar/

McDowell, I. (2006). *Measuring health: A guide to rating scales and questionnaires* (3rd ed.). New York: Oxford University Press.

Medicare Payment Advisory Commission. (2010). *Report to Congress: Aligning incentives in Medicare*. Washington, DC: Author. Retrieved from http://www.medpac.gov/documents/Jun10_EntireReport.pdf

Meenan, R. F., Mason, J. H., Anderson, J. J., et al. (1992, January). AIMS2: The content and properties of a revised and expanded Arthritis Impact Measurement Scales health states questionnaire. *Arthritis & Rheumatism, 35*(1), 1–10.

Monheit, A. C. (2010, Summer). Now the really hard part: Implementing health reform. *Inquiry, 47*(2), 97–102.

Morrisey, M. A. (2007). *Health insurance*. Chicago: Health Administration Press.

Mullner, R. M. (Ed.). (2009). *Encyclopedia of health services research* (2 vols.). Thousand Oaks, CA: Sage.

O'Brien, E. (2009). *Social Security Disability Insurance: A primer*. Washington, DC: AARP Public Policy Institute. Retrieved from http://assets.aarp.org/rgcenter/econ/i28_ssdi.pdf

Reis, J. P., Breslin, M. L., Iezzoni, L. I., et al. (2004). *It takes more than ramps to solve the crisis of healthcare for people with disabilities*. Chicago: Rehabilitation Institute of Chicago. Retrieved from http://www.dredf.org/healthcare/RIC_whitepaperfinal.pdf

Roessler, R. T. (2002, July-September). TWWIIA initiatives and work incentives: Return-to-work implications. *Journal of Rehabilitation, 68*(3), 11–16.

Sanchez, T. W., & Brenman, M. (2008). *The right to transportation: Moving to equity*. Chicago: American Planning Association.

Shortell, S. M., Casalino, L. P., & Fisher, E. S. (2010, May). *Implementing accountable care organizations*. Berkeley: Berkeley Center on Health Economics and Family Security, School of Law, University of California. Retrieved from http://www.law.berkeley.edu/files/chefs/Implementing_ACOs_May_2010.pdf

Social Security Administration. (2009). *SSI annual statistical report, 2008* (SSA Pub. No. 13-11827). Washington, DC: Author. Retrieved from http://www.socialsecurity.gov/policy/docs/statcomps/ssi_asr/2008/ssi_asr08.pdf

Stone, J., Baumrucker, E. P., Binder, C., et al. (2010). *Medicaid and the state Children's Health Insurance Program (CHIP) provisions in PPACA (R41210)*. Washington, DC: Congressional Research Service. Retrieved from http://www.crs.gov

Switzer, J. V. (2003). *Disabled rights: American disability policy and the fight for equality.* Washington, DC: Georgetown University Press.

Watts, M. O. (2009). *The Community Living Assistance Services and Supports (CLASS) Act* (Pub. #7996). Menlo Park, CA: Henry J. Kaiser Family Foundation. Retrieved from http://www.kff.org/healthreform/upload/7996.pdf

Williams, E. D., & Redhead, C. S. (2010). *Public health, workforce, quality, and related provisions in the Patient Protection and Affordable Care Act (PPACA)* (R41278). Washington, DC: Congressional Research Service. Retrieved from http://www.crs.gov

World Health Organization (2001). *International Classification of Functioning, Disability and Health: ICF.* Geneva: Author. Retrieved from http://apps.who.int/classification/icfbrowser

Three

Chronology of Critical Events

The histories of medicine, public health, and disability are old and intricately intertwined. The dates of some of the major milestones in those histories are listed below.

10000 BCE

With the early domestication of plants and animals, new human diseases arise, such as diphtheria, measles, and smallpox.

8000 BCE

Human skulls are found in both the New and Old World showing marks from trepanation, a surgical operation in which a small hole is drilled in the skull.

4500 BCE

Human skeletal remains from this era are found in the New and Old World that show traces of rheumatoid arthritis.

4000 BCE

The first urban centers are formed in Mesopotamia.

3000 BCE

Many Mesopotamian clay tablets document the practice of medicine, including prescriptions for medications for various diseases.

2600 BCE

The Egyptian scribe Hesy-Re is the earliest person identified as a dental practitioner. An inscription on his tomb includes the title "the greatest of those who deal with teeth, and of physicians."

1790 BCE

The Babylonian Code of Hammurabi, one of the first written codes of laws, describes how much a physician should be paid for successful surgery and cure of a patient (ten shekels), and what the punishment should be for the physician if the patient dies from the surgery (his hands will be cut off).

1500 BCE

The Egyptian Ebers Papyrus, the oldest most complete surviving medical textbook, describes a large number of medical conditions, including arthritis, diabetes, deafness, depression, and eye diseases.

The Egyptian Edwin Smith Papyrus, the oldest textbook on trauma surgery, describes the histories of 48 trauma cases beginning with head injuries and followed by thorax and spinal injuries. Treatment for each case is classified as being either favorable, uncertain, or an ailment not to be treated.

1403 BCE

An Egyptian stele depicts a priest with a paralysis and a withered lower right leg and foot—perhaps caused by polio—using a long pole as a walking aid.

650 BCE

Epilepsy is described in a Babylonian text.

600 BCE

The Indian surgeon Sushruta, one of the earliest surgeons of recorded history, describes various surgical operations including cataract surgery and rhinoplasty (nose surgery).

Massage and acupuncture are practiced in Japan.

500 BCE

Sick and afflicted pilgrims flock to the Grecian Temples of Asclepius to take part in a ritual called incubation. Acslepius, the ancient, kindly god of medicine in Greek mythology, is expected to visit them during a dream-state and either heal them or prescribe drugs, diet, and modes of treatment.

460–370 BCE

Hippocrates, the Greek physician who is considered the founder of Western Medicine, is the first to assert that epilepsy is a brain disorder and is not caused by a curse of the gods. The Hippocratic oath of medical ethics defines good medical practice and morals, and derivatives of the oath are still used today by many physicians as they begin their medical practice.

431 BCE

The first known hospital is established in Sri Lanka.

300 BCE

The oldest known artificial limb, a bronze leg dating from this era, is found in a tomb in Capua, Italy, in 1858.

131–201 CE

Galen of Pergamum, a Greek surgeon, anatomist, and physiologist who serves as a surgeon to a school of gladiators (and eventually as surgeon to the emperor) is the most famous physician in Roman times. Galen's numerous medical books are highly influential for centuries.

541

The first bubonic plague pandemic occurs.

549

In the wake of the plague, the Byzantine Emperor Justinian enacts a law to isolate people arriving from plague-infected regions.

583

The French Council of Lyons restricts lepers from freely associating with healthy persons.

600

China has a well-established quarantine policy detaining plague-stricken sailors and foreign travelers who arrive in Chinese ports.

910

Abu Bakr ar-Rhazi (c. 864–935), a Persian physician, is the first to distinguish between smallpox and measles, and to suggest blood as the cause of infectious disease.

1123

St. Bartholomew's Hospital is founded in London.

1200

Europe has about 19,000 leprosaria, or houses for leper patients.

1202

King John of England proclaims the first English food law, the Assize of Bread, which prohibits the adulteration of bread with such ingredients as ground peas and beans.

1284

Salvino D'Armato (1258–1312) of Florence is credited with inventing the world's first wearable eyeglasses.

1347

The Black Death bubonic plague begins in Europe. By the time it ends in 1351, the plague will kill an estimated 25% to 60% of the population of Europe.

1348

Venice establishes the world's first institutionalized system of quarantine, giving the city's council of three the authority to detain ships, cargoes, and individuals for up to 40 days.

1400

To prevent the Black Death, the city of Milan institutes a permanent health board.

1403

Venice establishes the world's first maritime quarantine station, or lazaretto, on an island in the Venetian lagoon.

1409

Spain becomes the cradle of humane psychiatry, establishing a number of asylums in which inmates are kept unchained, given games to use, provided with occupations, and given wholesome diets and hygiene.

1424

The first recorded regulations for midwives are established in Brussels.

1495

King Charles VIII's army is infected with syphilis during the siege of Naples; some believe the disease was brought from the New World by Columbus's sailors.

1518

The College of Physicians is formed in England; it later receives a royal charter and becomes the Royal College of Physicians.

1524

Theophrastus Bombastus von Hohenheim or Paracelsus (1493–1541), a Swiss alchemist, astrologer, and physician, writes the first book on an occupational disease, *On Miners' Consumption*.

1546

Girolamo Fracastoro (c.1483–1553), an Italian physician, writes *De Contagione et Contagiosis Morbis*, which presents an early version of the germ theory of disease.

1578

Guillaume de Baillou (1538–1616), a French physician and anatomist, is the first to use the word "rheumatism" to describe acute arthritis, a condition in which "the joints are wracked with pains so that neither foot, hand, nor finger can be moved without pain and protest."

1590

Dutch lens grinders Hans and Zacharias Janssen invent the compound microscope.

1595

The first known dedicated wheelchair, called an invalids chair, is made for King Phillip II of Spain.

1628

William Harvey (1578–1657), an English physician and anatomist, writes on the circulation of the blood in his book *An Anatomical Treatise on the Movement of the Heart and Blood in Animals*.

1643

Herman van der Huyden of Belgium publishes the first clear description of quinine as a remedy to suppress and prevent malaria; earlier Jesuit missionaries in Peru found quinine being used to treat fevers.

1647

The first New World epidemic of yellow fever begins in Barbados.

1658

Johann Jakob Wepfer (1620–1695), a Swiss physician who is considered one of the founders of neurology, publishes *Anatomical Observations on the Cadavers of Persons Carried Off by Apoplexy*. In the book, he is the first to hypothesize that the effects of a stroke are caused by bleeding in the brain.

1662

John Graunt (1620–1674), an English haberdasher, publishes *Natural and Political Observations Made Upon the Bills of Mortality*. Graunt analyzes the death records of London parishes and invents the first life table. He is considered to be the founder of demography and one of the founders of medical statistics.

1665

Robert Hooke (1635–1703), an English physicist, makes important contributions to the development of the microscope.

1674

Anton van Leeuwenhoek (1632–1723), a Dutch tradesman, invents a simple and inexpensive microscope with one lens. Using his microscope, he is the first person to describe bacteria.

1676

Thomas Sydenham (1624–1689), an English physician known as the founder of clinical medicine in Britain, is the first Western physician to use quinine in the treatment of malaria, laudanum in pain relief, and iron in the treatment of diseases of the blood.

1683

William Petty (1623–1687), an English physician and economist, is the first to apply quantitative reasoning to assess the benefits of physician practice and hospital care.

1701

Massachusetts passes a statute stipulating that all individuals suffering from plague, smallpox, and other contagious diseases must be isolated in separate houses.

1733

Stephen Hales (1677–1761), an English clergyman and physiologist, becomes the first to measure blood pressure when he measures the blood pressure of horses and other animals.

1736

Claudius Amyand (1681–1740), a French-born English surgeon, performs the world's first successful appendectomy.

1740

The Paris Academy of Sciences officially recommends mouth-to-mouth resuscitation for drowning victims. Mouth-to-mouth breathing dates to biblical times, when it was used by midwives to resuscitate newborns.

1747

James Lind (1716–1794), a Scottish naval surgeon, discovers that citrus fruits can prevent scurvy, a dreaded dietary-deficiency disease. Lind conducts his experiment by giving some sailors oranges and limes and comparing their health to other sailors whose diets remain free of citrus fruits. Based on the experiment, Lind is considered to be the founder of medical clinical trials.

1751

Thomas Bond (1712–1784), an American physician and surgeon, and Benjamin Franklin (1706–1790), an American inventor, statesman, and diplomat, establish the first hospital in the United States, the Pennsylvania Hospital, "to care for the sick-poor and insane who were wandering the streets of Philadelphia."

1752

William Smellie (1697–1763), a Scottish obstetrician, publishes his *Theory and Practice or Treatise on Midwifery*. Smellie is the first to apply a scientific approach to obstetrics.

1763

On April 25, Edmund Stone (1702–1768), a Church of England rector, reports to the Royal Society that he successfully treated 50 persons with rheumatic fever by giving them willow bark; the active ingredient in willow bark is later identified as salicin, which has an effect similar to that of the basic component in aspirin.

The first American medical society is founded in New London, Connecticut.

1765

John Morgan (1735–1789), an American physician, founds the first American medical school—the Medical College of Philadelphia, now the University of Pennsylvania College of Medicine.

1770

Robert Tucker, an American physician, receives the first medical degree in the United States. It is conferred upon him by King's College, now Columbia University's College of Physicians and Surgeons.

1773

The first hospital for the mentally ill in the United States is founded in Williamsburg, Virginia.

1741

Nicholas Andry (1658–1742), a French physician, publishes *Orthopaedia: Or, the Art of Correcting and Preventing Deformities in Children*, and coins the term orthopedics (from the Greek *ortho*, straight, and *paedeia*, child). Today, the medical specialty of orthopedics is concerned with the prevention and treatment of diseases and injuries to the musculoskeletal system, including bones, joints, and muscles.

1775–1783

The American Revolutionary War takes place, resulting in the deaths of 4,435 American soldiers and sailors. Another 6,188 American soldiers and sailors are wounded in the conflict.

1776

John Hunter (1728–1793), a Scottish surgeon who is considered the founder of scientific surgery because he applied a rational and scientific approach to surgery, is appointed surgeon to King George III.

1778

William Brown (1748–1792), a Scottish-born American, publishes the first American pharmacopoeia.

1779

Percivall Pott (1714–1788), an English surgeon, describes spinal deformity and paralysis associated with tuberculosis, now called Pott's disease or Pott's spine.

1780

Benjamin Franklin invents bifocal lenses.

Jean Andre Venel (1740–1791), a Swiss physician who is considered the founder of orthopedics and the first true orthopedist, establishes the world's first hospital dedicated to the treatment of crippled children's skeletal deformities.

1781

The Massachusetts Medical Society, a professional association of physicians, is founded; it is the oldest continuously operated medical society in the United States.

1785

William Withering (1741–1799), an English physician, introduces digitalis, derived from foxglove, to cure dropsy.

1793

Philippe Pinel (1745–1826), a French physician who is considered one of the founders of psychiatry, believes that mental patients should be treated humanely; acting on this conviction, he has the chains removed from patients in an insane asylum.

Benjamin Bell (1749–1806), a Scottish surgeon, determines the difference between gonorrhea and syphilis.

A yellow fever epidemic occurs in Philadelphia.

The first local health department with a permanent board of health is formed in Baltimore.

1794

Thomas Percival (1740–1804), an English physician, develops the first modern code of medical ethics, which he privately publishes.

1795

Alexander Gordon (1752–1799), a Scottish physician, publishes *A Treatise on the Epidemic Puerperal Fever of Aberdeen*, in which he shows that the cause of puerperal fever is the introduction of "putrid" (infected) material into the uterus by the midwife or physician; he recommends they wash their hands to prevent the spread of the disease. His work goes unnoticed.

1796

Edward Jenner (1749–1823), an English country physician, creates the world's first successful vaccination for a disease—smallpox.

The Boston Dispensary is founded; it is the forerunner of today's home care programs.

1797

The first medical journal in the United States, the *Medical Repository*, is published in New York City. The quarterly journal will continue to be published until 1824.

1798

On July 6, President John Adams signs an act establishing the Marine Hospital Service (MHS), the predecessor of the U.S. Public Health Service

(PHS). The MHS will form a network of hospitals to provide medical care for sick and disabled American merchant seamen.

1802

The world's first pediatric hospital, *L'Hopital des Enfants Malades*, is founded in France.

1803

The first permanent Marine hospital is authorized to be built in Boston.

1805

Frederick Serturner (1783–1841), a German chemist, isolates the chemical compound morphine (later named after Morpheus, the Greek god of dreams) from the opium poppy; despite being highly addictive, it will be widely used as a painkiller.

1806

New York passes the Medical Practices Act, the first physician licensing law in the nation. The act allows licensed physicians to recover their fees in court.

1807

Benjamin Waterhouse (1754–1846), an American physician and Harvard professor, is appointed physician in charge of the Boston Marine Hospital. Waterhouse is the first to introduce interns and residents into hospitals in the United States.

1811

The Massachusetts General Hospital is established in Boston.

1812–1815

The War of 1812 takes place, resulting in the death of 2,260 American soldiers and sailors and the wounding of another 4,505 American servicemen.

1812

American physician Benjamin Rush (1745–1813) publishes *Inquiries and Observations on Diseases of the Mind*, the first psychiatric textbook in the United States. Rush is considered to be the founder of American psychiatry.

The *New England Journal of Medicine and Surgery and the Collateral Branches of Science*, now the *New England Journal of Medicine*, is published; it is the world's oldest continuously published medical journal.

1816

Theophile Laennec (1781–1826), a French physician, invents the stethoscope to listen to sounds within the body to aid in diagnosis.

1817

The first school for deaf students in the United States is established in Hartford, Connecticut.

James Parkinson (1755–1824), an English physician, publishes his "Essay on the Shaking Palsy." Later, the neurodegenerative disease he described—Parkinson's Disease—is named after him.

1818

James Blundell (1790–1878), an English obstetrician, performs the world's first known human-to-human blood transfusion. Blundell performs a total of ten transfusions, four of which are successful.

1820

The U.S. Pharmacopeia, the first compendium of standard drugs for the United States, is established in Washington, D.C. It creates a system of standards, a system of quality control, and a national formulary.

1821

The Philadelphia College of Pharmacy, now the University of the Sciences of Philadelphia, is founded; it is the first college of pharmacy in North America.

Charles Bell (1774–1842), a Scottish anatomist and surgeon, describes facial paralysis. The disease eventually becomes known as Bell's palsy in recognition of his research work.

1823

On October 5, the first issue of the *Lancet* is published in England; the *Lancet* will become one of the world's leading medical journals.

1828

Johann Schonlein (1793–1864), a German physician, describes and coins the term hemophilia.

1829

Louis Braille (1809–1852), a Frenchman who lost his sight at three years of age, publishes a description of a raised dot reading system for the blind that he developed over the previous few years; this system comes to be known as Braille.

Dorothea Dix (1802–1887), an American philanthropist and social reformer, begins her 50-year effort to improve conditions for people with disabilities incarcerated in jails and poorhouses. Dix persuades prominent people to lobby their state legislatures to build mental hospitals. More than 32 state mental hospitals are credited to her efforts.

1832

On July 19, the British Medical Association is founded.

A cholera epidemic occurs in New York City and kills nearly 3,500 of the city's 250,000 residents.

1836

Pierre Louis (1787–1872), a French physician who has been called one of the founders of medical statistics, publishes *Researches on the Effects of Bloodletting in Some Inflammatory Diseases*, in which he concludes that there were "narrow limits to the utility" of bloodletting for the treatment of pneumonia. The medical practice of bloodletting, which was used to treat many diseases for thousands of years, eventually falls into disfavor.

The Library of the Office of the Surgeon General of the Army is established; it will eventually become the National Library of Medicine (NLM).

1837

William Farr (1807–1883), an English epidemiologist and physician, collects statistical data on mortality, morbidity, and disability. Farr, John Graunt, and Pierre Louis are considered the founders of medical statistics.

1838

Jean-Etienne Dominique Esquirol (1772–1840), a French psychiatrist, is the first to distinguish between mental illness and mental retardation.

1839

William Selpho of New York produces the first artificial limbs manufactured in the United States.

1840

On October 3, the *Provincial Medical and Surgeon Journal*, now *BMJ* (*British Medical Journal*), is published; *BMJ* is a widely read medical peer-reviewed journal.

The first attempt to measure the extent of mental illness and mental retardation in the United States occurs with the U.S. Census of 1840, which includes a category of "insane and idiotic."

The world's first college devoted exclusively to dentistry is opened in Baltimore.

Friedrich Henle (1809–1885), a German physician and pathologist, publishes *On Miasma and Contagia*, which provides the theoretical basis for the germ theory of disease.

1842

Edwin Chadwick (1800–1890), an English social reformer, publishes *Report on the Sanitary Conditions of the Labouring Population of Great Britain*.

1844

The American Psychiatric Association (APA) is founded; it is a specialty society representing American and international member physicians.

1846–1848

The Mexican-American War takes place, resulting in 13,283 dead and 4,152 wounded American soldiers and sailors.

1846

On October 16, William T. G. Morton (1819–1868), a Boston dentist, successfully uses ether as an anesthetic at the Massachusetts General Hospital.

B. Frank Palmer is granted the first U.S. patent for an artificial limb.

1847

On May 7, American physician Nathan Smith Davis (1817–1904) establishes the American Medical Association (AMA). The AMA will gradually extend its authority and become the single greatest influence on the organization and practice of medicine in the United States throughout much of the 20th century.

1848

On June 26, the U.S. Congress passes the Drug Importation Act, which requires U.S. Customs Service inspection to stop the entry of adulterated drugs from overseas.

Ignaz Semmelweis (1818–1865), a Hungarian obstetrician, discovers that the incidence of puerperal fever, an often fatal disease, could be drastically reduced by the use of hand washing by the hospital medical staff at the obstetric clinic of the Vienna General Hospital. Physicians at the clinic scoff at the idea.

1849

A cholera epidemic kills one of every 36 residents of Chicago.

1850

Lemuel Shattuck (1793–1859), an American bookseller, teacher, and statistician, publishes his report, *The Sanitary Survey of 1850*, and submits it to the Massachusetts Sanitary Commission. The influential report, which recommends Massachusetts establish a state board of health staffed by professional sanitary inspectors, will serve as a model for many other states.

Hermann von Helmholtz (1821–1894), a German physiologist and physicist, invents the ophthalmoscope, an instrument used for inspection of the interior of the eye.

1851

The first International Sanitary Conference is held in Paris, France; eventually it will become the World Health Organization (WHO).

1852

The American Pharmaceutical Association, now the American Pharmacists Association, is founded in Philadelphia.

1853

Charles Pravaz (1791–1853), a French surgeon, and Alexander Wood (1817–1884), a Scottish surgeon, independently invent the hypodermic syringe.

William Budd (1811–1880), an English physician, records an outbreak of typhoid fever in a Welsh inn. Noticing the close proximity of the local well to the inn's septic tank, Budd suggests that contaminated water may have been the source of the outbreak.

1854

John Snow (1813–1858), an English anesthesiologist and epidemiologist who is considered the founder of modern epidemiology, becomes convinced that contaminated water is the source of a cholera epidemic in

London. He subsequently convinces the authorities remove the pump handle from London's Broad Street public well, and the epidemic ends. Later, Snow further tests his hypothesis by conducting a statistical study of the cholera rates of London households that receive water from two different water companies; he confirms higher cholera rates in households that used water from the company that obtained its water from a more polluted part of the Thames River.

1855

The Government Hospital for the Insane is established in Washington, D.C.; it later becomes St. Elizabeth's Hospital.

James Marion Sims (1813–1883), an American physician, founds the first gynecologic hospital in the United States, the Hospital for Women's Diseases in New York City.

The Children's Hospital of Philadelphia, the nation's first hospital devoted exclusively to caring for children, is founded.

1857

New York City establishes the nation's first municipal pension fund providing disability and death benefits for the city's police.

The Columbia Institution for the Deaf, Dumb, and Blind is founded; it later becomes Gallaudet College.

1858

Florence Nightingale (1820–1910), an English nurse and hospital reformer, works with William Farr on a uniform reporting system for London hospitals and publishes *Notes on Matters Affecting the Health of the British Army.*

1859

On November 24, Charles Darwin (1809–1882), an English naturalist and founder of evolutionary biology, publishes *On the Origin of Species by Means of Natural Section, or the Preservation of Favoured Races in the Struggle for Life*. Darwin's theory of evolution by natural selection will have an enormous impact upon science, medicine, and society.

The American Dental Association (ADA) is founded.

1860

William Little (1810–1894), an English orthopedic surgeon, is the first to classify cerebral palsy as a specific disease.

Albert Niemann (1834–1861), a German chemist, isolates cocaine from the leaves of the Peruvian coca plant. At first cocaine is widely viewed as a miracle drug that could treat depression and cure heroin addiction; later it will be classified as a controlled substance.

The Florence Nightingale's Nursing School is founded at St. Thomas's Hospital, London.

1861–1865

The American Civil War takes place, resulting in approximately 625,000 deaths and 412,000 wounded among Northern and Confederate soldiers and sailors. There are about 60,000 amputations, with 60% involving upper extremities.

1861

On June 9, the U.S. Sanitary Commission is created to coordinate the volunteer efforts of women who want to contribute to the Union war effort. The commission, which is directed by American landscape architect Frederick Law Olmsted (1822–1903), helps staff field hospitals, provides supplies, and works to educate the military and government on matters of health and sanitation.

1862

The U.S. Congress passes a law providing the sum of $15,000 to supply limbs to disabled soldiers. Each "loyal" Union soldier is granted $75 to purchase a prosthetic leg. Ensuing laws increase the allowance and eligibility parameters of the program, assuring artificial limb makers of a market.

President Abraham Lincoln appoints Charles M. Wetherill as the first employee of the U.S. Department of Agriculture's Bureau of Chemistry, the predecessor of the U.S. Food and Drug Administration (FDA).

1864

The International Red Cross is founded in Geneva, Switzerland.

1865

The Willard State Hospital of New York, the first 1,000-bed mental hospital in the nation, opens. By the mid-20th century, some state mental hospitals will accommodate more than 10,000 beds.

1866

Gregor Mendel (1822–1884), a German monk who is considered the founder of modern genetics, publishes his paper "Experiments on Plant Hybridization." In the paper, he presents the underlying principles of heredity, but his work goes unnoticed for many decades.

John Langdon Down (1828–1896), an English physician, publishes the first description of what is later known as Down Syndrome.

Thomas Allbutt (1836–1925), an English physician, develops the clinical thermometer.

The New York State Legislature approves the creation of the Metropolitan Board of Health, now the New York City Department of Health and Mental Hygiene.

1867

Joseph Lister (1827–1912), an English surgeon and bacteriologist, publishes *On the Antiseptic Principle of the Practice of Surgery*, which shows that antiseptics reduce post-operative infections.

San Francisco passes the nation's first "ugly law" banning "diseased, maimed and deformed persons" from appearing in public; similar laws are passed in Chicago, Omaha, and Cleveland, and they will not be repealed until the 1960s and 1970s.

1868

Jean Martin Charcot (1825–1893), a French neurologist, is the first to categorize, describe, and document the disease multiple sclerosis (MS).

1872

Stephen Smith (1823–1922), a physician, attorney, and commissioner of New York City's Metropolitan Health Board, establishes the American Public Health Association (APHA) to advance sanitary science and promote the practical application of public hygiene.

The first formal school of nursing in the United States is established at the New England Hospital for Women and Children in Boston.

1873

William Budd publishes his classic paper on typhoid fever, "Typhoid Fever: Its Nature, Mode of Spreading, and Prevention."

1874

Louis Pasteur (1822–1895), a French chemist and microbiologist, suggests placing medical instruments in boiling water to sterilize them.

Andrew Taylor Still (1828–1917), a Missouri physician, creates osteopathic medicine. Still believes that illness is caused by a dislocation of bones in the spinal column and that a pathological condition in one of the body's organs affects other organs.

1876

The Provisional Association of American Medical Colleges, now the Association of American Medical Colleges (AAMC), is founded by representatives of 22 medical schools meeting in Philadelphia.

1878

On February 19, Louis Pasteur speaks before the French Academy of Medicine on his belief that disease, putrefaction, and fermentation are caused by microorganisms.

A major yellow fever epidemic occurs in the Mississippi Valley, resulting in 120,000 cases of the disease and 20,000 deaths.

1881

Carlos Finlay (1833–1915), a Cuban physician and epidemiologist, identifies the *Aedes aegypti* mosquito as the vector of yellow fever.

Warren Tay (1843–1927), an English ophthalmologist, is the first to describe the genetic disorder known today as Tay-Sachs; several years later Bernard Sachs (1858–1944), a New York neurologist, also describes the disorder. Tay-Sachs disease is a fatal disorder characterized by mental and motor deterioration.

Stephane Tarnier (1828–1897), a French obstetrician, introduces the world's first closed incubator for infants at a Paris hospital.

Clara Barton (1821–1912), an American nurse, establishes the American Red Cross in Washington, D.C.

The Chicago City Council enacts an "ugly law" that states: "No person who is diseased, maimed, mutilated or in any way deformed so as to be an unsightly or disgusting object or improper person to be allowed in or on the public ways or other public places in this city, or shall therein or thereon expose himself to public view, under penalty of not less than one dollar nor more than fifty dollars for each offense."

1882

Robert Koch (1843–1910), a German physician and bacteriologist, establishes criteria for identifying and confirming the microbiological cause of diseases. These criteria are known as Koch's Postulates.

1883

On July 14, the first issue of the *Journal of the American Medical Association* (*JAMA*) is published; the journal will disseminate the latest medical findings and greatly contribute to the prestige of the association.

Germany establishes the Sickness Insurance Funds, a program designed by Chancellor Otto von Bismarck that marks the beginning of the world's first national health insurance program.

Francis Galton (1822–1911), an English scientist and cousin of Charles Darwin, publishes *Inquiries into Human Faculty and Development* and coins the term eugenics (from the Greek *eu*, good or well, and the suffix *genes*, born), which he defines as "the science of improving the stock." Advocates of euthanasia begin making eugenics arguments to justify their position.

1885

On July 6, Louis Pasteur begins administering the world's first rabies vaccination to a nine-year-old boy who was bitten by a rabid dog.

1886

Because the U.S. government will only pay for the prosthetics of Union civil war veterans, the former states of the Confederacy must bear the costs of providing prosthetics to their veterans. Mississippi, for example, spends 20% of its state's revenues on artificial arms and legs.

1887

The National Institutes of Health (NIH), which will become the primary federal agency for conducting and supporting medical research in the United States, begins with the establishment of a one-room Laboratory of Hygiene at the Marine Hospital in Staten Island, New York.

The American Orthopaedic Association is founded.

1889

The U.S. Congress gives the Marine Hospital Service quarantine responsibilities.

The Mayo Clinic is founded in Rochester, Minnesota; it will become the largest integrated, nonprofit, group practice in the world

Under the leadership of Chancellor Otto von Bismarck, Germany formally establishes the world's first old-age social insurance program.

1890

Emil von Behring (1854–1917), a German bacteriologist, and Shibasaburo Kitasato (1856–1931), a Japanese bacteriologist, work together to develop vaccines against tetanus and diphtheria.

1892

Robert Koch discovers the tubercle bacillus, the cause of tuberculosis.

Jules Emile Pean (1830–1898), a French surgeon, performs the first total joint replacement, replacing an infected shoulder ball-and-socket joint with a shaft of platinum topped by a wax-coated black rubber ball. The operation is unsuccessful.

The first college of osteopathic medicine, the American School of Osteopathy, is founded in Kirksville, Missouri. The institution is now known as the Kirksville College of Osteopathic Medicine of the A. T. Still University of Health Sciences.

The American Psychological Association (APA) is founded; it will become the world's largest association of psychologists.

1893

The Johns Hopkins University Medical School, the first modern American medical school, opens in Baltimore.

The American Society of Superintendents of Training Schools, now the National League for Nursing (NLN), is founded.

1894

The first known polio epidemic in the United States occurs in Vermont.

Edward Trudeau (1848–1915), an American physician who has pulmonary tuberculosis, begins construction of the Adirondack Cottage Sanitarium at Saranac Lake, New York. This marks the beginning of the tuberculosis sanitarium movement in the United States.

William Halsted (1852–1922), an American surgeon who was the first surgeon-in-chief of Johns Hopkins Hospital, develops and introduces rubber surgical gloves.

1895

On November 8, Wilhelm Conrad Roentgen (1845–1923), a German physicist, discovers x-rays. The discovery marks the beginning of the modern medical specialty of radiology.

Daniel David Palmer (1845–1913), a Davenport, Iowa, healer, develops the chiropractic approach to healing. Chiropractic (from the Greek *cheir*, hand, and *praxis*, practice, or done by hand), which is considered to be complementary and alternative medicine (CAM), involves treating patients by manipulating bones in the spinal column.

The National Medical Association (NMA) is founded; it promotes the collective interests of physicians and patients of African descent and other minority and underserved populations in the nation.

1896

Scipione Riva-Rocci (1863–1937), an Italian physician, develops the modern sphygmomanometer, an instrument that measures blood pressure.

Antoine Henri Becqueral (1852–1908), a French physicist, discovers radioactivity.

The Nurses Associated Alumnae, now the American Nurses Association (ANA), is founded; it is a professional society representing registered nurses (RNs).

The first U.S. life insurance company, Fidelity Mutual Life Insurance, provides disability benefits.

1897

Ronald Ross (1857–1932), an English physician and parasitologist, locates the malaria parasite in the Anopheles mosquito.

The American Association for the Advancement of Osteopathy, now the American Osteopathic Association (AOA), is founded in Kirksville, Missouri.

Minnesota passes the first state law to provide medical and surgical aid for crippled children.

1898–1901

The Spanish-American War takes place, resulting in 2,446 dead and 1,662 wounded American soldiers and sailors.

1898

Marie Sklodowska Curie (1867–1934), a Polish-born French physicist, and her husband Pierre Curie (1859–1906), a French physical chemist, discover the radioactive element radium. Radium will be used to treat cancer and other diseases, but it will eventually be replaced by the use of x-rays.

Ohio passes the first state law in the nation providing pensions for the blind.

1899

The Association of Hospital Superintendents is founded; the organization is now known as the American Hospital Association (AHA).

1900

Infectious diseases are common in the United States. The three leading causes of death in the nation at this time are pneumonia, tuberculosis, and diarrhea and enteritis.

To prevent contamination of Lake Michigan drinking water, sanitary engineers in Chicago reverse the flow of the polluted Chicago River, creating the world's only river that "runs backward." The flow of the river is diverted into the Illinois River, which flows into the Mississippi River.

The U.S. Army Commission on Yellow Fever is established in Cuba under the direction of American physician Major Walter Reed (1851–1902) to test whether mosquitoes are the vector for yellow fever. To test the theory, healthy volunteers are subjected to mosquitoes that had previously bitten yellow fever patients.

Sigmund Freud (1856–1939), an Austrian psychoanalyst, publishes *The Interpretation of Dreams*. Freud's new theories and treatment approaches are adopted by prominent psychiatrists, and psychoanalysis becomes the leading therapy throughout the 20th century in the United States.

1901

Karl Landsteiner (1868–1943), an Austrian-born American biologist, discovers human blood groups and names them A, B, AB, and O. His discovery makes blood transfusion safer.

1902

Alexis Carrel (1873–1944), a French physician, develops a technique to suture blood vessels; in 1912 Carrel, who worked at the Rockefeller Institute for Medical Research, New York, for many years, will become the first scientist working in the United States to receive the Nobel Prize in physiology or medicine.

The Marine Hospital Service is reorganized into the U.S. Public Health and Marine Hospital Service.

The First International Sanitary Convention of the American Republics establishes the International Sanitary Bureau, now the Pan American Health Organization (PAHO), in Washington, D.C. PAHO works with all countries of the Americas to improve health and raise living standards.

A psychiatric unit is established in the Albany General Hospital of New York; other community hospitals across the United States will add similar units.

The first state workmen's compensation law is enacted in Maryland. However, the law is declared unconstitutional in 1904.

1903

Willem Einthoven (1860–1927), a Dutch physician and physiologist, invents the electrocardiogram (EKG), a machine that produces a graphic record of the electrical activity of a patient's heartbeat.

Illinois passes a law authorizing special pensions for the blind.

Helen Keller (1880–1968), a blind and deaf American author, political activist, and lecturer, publishes her autobiography, *The Story of My Life*.

1904

Winifred Holt Mather (1870–1945), an American social worker, establishes Lighthouse No. 1 for blind people in New York City, the first of many such institutions throughout the world.

The National Tuberculosis Association, now the American Lung Association, is founded.

The American Medical Association (AMA) creates the Council on Medical Education (CME) to restructure medical education.

1905

John B. Murphy (1857–1916), a Chicago surgeon, develops the first artificial hip joints.

The Milbank Memorial Fund is established in New York City; it works to improve health by helping decision makers acquire and use the best evidence to inform healthcare policy and population health.

1906

On June 30, President Theodore Roosevelt signs the Pure Food and Drug Act into law. This legislation prohibits interstate commerce in misbranded and adulterated foods, drinks, and drugs; prohibits the addition of color additives to conceal inferiority; and prohibits the use of "poisonous" colors in confectionary.

The University of Michigan establishes a psychiatric hospital for research, training, and treatment; other universities will establish similar hospitals.

Alois Alzheimer (1864–1915), a German physician, is the first to describe the brain disorder that is named after him.

1907

Mary Mallon, better known as Typhoid Mary, is quarantined on North Brother Island in New York's East River; Mallon, a cook who is known to have infected 53 people (five of whom died), will spend a total of 26 years in quarantine until her death in 1938.

Indiana is the first state in the nation to implement a eugenic sterilization law; 31 other states will pass similar laws. In some states prisoners as well as "feebleminded" individuals were targeted for sterilization.

1908

Clifford Beers (1876–1943), an American mental health advocate, publishes his book *The Mind That Found Itself: An Autobiography*. The harrowing book, which documents the author's three-year confinement in an asylum, creates a storm of protest and public concern. The book's release marks the beginning of the modern mental health movement in the United States.

A workmen's compensation system is established for civilian employees of the federal government.

The Chicago Medical Society and Hull House sponsor a birth record survey to document the role of midwifery in childbirth.

1909

On January 25, President Theodore Roosevelt sponsors the first White House Conference on Children. The conference opposes the institutionalization of dependent and neglected children.

On February 5–26, with the support of President Roosevelt, the International Opium Commission convenes in Shanghai, China. This event is the first multinational drug-control initiative.

On May 1, the U.S. Army's Walter Reed General Hospital, now Walter Reed Army Medical Center, opens in Washington, D.C.

As part of President Roosevelt's National Conservation Commission, Yale University's Professor Irving Fisher (1867–1947) compiles an inventory of medical care in the United States. His inventory is published in *A Report on National Vitality, Its Wastes and Conservation*.

Ignatz Nascher (1863–1945), an Austrian-born American physician who is considered the founder of geriatric medicine, coins the word geriatrics (from the Greek *geras,* old age, and *intrikos,* medical treatment); Nascher believes that physicians pay insufficient attention to the ill-health of older people, and that their health could be improved by better diet, exercise, and mental stimulation.

Clifford Beers helps establish the National Committee for Mental Hygiene, now Mental Health America.

To prevent infectious disease, Chicago becomes the first city in the United States to adopt a compulsory milk pasteurization ordinance.

1910

Paul Ehrlich (1854–1915), a German medical scientist, announces his discovery of Salvarsan, also known as 606, the first effective treatment against syphilis; this breakthrough is regarded as the beginning of modern chemotherapy.

James Herrick (1861–1954), a Chicago physician, is the first to describe the genetic disease sickle-cell anemia; Herrick reports the case of a 20-year-old West Indies dental student with peculiar elongated sickle-shaped red blood cells.

Ernest Amory Codman (1869–1940), a Boston surgeon, begins studying hospital outcomes, or "end results," to determine how they can be improved. His work anticipates contemporary approaches to medical quality monitoring and assurance.

The Carnegie Foundation publishes its *Bulletin Number Four,* more commonly referred to as the Flexner Report. The report, compiled by Abraham Flexner (1866–1959), an American teacher and researcher, is highly critical of American medical education and recommends that many of the nation's poor quality medical schools be closed.

1911

The American Public Health Association (APHA) begins publishing the *Journal of the American Public Health Association.*

William Hill (1858–1928), an English physician, develops the modern gastroscope, a tube swallowed by a patient so that the physician can look at the inside of the patient's stomach.

1912

Running for president as the nominee of the Progressive Party, former President Theodore Roosevelt proposes that America adopt national health insurance. He is the first president (sitting or former) to propose such a system.

Isaac Adler (1849–1918), a New York physician, is the first to propose a link between cigarette smoking and lung cancer; Adler presents his hypothesis in his medical monograph *Primary Malignant Growths of the Lungs and Bronchi.*

Casimir Funk (1884–1967), a Polish-born American biochemist, introduces the term vitamin.

The U.S. Public Health Service is reorganized and given added responsibility for medical research beyond communicable disease.

D. W. Dorrance, who lost his right hand in an industrial accident, patents the first split hook mechanical hand. He brings the two halves together by hinges, adds a thumb, and applies rubber bands for closure.

1913

The American College of Surgeons (ACS) is founded in Chicago.

The American Society for the Control of Cancer (ASCC), now the American Cancer Society (ACS), is founded in New York City.

John Jacob Abel (1857–1938), an American biochemist and pharmacologist, develops the first artificial kidney.

1914–1918

On July 28, World War I begins in Europe. The war results in an estimated total of between 8 and 16 million military and civilian deaths.

1914

Margaret Sanger (1879–1966), an American activist and founder of Planned Parenthood, coins the term "birth control" in the June issue of *The Woman Rebel.*

On December 17, President Woodrow Wilson signs the Harrison Narcotics Act into law. The act, which marks the beginning of "America's War on Drugs," requires prescriptions for products exceeding the allowable limit of narcotics and mandates increased recordkeeping for physicians and pharmacists who dispense narcotics.

Joseph Goldberger (1874–1929), a U.S. Public Health Service physician, conducts an epidemiological study that identifies the cause of the dietary disease pellagra, which is a scourge of poor Southerners.

Chicago's Michael Reese Hospital opens the nation's first incubator unit for the treatment of premature infants.

Ignatz Nasher (1863–1944) publishes the first textbook on geriatric medicine, *Geriatrics: The Diseases of Old Age and Their Treatment.*

1915

The National Board of Medical Examiners (NBME) is founded; its function is to administer a standardized licensing examination to physicians.

The Association for the Prevention and Relief of Heart Disease is established in New York City.

1916

On September 1, President Woodrow Wilson signs the Keating-Owen Child Labor Act into law. The act is the first federal statute to impose restrictions on child labor, but the U.S. Supreme Court declares it unconstitutional.

A polio epidemic occurs in New York; it kills more than 2,300 mostly young New Yorkers.

The first school of public health in the United States is founded at Johns Hopkins University.

1917

On April 6, the United States enters World War I. More than 116,500 American soldiers and sailors are killed in the conflict, and another 204,000 are wounded. The war creates an enormous need for physical reconstruction services to improve the functional restoration of the injured.

Major Frank B. Granger is designated director of the physiotherapy service of the reconstruction division of the U.S. Army Medical Corps. He establishes reconstruction units in 35 general hospitals and 18 base hospitals throughout the United States.

The International Center for the Disabled (ICD) is founded in New York City; it is the first comprehensive outpatient rehabilitation center in the nation.

The Artificial Limb Manufacturers and Brace Association, now known as the American Orthotic and Prosthetic Association (AOPA), is founded.

The National Society for the Promotion of Occupational Therapy, the predecessor of the American Occupational Therapy Association (AOTA), is founded.

1918–1920

The Great Influenza Pandemic occurs, resulting in 50 million to 100 million deaths worldwide, including almost 700,000 deaths in the United States. It is the largest, deadliest epidemic in modern history.

1918

Ernest Amory Codman publishes *A Study in Hospital Efficiency: As Demonstrated by the Case Report of the First Five Years of a Private Hospital*.

The Commonwealth Fund, a philanthropic foundation, is established with the broad charge to enhance the common good, it later conducts important research in many areas of medicine and public health.

1919

The Treaty of Versailles, which officially ends World War I, establishes the League of Nations, the forerunner of the United Nations (UN).

The American Medical Association (AMA) conducts one of the first national surveys of hospitals and state boards of health.

Edgar Allen, an Ohio businessman, establishes the National Society for Crippled Children, the predecessor of Easter Seals.

1920

Disabled American Veterans of the World War, now the Disabled American Veterans (DAV), is founded.

1921

President Warren Harding signs the Sheppard-Towner Act, also known as the Maternity and Infancy Act, into law on November 23. The act authorizes federal aid to states for maternity, child health, and welfare programs.

The American Foundation for the Blind (AFB) is founded in New York City.

The American Women's Physical Therapeutical Association, now the American Physical Therapy Association (APTA), is founded.

The U.S. Veterans Bureau is established, and the U.S. Public Health Service transfers the responsibility for the medical care of all returning veterans to it.

Franklin Roosevelt (1882–1945), who will later become president of the United States, contracts polio at the age 39; the disease inspires his interest in medical philanthropy.

Edgar Sydenstricker (1881–1936), an American public health statistician and economist, begins the Hagerstown, Maryland, Morbidity Survey.

The survey, which gathers data on the incidence of illness, is a precursor of the U.S. National Health Survey.

Fredrick Banting (1891–1941) and Charles Best (1899–1978), Canadian physiologists, isolate insulin and use it to treat diabetes. At the time diabetes is a feared disease that often results in death. The widespread use of insulin will eventually enable diabetics to live normal lives.

1922

Rehabilitation International (RI) is founded in New York City; RI evolves into a global network of experts, professionals, and advocates working to empower persons with disabilities.

Julius Hess (1876–1955), an American physician, publishes *Premature and Congenitally Diseased Infants*, the first American textbook on prematurity.

1923

Henry Kessler (1896–1978), an American physician and pioneer in rehabilitation medicine, initiates surgical techniques that allow muscular control of artificial limbs.

Elliott Cutler (1888–1947), an American surgeon, performs the first successful surgical operation for mitrial valve stenosis at a time when cardiac surgery is in its infancy.

Montana and Nevada enact the nation's first old-age pension laws.

The first issue of the *Milbank Memorial Fund Quarterly Bulletin*, now *Milbank Quarterly*, is published; it addresses population health and health policy.

The American College of Radiology and Physiotherapy, now the American Congress of Rehabilitation Medicine, is founded.

1924

The American Heart Association (AHA) is founded.

1925

American physician Alice Hamilton (1869–1970) documents workplace hazards and publishes *Industrial Poisons in the United States*. Hamilton, the first woman professor at Harvard Medical School, is considered to be the founder of occupational medicine.

1927

On May 2, the U.S. Supreme Court rules in *Buck v. Bell* that states can forcibly sterilize residents in order to prevent "feebleminded and socially inadequate" people from having children; it is the only time the Supreme Court endorses surgery as a tool of government policy.

Philip Drinker (1894–1972) and Louis Shaw (1886–1940), American bioengineers at Harvard University, invent the first modern and practical respirator. The tank respirators, or "iron lungs," will eventually be used by thousands of polio victims suffering from chest paralysis.

The Committee on the Costs of Medical Care (CCMC) is established. The privately funded committee will publish numerous reports on healthcare costs and distribution.

1928

Alexander Fleming (1881–1955), a Scottish bacteriologist, makes a chance discovery of penicillin in a mould while working at St. Mary's Hospital in London. Starting in World War II, penicillin will become one of the most widely used antibiotics.

1929–1942

The Great Depression takes place, spurring major social reforms in health care and other policy areas.

1929

Werner Forssmann (1904–1979), a German physician, is the first to insert a catheter into his heart and x-ray it to document its location; for his self-experimentation, Forssmann is fired from the hospital where he works and denounced by the medical establishment.

Justin Ford Kimball (1872–1956), an educator and vice president of Baylor University, develops an insurance plan whereby Dallas schoolteachers can prepay for hospital care at Baylor Hospital. Kimball's insurance plan ultimately leads to Blue Cross and Blue Shield plans.

Dorothy Harrison Eustis and Morris Frank found Seeing Eye, the first guide dog training school in the United States.

1930

Enactment of the Ransdell Act on May 26 transforms the Hygienic Laboratory into the first National Institute of Health, later the National Institutes of Health (NIH). The act establishes fellowships in basic biological and medical research.

On July 21, the Veterans Affairs Consolidation Act creates the Veterans' Administration.

The U.S. Public Health Service (PHS) establishes the Narcotics Division, later renamed the Division of Mental Hygiene, bringing together research and treatment programs to combat drug addiction and study the causes, prevalence, and means of preventing and treating nervous and mental disease.

The W. K. Kellogg Foundation is founded; it will fund research on various areas of healthcare.

The American Academy of Pediatrics (AAP) is founded.

1932

The Committee on the Costs of Medical Care (CCMC) publishes its final report, *Medical Care for the American People*.

The National Labor Relations Act, requiring management to bargain with labor over wages and conditions, is enacted. The act will become a catalyst for employer-based health benefits.

The U.S. Public Health Service (PHS), working with the Tuskegee Institute, begins a study to record the natural history of syphilis. It is called the "Tuskegee Study of Untreated Syphilis in the Negro Male."

Harry Jennings, an American mechanical engineer, designs the first sturdy, transportable, folding, tubular steel wheelchair for a paraplegic patient named Herbert Everest; the new wheelchair weights 50 pounds, compared to the usual 90 pounds.

1933

Albert S. Hyman (1893–1972), a New York City cardiologist, invents the world's first artificial pacemaker to resuscitate patients whose hearts have stopped. He and his brother Albert, who helped design the machine, are granted the first U.S. patent for an artificial heart pacemaker.

The American Academy of Orthopedic Surgeons (AAOS) is founded in Chicago.

The American College of Hospital Administrators, now the American College of Healthcare Executives (ACHE), is founded in Chicago.

1934

The first master's level professional degree program in hospital administration is created at the University of Chicago.

1935

On August 14, President Franklin Roosevelt signs the Social Security Act into law. The act provides federal old age benefits and grants to the states for assistance to blind people and children with disabilities.

The U.S. Public Health Service (PHS) conducts the first National Health Survey (NHS). It surveys 800,000 families in selected cities and rural areas in 19 states.

Gerhard Domagk (1895–1964), a German bacteriologist, announces the discovery of the first sulfa drug to treat streptococcal infection.

1936

Frank Krusen (1898–1973), an American physician, establishes the nation's first Department of Physical Medicine at the Mayo Clinic and the nation's first residency program in physical medicine. Krusen is considered the founder of American physical medicine.

1937

On August 5, President Franklin Roosevelt signs into law the National Cancer Institute Act, which creates the National Cancer Institute (NCI). Originally, the NCI is an independent research institute, but it will become part of the National Institutes of Health (NIH) in 1944.

The National Cancer Institute (NCI) conducts the First National Cancer Survey.

Bernard Fantus (1874–1940), a Hungarian-born American physician, establishes a blood bank at Cook County Hospital in Chicago. Fantus, who first coined the term "blood bank," popularizes the concept, and soon other hospitals across the nation establish them.

1938

Frank Krusen coins the term "physiatrist" to identify physicians who specialize in physical medicine. The name is derived from the Greek words *physis*, pertaining to physical phenomena, and *iatreia*, referring to healer or physician.

The American Academy of Physical Medicine and Rehabilitation (AAPM&R) is founded.

The National Foundation for Infantile Paralysis, later renamed the March of Dimes, is founded.

Philip Wiles (1899–1966), an English orthopedic surgeon, develops the first total artificial hip replacements, using stainless steel.

James Allison Glover (1874–1963), an English physician and public health officer, documents variations in tonsillectomy rates among school districts in England. Glover suggests that the differences are the result of medical practice preferences by physicians. His work marks the beginning of small area analysis.

1939

Edmund Cowdry (1888–1975), a Canadian-born American anatomist who is considered a founder of scientific gerontology, publishes *Problems of*

Ageing: Biological and Medical Aspects. The work is considered a classic in gerontology.

The National Foundation for Infantile Paralysis begins the mass distribution of iron lungs for polio victims.

German dictator Adolf Hitler initiates the T-4 Euthanasia Program to kill the incurably ill, physically or mentally disabled, and elderly people. The T-4 program, which is directed by Hitler's personal physician, Karl Brandt (1904–1948), is officially discontinued in 1941. However, the killings continue covertly until the military defeat of Nazi Germany in 1945.

1939–1945

World War II begins in Europe when Nazi Germany invades Poland on September 1, 1939. The war will be the deadliest military conflict in history, resulting in 50 million to 70 million military and civilian deaths.

During the war, millions of Nazi concentration camp prisoners are murdered and more than 1.5 million prisoners die of typhus, a preventable disease.

1940

Elizabeth Kenny (1886–1952), an Australian physical therapist, comes to the United States. Kenny's pioneering methods of treating polio using hot-pack applications, stretching exercises, and muscle message are unconventional and controversial but eventually become standard elements of care for the disease.

The National Federation of the Blind (NFB) is founded; it will become the largest membership organization of blind people in the United States.

Howard Florey (1898–1968), an Australian experimental pathologist, and Ernst Chain (1906–1979), a German-born British biochemist, develop penicillin as an antibiotic.

Karl Landsteiner (1868–1943), an Austrian-born American biologist, and Alexander Wiener (1907–1976), a New York physician, discover the

Rh Factor or "Rhesus Factor" in blood. This discovery helps make blood transfusions safer.

The American Diabetes Association is founded.

Less than 10% of the U.S. population has health insurance coverage.

1941

On December 8, the United States enters World War II. The war results in 405,000 deaths and 670,000 wounded among American soldiers and sailors. It causes an enormous need for physical medicine and rehabilitation services.

Norman Gregg (1892–1966), an Australian ophthalmologist, links rubella (German measles) in pregnancy to the occurrence of cataracts and other abnormalities in children.

Dickinson Richards (1895–1973), an American physician, and Andre Cournand (1895–1988), a French-born American physician, begin a series of experiments using cardiac catheterization at New York's Bellevue Hospital. Their work will revolutionize cardiopulmonary medicine, opening new vistas of diagnosis and treatment.

1942

Elizabeth Kenny establishes the Sister Kenny Rehabilitation Institute in Minneapolis, now part of Abbott Northwestern Hospital.

The American Geriatrics Society is founded.

1943

The Baruch Committee on Physical Medicine is formed by New York philanthropist Bernard Baruch. The committee will have a major impact on expanding the field of physical medicine.

Selman Waksman (1888–1973), a Ukrainian-born American microbiologist at Rutgers University, discovers the antibiotic streptomycin, which will later be used in the treatment of tuberculosis and other diseases.

Willem Kolff (1911–2009), a Dutch-born American physician, develops the first kidney dialysis machine in Nazi-occupied Holland.

Alice Hamilton publishes *Exploring the Dangerous Trades: The Autobiography of Alice Hamilton, M.D.*

Leo Kanner (1894–1981), an Austrian-born psychiatrist and Johns Hopkins University professor considered to be the founder of child and adolescent psychiatry, publishes the paper "Autistic Disturbances of Affective Contact." His paper, together with the work of Austrian pediatrician Hans Asperger (1906–1980), will form the basis of the modern study of autism.

1944

During World War II, price and wage controls are strictly enforced in the United States. To compete for workers, employers begin offering health insurance benefits, giving rise to the employer-based health insurance system that is still largely in place today.

The American Hospital Association (AHA) forms the Commission on Hospital Care to survey hospital needs. The survey results will influence the federal government to provide funds for new hospital construction.

1945

On October 24, the United Nations (UN) is formally founded in New York City.

President Harry Truman proposes the creation of national health insurance. Truman is the first sitting president to do so.

Henry Kaiser (1882–1967), an American industrialist, and Sidney Garfield (1906–1984), an American physician, establish an integrated managed care organization called Kaiser Permanente in Oakland, California.

Water fluoridation to prevent tooth decay begins in the cities of Newburgh, New York, and Grand Rapids, Michigan, and it soon is used by many other cities across the nation. The decline in tooth decay (dental caries) resulting from the fluoridation of community drinking water is considered to be one of the ten greatest achievements of American public health in the 20th century.

The Gerontological Society of America (GSA) is formally established to "promote the scientific study of aging."

1946

On July 1, the Communicable Disease Center, now the Centers for Disease Control and Prevention (CDC), is established in Atlanta, Georgia. It initially focuses on fighting malaria by killing mosquitoes.

On July 3, President Harry Truman signs the National Mental Health Act into law. The act establishes the National Institute for Mental Health (NIMH) and, for the first time, provides federal funds for research into mental disorders, training of mental health professionals, and community psychiatric services.

On August 13, President Truman signs the Hospital Survey and Construction Act, or Hill-Burton Act, into law, providing federal grants to the nation's non-profit hospitals to modernize their physical plants. In exchange for these grants, hospitals are required to provide charity care or discount the cost of care for those who cannot afford it.

Paralyzed Veterans of America (PVA) is established in Washington, D.C.; it is the only congressionally chartered service organization dedicated solely to serving the needs of veterans with spinal cord injury or spinal cord dysfunction.

The first medical clinical trial using randomized treatment and control groups is carried out by the Medical Research Council in England; this pioneering trial involves the use of streptomycin to treat pulmonary tuberculosis.

Saskatchewan becomes the first Canadian province to introduce near universal healthcare coverage. This milestone marks the beginning of Canada's national healthcare system.

1947

Penicillin becomes the drug of choice to treat syphilis. However, researchers conducting the U.S. Public Health Service's Tuskegee Syphilis Study do not offer the drug to the infected men in the study, and they discourage local physicians and public health departments from providing the drug to them.

1948

The United Nations (UN) issues the Universal Declaration of Human Rights. The declaration includes assurance that "everyone has the right to a standard of living adequate for the health and well-being of himself and of his family, including food, clothing, housing and medical care."

The World Health Organization (WHO) is formed as part of the United Nations (UN). Headquartered in Geneva, Switzerland, the WHO is the world's coordinating authority on international public health. In its constitution, the WHO broadly defines health as "a state of complete physical, mental and social well-being and not merely the absence of disease or infirmity."

The U.S. Congress establishes the National Heart Institute, now the National Heart, Lung, and Blood Institute (NHLBI), which is part of the National Institutes of Health (NIH).

The Framingham Heart Study begins in the small town of Framingham, Massachusetts. The world-famous study, which continues today, studies cohorts of individuals to determine the risk factors such as smoking, diet, and exercise that are associated with heart disease and stroke.

The U.S. Congress authorizes the Veterans Administration, now the U.S. Department of Veterans Affairs (VA), to undertake rehabilitation research and engineering projects with an initial emphasis on prosthetics.

David Karnofsky (1914–1969), an American oncologist, creates the Performance Status Scale (Karnofsky Scale) to measure the outcome of cancer treatment. The scale classifies the functional impairment of cancer patients.

Philip Hench (1896–1965), the first rheumatologist at the Mayo Clinic of Rochester, Minnesota, and Edward Kendall (1886–1972), a biochemist, discover that cortisone can be used to treat rheumatoid arthritis.

John Enders (1897–1985), an American bacteriologist, discovers a process to grow the poliovirus in a laboratory. This breakthrough will quickly lead to the development of the first successful polio vaccine.

The American Society of Human Genetics (ASHG) is established.

The Arthritis and Rheumatism Foundation, now the Arthritis Foundation, is founded.

The National Spinal Cord Injury Association is founded.

The Henry J. Kaiser Family Foundation (KFF) is founded; it addresses the unmet healthcare needs of the citizens of the United States.

The United Kingdom establishes its National Health Service (NHS), a national health program.

1949

On April 15, the National Institute of Mental Health (NIMH), one of the first four National Institutes of Health (NIH), is formally established.

Researchers discover that lithium can be used to treat and reduce the symptoms of bipolar disorder.

The United States is declared free of malaria as a significant public health problem.

The United Cerebral Palsy Association is founded, uniting all local cerebral palsy organizations in the United States.

1950–1953

The Korean War takes place, claiming the lives of 33,739 American soldiers and sailors and wounding another 103,284 servicemen.

1950

The U.S. Congress creates a grant-in-aid program for state public assistance programs for the disabled.

The National Institute of Neurological Disorders and Stroke (NINDS) is established as part of the National Institutes of Health (NIH).

Howard Rusk (1901–1989), an American physician who is considered to be the founder of rehabilitation medicine, opens the Institute of Rehabilitation Medicine, now the Howard A. Rusk Institute of Rehabilitation Medicine, at the New York University Medical Center in New York City.

The American Dental Association (ADA) endorses the use of fluoridation to prevent tooth decay.

The National Association for Retarded Citizens, now The Arc, is founded.

The Pan American Health Organization (PAHO) undertakes a hemisphere-wide smallpox eradication program.

1951

John Gibbon, Jr. (1903–1973), an American surgeon, develops the first heart-lung machine.

The Joint Commission on Accreditation of Hospitals (JCAH), now the Joint Commission, an independent not-for-profit organization whose primary purpose is to provide voluntary accreditation, is jointly formed by the American College of Physicians (ACP), American College of Surgeons (ACS), American Hospital Association (AHA), American Medical Association (AMA), and the Canadian Medical Association (CMA).

Talcott Parsons (1902–1978), a Harvard University sociologist, introduces the concept of the sick role in his book *The Social System*. The book becomes a standard textbook in sociology—and particularly in medical sociology.

1952

The worst polio epidemic in U.S. history occurs, with a total of 57,628 reported cases.

Jonas Salk (1914–1995), an American virologist, develops the first success-ful polio vaccine. His vaccine uses a nonliving poliovirus.

Chlorpromazine (Thorazine), one of the first psychotropic drugs, is discov-ered to improve the condition of individuals with psychosis and delusion.

Virginia Apgar (1909–1974), an American obstetrical anesthesiologist, devises the first standardized method of assessing a newborn infant's health. The quick and simple method is today known as the Apgar Score.

Douglas Bevis (1919–1994), an English obstetrician and gynecologist, pub-lishes "The Antenatal Prediction of Hemolytic Disease of the Newborn." The article leads to the wide use of amniocentesis to detect various genetic diseases and conditions in newborns.

1953

Englishman Francis Crick (1916–2004) and American James Watson (1928–) discover the double-helix structure of deoxyribonucleic acid (DNA), the chemical compound that contains the genetic instructions for building, running, and maintaining living organisms.

The U.S. Department of Health, Education, and Welfare (HEW) is established.

Osteopathic medicine is recognized by the American Medical Association (AMA).

The Association of Schools of Public Health (ASPH) is founded; it repre-sents deans, faculty, and students of accredited and associate schools of public health.

1954

On December 23, Joseph E. Murray (1919–), a Boston surgeon at the Peter Bent Brigham Hospital, conducts the world's first successful kidney transplantation; he uses a set of identical twins as donor and recipient.

The Rehabilitation Institute of Chicago (RIC) is founded; it will become one of the nation's leading providers of physical medicine and rehabilita-tion services.

The Presidential Commission on Health Needs issues *Building America's Health*. Citing a national shortage of physicians, the commission urges increased training of physicians and other medical specialists.

1955

On July 3, President Harry Truman signs the Mental Health Study Act into law. The act authorizes the National Institute of Mental Health (NIMH) to create a Joint Commission on Mental Health and Illness to study and make recommendations on mental health and mental illness issues facing the nation.

Psychoactive drugs are introduced in the United States, and their widespread use will eventually lead to increased discharges of patients from mental hospitals.

The Indian Health Service (IHS), which is responsible for providing federal healthcare services to American Indians and Alaska Natives, is founded.

Howard Rusk establishes the World Rehabilitation Fund in New York City; it is devoted to the development and implementation of rehabilitation programs for people with disabilities throughout the world.

The first antihypertensive drug is used in the United States to lower elevated blood pressure in hypertensive emergencies.

Nearly 70% of the U.S. population has health insurance coverage.

1956

On July 4, President Dwight Eisenhower signs the National Health Survey Act into law. The act mandates the U.S. Public Health Service to conduct research and statistical analysis (including special sickness and disability studies) on the health needs of Americans.

On August 1, President Eisenhower signs the Social Security Act Amendment. The amendment provides monthly benefits to permanently and totally disabled workers aged 50–64 and to adult children of deceased or retired workers who became disabled before age 18.

The National Library of Medicine (NLM) is established; it will become the world's largest medical library.

American physician E. Donnall Thomas (1920–) performs the first successful bone marrow transplant between identical twins. The recipient, a patient with leukemia, accepts the donated marrow from his healthy twin, which is used to make new, healthy blood cells and immune system cells. Bone marrow transplantation will make it possible to treat many diseases that were once thought to be incurable.

American physicians Peter Safar (1924–2003) and James Elam (1918–1995) invent a mouth-to-mouth resuscitation method to revive unresponsive victims.

1957

Albert Sabin (1906–1993), an American microbiologist, develops the oral polio vaccine. His vaccine uses a live attenuated (weakened) poliovirus. The Sabin oral vaccine, which is cheaper to produce than the Salk vaccine, becomes widely used in the prevention of polio.

The National Health Interview Survey (NHIS) begins. The NHIS, which continues to this day, is the principal source of information on the health of the civilian population of the United States.

1958

The world's first modern intensive care unit (ICU) is established at the Baltimore City Hospital.

Clarence Lillehei (1918–1999), a pioneering American heart surgeon, develops the world's first small, external, portable, battery-powered heart pacemaker.

Ian Donald (1910–1987), a Scottish obstetrician, uses ultrasound to diagnosis disorders of the fetus.

The Pharmaceutical Manufacturers Association (PMA), now the Pharmaceutical Research and Manufacturers of America (PhRMA), is founded in Washington, D.C.

1959

The World Health Assembly adopts the goal of eradicating smallpox.

1960

On May 11, the U.S. Food and Drug Administration (FDA) approves the first birth control pill, the first drug in history to be given to a healthy person for long-term use. The "pill" would lead to enormous demographic and societal changes.

The Social Security Act is amended to allow people less than 50 years of age to qualify for Social Security Disability Insurance.

The National Center for Health Statistics (NCHS) is created through a merger of the National Office of Vital Statistics and the National Health Survey.

Robert Guthrie (1916–1995), an American microbiologist, develops a test for phenylketonuria (PKU), a rare but treatable genetic disorder that can lead to developmental disabilities. The inexpensive test will eventually be used around the world in mass screening programs for the disorder.

1961

On January 9, President John Kennedy hosts the first White House Conference on Aging. The conference issues its report *The Nation and Its Older People*, which is concerned with the provision of medical care to the elderly.

The Joint Commission on Mental Illness and Health issues its final report, *Action for Mental Health*. The report provides background for President Kennedy's message to the U.S. Congress on mental illness.

1962

The U.S. Food and Drug Administration (FDA) keeps the drug Thalidomide from being sold in the United States. The new drug, which is used in

Europe and Canada by some pregnant women to treat morning sickness, is later found to cause severe birth defects such as missing or shortened limbs; researchers later estimate that the drug caused more than 10,000 children to be born with major malformation.

Lasers are first used in eye surgery.

1963

On January 30, the National Institute of Child Health and Human Development (NICHD) is established as part of the National Institutes of Health (NIH).

On October 31, President John Kennedy signs the Mental Retardation Facilities and Community Mental Health Center Construction Act into law. The act provides grants to states to establish local mental health centers, and it also increases the deinstitutionalization of mental health patients.

The tranquilizer Valium is introduced in the United States; it quickly becomes the standard drug for the treatment of anxiety.

Massachusetts becomes the first state in the nation to mandate screening for phenylketonuria (PKU). Other states soon follow.

Sidney Katz (1924–), an American gerontologist physician, develops the first indices of activities of daily living (ADLs) to measure changes in physical function.

The American Heart Association formally endorses cardiopulmonary resuscitation (CPR).

Measles vaccine is licensed for general use in the United States.

Erving Goffman (1922–1982), a Canadian-born American sociologist, publishes *Stigma: Notes on the Management of Spoiled Identity*. The seminal work conceptualizes and creates a framework for the study of stigma.

1964–1973

The Vietnam War takes place between North Vietnam and the United States. The war results in 58,220 deaths and 303,644 wounded among American soldiers and sailors. During the war, surgeons perfect vascular injury repair, resulting in fewer deaths from serious wounds than in previous wars.

1964

On July 2, President Lyndon Johnson signs the Civil Rights Act into law. The landmark act will significantly impact subsequent disability rights legislation.

The Surgeon General's report *Smoking and Health* is published. The report, which focuses on the adverse health risks of smoking, prompts national changes in social norms and increased public awareness of the fatal consequences of continued tobacco use.

Home kidney dialysis is introduced in the United Kingdom and the United States.

The National Library of Medicine's Medical Literature Analysis and Retrieval System (MEDLARS) becomes operational. It is a large biomedical database that will eventually be put online.

1965

On July 14, President Lyndon Johnson signs the Older Americans Act into law; the act establishes the Administration on Aging (AoA) and provides a wide array of service programs through a network of state units on aging.

On July 30, President Johnson signs Medicare (Title XVIII of the Social Security Act) and Medicaid (Title XIX of the Social Security Act) into law; Medicare provides health care to the elderly, while Medicaid provides healthcare to the nation's poor.

Saad Nagi, an Egyptian-born American sociology professor at Ohio State University, develops one of the first models of disability based on his research on rehabilitation outcomes. The influential model is used by the Social Security Administration (SSA).

The Autism Society of America is founded.

1966

The United Nations (UN) issues the International Covenant on Economic, Social, and Cultural Rights, which decrees that every nation is responsible for "the creation of conditions which would assure, to all, medical service and medical attention in the event of sickness."

The Centers for Disease Control (CDC) announces a national measles eradication campaign.

The Commission on Accreditation of Rehabilitation Facilities (CARF) is founded. It currently accredits more than 5,500 rehabilitation service providers.

The Federation of American Hospitals (FAH) is founded. The FAH represents for-profit hospitals and managed community hospitals and health systems.

Irwin Rosenstock, an American health education professor, develops the Health Belief Model. The widely used model attempts to explain health-related behavior.

1967

On December 3, Christiaan Barnard (1922–2001), a South African surgeon, performs the world's first successful human heart transplant.

Rene Favaloro (1923–2000), an Argentinean cardiovascular surgeon, develops the coronary bypass operation.

Thomas Starzl (1926–), a Denver surgeon, performs the world's first successful human liver transplant.

Mammography for detecting breast cancer is introduced.

1968

On August 12, President Lyndon Johnson enacts the federal Architectural Barriers Act (ABA). The ABA, which takes the view that accessibility is a basic civil right for all, requires that all buildings designed, built, altered, or leased with federal funds be equipped with ramps, curb cuts, and other features that guarantee access to all facilities.

On December 26, the National Eye Institute is created as part of the National Institutes of Health (NIH).

Patrick Steptoe (1913–1988), an English gynecologist, and Robert Edwards (1925–), an English physiologist, fertilize a human egg outside of the woman's body. This marks an important step of in vitro fertilization.

The Association of Academic Health Centers (AAHC) is founded.

1970

On January 1, President Richard Nixon signs the National Environmental Policy Act into law. The act leads to the creation of the U.S. Environmental Protection Agency (EPA).

On December 29, President Nixon signs the Occupational Safety and Health Act. The landmark employee safety act creates the Occupational Safety and Health Administration (OSHA) and the National Institute for Occupational Safety and Health (NIOSH).

The National Institute on Alcohol Abuse and Alcoholism (NIAAA) is established. The NIAAA will lead national efforts to reduce alcohol-related problems.

The Institute of Medicine (IOM) is established as part of the National Academy of Sciences to advise the U.S. Congress on healthcare trends and policy. The IOM will publish many influential reports on various medical, public health, and disability topics.

Judith Heumann (1947–), a disability activist, organizes Disabled in Action in New York City.

1971

On December 2, the White House Conference on Aging recommends creating a National Institute on Aging.

On December 23, President Richard Nixon signs the National Cancer Act into law. The act strengthens the National Cancer Institute (NCI) in order to more effectively carry out the national effort against cancer.

The National Center for Health Statistics (NCHS) conducts the first National Health and Nutrition Examination Survey to determine the health status of Americans.

The National Library of Medicine (NLM) introduces MEDLINE (Medical Literature Analysis and Retrieval System Online) to provide online access to a subset of references in the MEDLARS (Medical Literature Analysis and Retrieval System) database. MEDLINE is a large database managed by NLM containing bibliographic references to millions of biomedical journal articles published in the United States and many foreign countries.

1972

On October 30, President Richard Nixon signs the Social Security Amendments into law. The amendments create the Supplemental Security Income (SSI) program. Medicare coverage is also expanded to include disabled and inpatient rehabilitation.

The U.S. Congress establishes the Congressional Office of Technology Assessment (OTA) to evaluate new and emerging technologies. However, the OTA is closed in 1995.

An Associated Press story about the U.S. Public Health Service's Tuskegee Syphilis Study causes a public outcry and the study ends.

Computerized axial tomography (CAT) is introduced commercially for medical imaging in the United States.

Edward Roberts (1939–1995), a disability activist, establishes the Center for Independent Living in Berkeley, California. The center quickly becomes a symbol of the Independent Living Movement emerging throughout the nation and the world.

1973

On September 26, President Richard Nixon signs the Rehabilitation Act into law. The act prohibits discrimination on the basis of disability in programs conducted by federal agencies, in programs receiving federal financial assistance, in federal employment, and in the employment practices of federal contractors.

On December 29, President Nixon signs the Health Maintenance Organization Act into law. The act provides federal grant and loan money to help support the startup of HMOs.

The U.S. Access Board is founded. The board is an independent federal agency devoted to ensuring accessibility for people with disabilities.

The International Association for the Study of Pain (IASP) is founded; it will become the world's largest multidisciplinary organization focused specifically on pain research and treatment.

1974

On May 31, President Richard Nixon signs the Research on Aging Act. The act creates the National Institute on Aging (NIA).

The Health Care Financing Administration (HCFA), now the Centers for Medicare and Medicaid Services (CMS), is established to manage the nation's Medicare and Medicaid programs.

The Robert Wood Johnson Foundation (RWJF) becomes a national philanthropy. Today, the RWJF is the nation's largest philanthropy exclusively dedicated to improving the health and health care of all Americans.

1975

On December 2, President Gerald Ford signs the Education for All Handicapped Children Act, later known as the Individuals with Disabilities Education Act (IDEA), into law. The landmark act makes it possible for states and localities to receive federal funds to assist in the education of children with disabilities.

1976

The World Health Organization (WHO) makes a three-fold distinction between impairment, disability, and handicap. According to the WHO, "impairment is any loss or abnormality of psychological, physiological or anatomical structure or function; a disability is any restriction or lack (resulting from an impairment) of ability to perform an activity in the manner or within the range considered normal for a human being; a handicap is a disadvantage for a given individual, resulting from an impairment or a disability, that prevents the fulfillment of a role that is considered normal (depending on age, sex and social and cultural factors) for that individual."

The National Center for Health Statistics (NCHS) publishes the first *Health, United States*. This annual report documents the health status of the nation.

1977

The first MRI (magnetic resonance imaging) body examination is performed.

1978

On July 25, the world's first successful "test-tube" baby, Louise Joy Brown, is born in England.

The Congressional Office of Technology Assessment (OTA) publishes *Assessing the Efficacy and Safety of Medical Technologies*. The influential report identifies many medical technologies that have not been thoroughly tested, and warns that others have only undergone flawed testing procedures.

The National Institute on Disability and Rehabilitation Research (NIDRR) is established. The NIDRR is a component of the Office of Special Education and Rehabilitation (OSERS) at the U.S. Department of Education.

1979

The World Health Organization (WHO) officially certifies the worldwide eradication of smallpox. This is the first disease in history to ever have been eradicated.

The U.S. Department of Health and Human Services (HHS) is created from the U.S. Department of Health, Education, and Welfare (HEW), with education responsibilities transferred to the newly created U.S. Department of Education (ED).

The U.S. Surgeon General publishes *Healthy People: The Surgeon General's Report on Health Promotion and Disease Prevention.* This landmark report lays the foundation for a national disease prevention program.

The American College of Epidemiology (ACE) is founded; the organization addresses the professional concerns of epidemiologists and develops criteria for their professional recognition.

The National Alliance for the Mentally Ill (NAMI) is founded in Wisconsin. NAMI will become one of the nation's largest grassroots health organizations.

The National Society of Genetic Counselors (NSGC) is founded.

1980

The World Health Organization (WHO) publishes the *International Classification of Impairment, Disabilities and Handicaps (ICIDH)*, which makes a clear distinction between impairment, disability, and handicap. However, some criticize the definition of disability as being too medical, too centered on the individual, and insufficiently focused on the interaction between the individual and society.

The World Health Assembly recommends that all countries cease routine smallpox vaccination.

1981

On June 5, the Centers for Disease Control's *Morbidity and Mortality Weekly Report* (MMWR) publishes a brief item about a strange cluster of *Pneumocystis carinii* pneumonia cases at three California hospitals involving five otherwise healthy gay men, two of whom died. This is considered the first mention of what would later be called AIDS (Acquired Immune Deficiency Syndrome).

The United Nations (UN) designates this year as the International Year of Disabled Persons.

Bruce Reitz, an American cardiac surgeon at Stanford University, performs the world's first successful heart-lung transplant.

1982

Robert Jarvik (1946–), an American physician and biomedical engineer, invents the first permanently implantable artificial heart, the Jarvik 7.

The American Association on Health and Disability (AAHD) is founded.

The American Paralysis Association, now the Christopher and Dana Reeve Foundation, is founded.

The American Society of Transplantation (AST) is founded.

1983

On January 4, President Ronald Reagan signs the Orphan Drug Act (ODA) into law. The ODA provides incentives to pharmaceutical companies to develop therapies for rare diseases.

Luc Montagnier (1932–), a French physician at the Pasteur Institute, discovers the human immunodeficiency virus (HIV), which causes AIDS. This discovery will lead to the development of a test detecting the presence of HIV in blood samples.

The Health Care Financing Administration (HCFA), now the Centers for Medicare and Medicaid Services (CMS), begins paying the nation's community hospitals for inpatient Medicare services using a prospective payment system based on diagnosis-related groups (DRGs); many hospitals react to the change in payment by releasing patients "quicker and sicker."

The National Institute of Mental Health (NIMH) begins publishing *Mental Health, United States*. This annual report will continue until 2006.

The world's first successful human embryo transfer, a key to in vitro fertilization, is performed at the University of California at Los Angeles School of Medicine.

The American Association of Preferred Providers Organizations (AAPPO) is founded.

1984

On April 1, the Canadian Health Act receives Royal Assent; it specifies the conditions and criteria that each Canadian province and territory must conform to in order to receive federal funds for health care. The act is designed to ensure accessibility, comprehensiveness, universality, portability, and public administration of Canada's health care.

On October 9, President Ronald Reagan signs the Social Security Disability Benefits Reform Act into law.

On October 19, President Reagan signs the National Organ Transplant Act into law, banning the buying and selling of human organs; the act will be amended in 1988 and 1990.

1985

The Blue Cross and Blue Shield Association establishes the Technology Evaluation Center (TEC); it will pioneer the development of scientific criteria for assessing medical technologies.

The Institute of Medicine (IOM) publishes *Injury in America, a Continuing Health Problem.*

The American Foundation for AIDS Research (amfAR) is founded.

1986

On April 7, President Ronald Reagan signs the Consolidated Omnibus Reconciliation Act (COBRA) of 1985 into law. The legislation contains the Emergency Medical Treatment and Active Labor Act (EMTALA), also known as the Patient Anti-Dumping Act, which requires all hospitals that receive

Medicare funds to admit and treat anyone who is facing severe risk of death, or who is in active labor, until the patient's medical condition is "stabilized."

On August 27, President Reagan signs the Temporary Child Care for Handicapped Children and Crisis Nurseries Act, which is part of the Children's Justice Act, into law. The act includes provisions to fund (1) temporary child care for children who have a disability or chronic illness and (2) crisis nurseries for children at risk of abuse or neglect.

The gene for duchenne muscular dystrophy is discovered.

1987

AZT (azidothymidine), the first and best-known anti-HIV drug, is approved by the U.S. Food and Drug Administration (FDA). Other drugs will follow, transforming HIV/AIDS from a death sentence to a chronic disease.

The World Health Organization (WHO) launches the Global Program on AIDS.

The Children and Adults with Attention-Deficit/Hyperactivity Disorder (CHADD) organization is founded.

1988

On December 1, the first World AIDS Day is held to raise awareness about HIV/AIDS.

The World Health Organization (WHO), Rotary International, the Centers for Disease Control (CDC), and UNICEF start the Global Polio Eradication Initiative.

The Institute of Medicine (IOM) publishes *The Future of Public Health*. The influential report concludes that the nation's public health system is in disarray, and it calls for a complete overhaul and refocus of governmental public health functions and organization.

The CDC establishes the National Center for Chronic Disease Prevention and Health Promotion.

The Federal Fair Housing Act is amended to include people with disabilities.

1989

On March 15, the Veterans Administration becomes a cabinet-level agency called the U.S. Department of Veterans Affairs (VA).

On November 27, Christoph Broelsch, a German transplant surgeon, performs the first successful living-donor liver transplant at the University of Chicago, with a one-year-old girl receiving part of her mother's liver.

1990–1991

The first Persian Gulf War results in the death of 382 American soldiers and sailors; an additional 467 American soldiers and sailors are wounded in the conflict.

1990

On July 26, President George H. W. Bush signs the Americans with Disabilities Act (ADA) into law. The ADA is landmark civil rights legislation that creates broad legal protections for people with disabilities.

On August 18, President Bush signs the Ryan White Comprehensive AIDS Resources Emergency (CARE) Act into law. The act assists local health-care systems in providing care for people with HIV/AIDS who do not have adequate health insurance or other resources.

The U.S. Congress establishes the National Center for Medical Rehabilitation Research (NCMRR) as part of the National Institute of Child Health and Human Development (NICHD) at the National Institutes of Health (NIH). The mission of the NCMRR is to enhance the quality of life for people with disabilities.

The Human Genome Project (HGP) begins. To conduct the enormous project, the National Institutes of Health (NIH) and the U.S. Department of Energy join with international partners to sequence all 3 billion letters, or base pairs, in the human genome, which is the complete set of DNA in the human body.

The National Committee for Quality Assurance (NCQA) is founded; it accredits managed care organizations and health plans.

1991

The Institute of Medicine (IOM) publishes *Disability in America: Toward a National Agenda for Prevention*. The seminal report identifies disability as a significant social, public health, and moral issue that affects every individual, family, and community across America.

The National Society of Genetic Counselors (NSGC) is founded.

1992

The World Health Organization (WHO) and Harvard University conduct the Global Burden of Disease Project (GBDP). The GBDP finds that in 1990 the most important causes of disability in all regions of the world were neuropsychiatric illnesses for adults.

The National Academy of Sciences publishes *Emerging Infections: Microbial Threats to Health in the United States*, which identifies the emergence of new and virulent diseases that are resistant to antibiotics.

The Centers for Disease Control (CDC) changes its official name to the Centers for Disease Control and Prevention.

1993–1994

President Bill Clinton proposes a universal healthcare plan, the Health Security Act. The plan fails to garner the necessary political support and never passes out of committee for a vote.

1993

The U.S. Congress creates the National Information Center on Health Services Research and Health Care Technology (NICHSR) at the National Library of Medicine (NLM). NICHSR becomes an important national resource for health services research and evidence-based medical practice guidelines.

The Cochrane Collaboration is founded in England; it will become a global network of volunteers dedicated to making information about the effects of health care available.

A gene for familial Amyotrophic Lateral Sclerosis (ALS), often referred to as Lou Gehrig's disease, is discovered. The gene coordinates the manufacture of a specific protein called superoxide dismutase 1 (SOD-1), whose function is to clean the cell of the waste products of cell metabolism known as free radicals.

1994

North and South America are declared to be free of polio.

1995

The American Association of People with Disabilities (AAPD) is founded; it will become the nation's largest cross-disability membership organization.

The Milbank Foundation for Rehabilitation is founded in New York City.

1996

On August 21, President Bill Clinton signs the Health Insurance Portability and Accountability Act (HIPAA) into law. The act helps protect health insurance coverage for workers who lose their jobs, requires the establishment of national standards for electronic healthcare transactions, and sets privacy rules for medical records.

The Social Security Administration (SSA) terminates payments for Supplemental Security Income (SSI) and Social Security Disability Income (SSDI) to persons listed as having a substance abuse disorder that is a primary cause of the disability under which they initially qualified for coverage.

David Sackett (1934–), an American-born Canadian physician who is considered to be one of the founders of evidence-based medicine (EBM), publishes his landmark paper "Evidence Based Medicine: What It Is and What It Isn't."

1997

On May 16, in a White House ceremony with the surviving members of the U.S. Public Health Service's Tuskegee Syphilis Study, President Bill Clinton apologizes for the study on behalf of the nation.

On August 5, President Clinton signs the State Children's Health Insurance Program (SCHIP) into law as part of the Balanced Budget Act of 1997. The goal of SCHIP, which is part of Title XXI of the Social Security Act, is to increase the medical coverage of low-income, uninsured children up to the age of 19 by extending eligibility for public insurance to children in families that earn too much to qualify for Medicaid yet earn too little to afford private health insurance.

The Institute of Medicine (IOM) publishes *Enabling America: Assessing the Role of Rehabilitation Science and Engineering*, which stresses the importance of recognizing rehabilitation science and rehabilitation engineering as legitimate scientific fields of study.

1998

On March 13, President Bill Clinton establishes by Executive Order the Presidential Task Force on the Employment of Adults with Disabilities (PTFEAD).

On April 21, President Clinton signs the Birth Defects Prevention Act into law. The act authorizes the Centers for Disease Control and Prevention (CDC) to collect and analyze birth defects data, operate regional centers for research on the prevention of birth defects, and educate the public about the prevention of birth defects.

On November 13, President Clinton signs the Assistive Technology Act (ATA) into law. The ATA provides grants to states to help bring about systems change to increase the availability of, access to, and funding for assistive technology.

The American Institute for Stuttering (AIS) is founded in New York City.

1999

On June 7, the first White House Conference on Mental Health is held.

On June 22, the U.S. Supreme Court decides in *Olmstead v. L.C. and E.W.* that individuals with disabilities must be offered services in the "most integrated setting."

On December 6, President Bill Clinton signs the Healthcare Research and Quality Act into law. The act directs the Agency for Healthcare Research and Quality (AHRQ) to publish annual reports on the state of healthcare quality and healthcare disparities in the nation.

On December 17, President Clinton signs the Ticket to Work and Work Incentives Improvement Act (TWWIIA) into law. The TWWIIA removes many of the disincentives that made it more difficult for people with disabilities who received Supplemental Security Income (SSI) or Social Security Disability Insurance (SSDI) benefits to return to full-time employment.

The Surgeon General publishes *Mental Health: A Report of the Surgeon General*. This publication, the first ever Surgeon General's report on mental health, seeks to end the stigma surrounding mental health problems and encourage the use of pharmaceuticals and psychotherapy treatments.

The Centers for Disease Control and Prevention (CDC) publishes a series of articles in *Morbidity and Mortality Weekly Report (MMWR)* describing the ten greatest public health achievements in the United States during the 20th century. The highlighted achievements are vaccination; motor-vehicle safety; safer workplaces; control of infectious diseases; decline in deaths from coronary heart disease and stroke; safer and healthier foods; healthier mothers and babies; family planning; fluoridation of drinking water; and the recognition of tobacco use as a health hazard.

2000

October 17, President Bill Clinton signs the Children's Health Act into law. The act expands research and services for a variety of child health programs including Safe Motherhood, a Centers for Disease Control and

Prevention (CDC) program developed to better understand the burden of maternal complications and mortality.

The U.S. Department of Health and Human Services publishes *Healthy People 2010*, a comprehensive, nationwide health promotion and disease prevention initiative. It contains the goal to "Promote the health of people with disabilities, prevent secondary conditions, and eliminate disparities between people with and without disabilities in the U.S. population."

The National Library of Medicine (NLM) creates the Web site ClinicalTrials .gov, an online resource designed to give the public easy access to information about ongoing medical research studies.

The Institute of Medicine (IOM) publishes its landmark report *To Err Is Human: Building a Safer Health System*. The report estimates that between 44,000 to 98,000 people die in a given year from medical errors that occur in the nation's hospitals.

The U.S. Census Bureau estimates that more than 38 million people in America lack health insurance coverage.

The William H. Gates Foundation merges with the Gates Learning Foundation and is renamed the Bill and Melinda Gates Foundation (B&MGF). The foundation's main initiatives include global health, education, libraries, and the Pacific Northwest.

Chronic diseases are common in the United States. The three leading causes of death in the nation are heart disease, cancer, and stroke.

2001

On September 11, terrorists attack the World Trade Center in New York City and the Pentagon in Washington, D.C.

On October 7, the war in Afghanistan, known as Operation Enduring Freedom, begins with the bombing and eventual occupation of Afghanistan by U.S. troops and a multinational force. The occupation of Afghanistan continues to the present.

The World Health Organization (WHO) publishes *The International Classification of Functioning, Disability and Health (ICF)*, which is officially endorsed by all WHO Member States.

The Social Security Advisory Board (SSAB) publishes *Charting the Future of Social Security's Disability Program: The Need for Fundamental Change*.

The President's Council on Bioethics is established.

2002

The Social Security Administration (SSA) updates its rules to better reflect the state of medical science. New SSA regulations take effect regarding the evaluation of disabilities based on problems of the musculoskeletal system (the most common type of disability under Social Security).

The Institute of Medicine (IOM) publishes *The Dynamics of Disability: Measuring and Monitoring Disability for Social Security Programs*. The report recommends monitoring, measuring, and evaluating the growth in the Social Security Administration's disability programs on a regular basis.

The Institute of Medicine (IOM) publishes *The Future of the Public's Health in the 21st Century*, which calls for strengthening of the government's public health infrastructure and the creation of a broader system of public-private collaboration to ensure the health of the nation's population.

The World Health Organization (WHO) publishes *Innovative Care for Chronic Conditions: Building Blocks for Action*, which makes the case for restructuring or developing primary care systems capable of providing high-quality chronic illness care.

2003

On March 19, the Iraq War, also sometimes known as the Second Gulf War, begins with the invasion of Iraq by U.S. troops and a multinational force. After a quick military victory, the United States and other forces occupy Iraq.

On April 14, scientists announce the completion of the Human Genome Project (HGP).

On October 25, President George W. Bush signs the Improving Access to Assistive Technology for Individuals with Disabilities Act into law. The legislation reauthorizes the Assistive Technology Act of 1998.

On December 8, President Bush signs the Medicare Prescription Drug Improvement and Modernization Act (MMA) into law. The MMA is a major overhaul of Medicare that includes the establishment of Medicare Part D, the prescription drug benefit.

The Social Security Advisory Board (SSAB) publishes *The Social Security Definition of Disability*.

The world's first SARS (Severe Acute Respiratory Syndrome) outbreak occurs in Asia and spreads to Canada and other countries; about 8,000 cases are documented globally, with 780 deaths.

America's Health Insurance Plans (AHIP), a large national trade association representing members providing health benefits, is established in Washington, D.C., through the merger of the Health Insurance Association of America (HIAA) and the American Association of Health Plans (AAHP).

2005

On July 26, the U.S. Surgeon General releases the *Call to Action to Improve the Health and Wellness of Persons With Disability*. This first-ever Surgeon General's Call to Action is issued on the 15th anniversary of the passage of the Americans with Disabilities Act.

Rubella is eliminated in the United States.

2006

On June 8, the U.S. Food and Drug Administration (FDA) approves the nation's first anticancer vaccine, the Human Papillomavirus (HPV) vaccine.

On December 19, President George W. Bush reauthorizes the Ryan White Act by signing the Ryan White HIV/AIDS Treatment Modernization Act into law.

2007

The Institute of Medicine (IOM) publishes *The Future of Disability in America*. The report argues that concerted action is essential for the nation to improve the lives of people with disabilities.

Scientists discover how to use human skin cells to create embryonic stem cells.

Worldwide there are an estimated 33.2 million people living with HIV/AIDS.

2008

The National Institute of Child Health and Human Development (NICHD) is renamed the Eunice Kennedy Shriver National Institute of Child Health and Human Development.

The U.S. Census Bureau estimates that 45.7 million people in the nation lack health insurance coverage.

The H1N1 Swine Flu Pandemic begins in Mexico and quickly spreads to other countries.

The American Heart Association (AHA) changes its guidelines on cardio-pulmonary resuscitation (CPR). A simpler form of CPR is promoted that requires hands-only and not mouth-to-mouth resuscitation.

2009

On February 4, President Barack Obama signs the Children's Health Insurance Reauthorization Act into law. The act expands the State Children's Health Insurance Program (SCHIP) to an additional 4 million children and pregnant women, including legal immigrants who previously were subject to a waiting period.

On February 19, President Obama signs the American Recovery and Reinvestment Act of 2009 (Recovery Act) into law. It includes several provisions concerning people with disabilities, including $500 million to help the Social Security Administration (SSA) reduce its backlog in processing disability applications; $12.2 billion to fund the Individuals with Disabilities Education Act (IDEA); $87 billion to states to bolster their Medicaid programs; and over $500 million to fund vocational rehabilitation services to help with job training, education, and placement.

On May 27, the U.S. Department of Veterans Affairs (VA) announces the beginning of a three-year study of a highly advanced artificial arm that easily allows users to pick up a key or hold a pencil.

On July 9, the National Institutes of Health (NIH) hosts the White House's H1N1 Influenza Preparedness Summit to discuss how to investigate, monitor, and slow the spread of the influenza outbreak.

On July 24—only two days before the 19th anniversary of the signing of the Americans with Disabilities Act (ADA)—President Obama signs the United Nation's Convention on the Rights of Persons with Disabilities (CRPD).

On September 9, President Obama outlines his health insurance reform proposal in an address to a Joint Session of Congress.

On October 30, President Obama reauthorizes the Ryan White Act by signing the Ryan White HIV/AIDS Treatment Extension Act into law.

2010

On February 17, an issue of the *Journal of the American Medical Association* (J. Van Cleave, et al., "Dynamics of Obesity and Chronic Health Conditions Among Children and Youth") reports that the rate of chronic health conditions such as obesity, asthma, and behavior/learning problems increased from 12.8% of U.S. children in 1994 to 26.6% in 2006.

On March 23, President Barack Obama signs the Patient Protection and Affordable Care Act into law. The sweeping new law greatly expands the role of the federal government in health care. Specifically, the act requires that all Americans have health insurance; bars health insurance companies from discriminating based on pre-existing medical conditions, health status, or gender; prohibits lifetime limits on coverage; prohibits rescission (dropping) of customers by insurers; creates insurance exchanges; requires employers with 50 workers or more to offer health insurance benefits or pay a fee; expands Medicaid and provides premium assistance; and creates temporary insurance pools for consumers with pre-existing conditions until insurance exchanges open in 2014.

Four

Biographies of Key Contributors in the Field

A large number of individuals have made significant discoveries and contributions to the fields of medicine, public health, and disability. The biographical sketches in this chapter, presented in alphabetical order, profile some of those individuals.

Frederick Banting (1891–1941)

Canadian researcher who co-discovered
insulin treatment for diabetes

Frederick Grant Banting was born on November 14, 1891, in Alliston, Ontario, Canada. He was the youngest of five children born to William Thompson Banting, a prosperous farmer, and Margaret Grant. After earning a bachelor's degree in medicine from the University of Toronto medical school in 1916, Banting joined the Canadian Army Medical Corps. He served his country in World War I in France, where he was wounded at the battle of Cambrai in 1918. One year later he was awarded the Military Cross for heroism under fire.

When the war ended, Banting returned to Canada and resumed his medical studies, completing an internship at Toronto's Hospital for Sick Children. Banting then opened his own short-lived private practice in London, Ontario, where he also taught orthopedics at the University of Western Ontario. In 1922 he earned his doctorate in medicine.

Banting's pioneering work on diabetes began in 1920, when he developed a theory for the isolation and extraction of pancreatic cells—protein hormones that came to be known as insulin—that were capable of combating diabetes. He convinced John MacLeod, the head of the University of Toronto's physiology department, of the merits of his idea, and MacLeod supplied him with facilities and other resources to conduct his experiments. Importantly, MacLeod assigned a gifted medical student named Charles Best to serve as Banting's assistant. The two young researchers established a rapport, and their collaborative efforts quickly bore fruit. By mid-1921, experiments they conducted on dogs confirmed Banting's hypothesis about the powers of insulin to control diabetes. Delighted by these results, MacLeod formally added Banting to his staff and arranged for biochemist James Collip to provide help to Banting and Best.

In 1922 the researchers tested insulin on Leonard Thompson, a 14-year-old youth suffering from diabetes. Thompson's health quickly improved, and reports of the exciting new diabetes treatment spread rapidly. The fame of Banting and Best surged again in the fall of 1922, when they successfully treated the adolescent daughter of U.S. Secretary of State Charles Evans Hughes for her diabetes. Heartened by these and other successes, the researchers arranged with the Eli Lilly pharmaceutical company for the production of commercial levels of insulin.

In 1923 Banting and MacLeod were awarded the Nobel Prize in Physiology or Medicine for their groundbreaking research efforts. Distressed that Best's contribution was not recognized by the Nobel Committee, Banting shared his cash prize with his colleague. That same year, the Ontario Legislative Assembly established the Banting and Best Institute, a new research facility within the University of Toronto's Department of Medical Research. Banting spent the next several years at the institute conducting research into cancer and silicosis, among other subjects. He also received a generous annuity from the Canadian government, as well as numerous honorary degrees and memberships from universities and scientific institutions around the world.

In 1924 Banting married Marion Robertson, with whom he had one son, named William. His first marriage ended in divorce after eight years, and in 1937 he married Henrietta Ball. Banting returned to active military service in 1939, when World War II erupted across Europe. He served as a liaison officer between Canadian and British military medical services until February 21, 1941, when he died in a plane crash on the coast of Newfoundland.

Further Reading

Bliss, M. (1984). *Banting: A biography*. Toronto, Canada: McClelland and Stewart.
Sir Frederick Grant Banting. Banting and Best Department of Medical Research,
University of Toronto. Retrieved from http://www.utoronto.ca/bandb/
banting.htm

Charles Best (1899–1978)

*Canadian researcher who co-discovered
insulin treatment for diabetes*

Charles Herbert Best was born on February 27, 1899, in West Pembroke, Maine, to Canadian expatriates Luella Fisher Best and Herbert Huestis Best, who worked as a physician. He moved to Canada in 1915 to attend college, but when World War I broke out, he enlisted in the Canadian Army, where he rose to the rank of sergeant. After the war, Best returned to Canada and earned a bachelor's degree in physiology and biochemistry from the University of Toronto in 1921.

Shortly before graduating, Best was asked by John MacLeod, director of the University of Toronto's physiology department, if he would be interested in assisting Frederick Banting with a new research project designed to determine whether a pancreatic hormone—soon to be known as insulin—could be used to treat diabetes. Best agreed, and by the end of 1921 he, Banting, and biochemist James Collip had developed an effective and safe program of insulin treatments for people suffering from diabetes. The first beneficiary of this treatment was Leonard Thompson, a 14-year-old Canadian youth, but the most famous of the patients successfully treated by Banting and Best was the daughter of U.S. Secretary of State Charles Evans Hughes.

In the spring of 1922, Banting and Best devised a methodology for large-scale production of insulin by the Eli Lilly pharmaceutical company. Best directly supervised these early rounds of insulin production, and he continued these duties even after enrolling in the University of Toronto Medical School in the fall of 1922. Less than one year later, Ontario legislators passed the Banting and Best Medical Research Act, which provided funding for a new medical research facility—the Banting and Best Institute—at the University of Toronto. Banting was named the institute's first director, while Best became its most prominent medical researcher. In October 1923, Banting and MacLeod were awarded the Nobel Prize in

Physiology or Medicine in recognition of the insulin discovery. Banting was so upset about Best's exclusion from this honor that he insisted on splitting his Nobel Prize money with his younger colleague.

In September 1924, Best married Margaret Mahon, and a year later he graduated from medical school with top honors. The newlyweds then relocated to England, where Best earned a Doctor of Sciences degree from the University of London. In 1928 he returned to Toronto to take over for the retiring MacLeod at the University of Toronto's physiology department. It was in this capacity that Best spearheaded important research into the use of heparin, a blood anticoagulant, in intensive surgical procedures.

After Banting's tragic death in a plane crash in February 1941, Best was asked to take the place of his old friend and colleague as director of the Banting and Best Department of Medical Research in Toronto. One year later, he became a high-ranking officer with the Royal Canadian Navy. Best's post–World War II career included a turn as a writer of physiology textbooks. He also received numerous honors, awards, and tributes during this time for his many scientific contributions, and in 1953 the University of Toronto named a new building for medical research in his honor. That same year, he became the first president of the International Union of Physiological Sciences. Best retired in 1965 and spent the next several years traveling the world with his wife. He died in Toronto on March 31, 1978.

Further Reading

Best, H. B. M. (2003). *Margaret and Charley: The personal story of Dr. Charles Best, co-discoverer of insulin.* Toronto, Canada: Dundurn Press.
Charles Herbert Best. Banting and Best Department of Medical Research, University of Toronto. Retrieved from http://www.utoronto.ca/bandb/best.htm

Ernest Amory Codman (1869–1930)

American orthopedist and quality assurance advocate for hospital care

Ernest Amory Codman was born in Boston, Massachusetts, on December 30, 1869. His parents were Elizabeth Hurd Codman and William Coombs Codman, a wealthy local businessman. An 1895 graduate of Harvard Medical School, Codman joined the staff of Massachusetts General Hospital as an assistant surgeon. Four years later, he married fellow Bostonian Katherine P. Bowditch, who later became a prominent activist in the women's suffrage movement. In 1900 he joined the staff of Harvard Medical

School, where he lectured and taught about surgery until 1915. It was during this period that Codman became a nationally recognized authority on tumors and diseases of the shoulder.

During the mid-1910s, however, Codman's reputation as an expert on shoulder physiology was eclipsed by his unrelenting efforts to reform surgical practices and impose new performance standards on American hospitals. The centerpiece of Codman's crusade was his enthusiasm for what he called "end result systems." These follow-up studies of hospital patients would monitor the post-operative or post-treatment health of patients—and thus give hospital administrators, surgeons, and other medical professionals much-needed documentation to gauge the efficacy of different treatments.

Codman and other like-minded reformers believed that an increased emphasis on clinical science techniques could bring about more uniform regulation of American healthcare. He preached this message tirelessly from his seat on the Committee on the Standardization of Hospitals, a board established by the American College of Surgeons (which he had helped found). But many surgeons and physicians were leery of a number of Codman's evaluation and standardization ideas, such as his suggestion that survey results be used to publicly rank surgeons.

Codman's campaign for nationwide adoption of the end-result system—including his decision to open his own private "End Result Hospital" in 1911—alienated many of his hometown's most prestigious physicians. He lost his affiliations with both Massachusetts General Hospital and Harvard Medical School by 1915, but he remained a tireless promoter of his standardization ideas. In 1916, in fact, Codman published *A Study in Medical Efficiency*, in which he reported on the progress of 337 patients who had been treated and discharged at his hospital from 1911 to 1916. This early effort to systematically track patient outcomes has been widely described as a forerunner to today's "morbidity and mortality" studies. Codman remained a fierce advocate of his hospital reform ideas until his death on November 23, 1940, in Ponkapog, Massachusetts.

Further Reading

Mallon, B. (2000). *Ernest Amory Codman. The end result of a life in medicine*. Philadelphia, PA: W. B. Saunders.

Neuhauser, D. (2002). Heroes and martyrs of quality and safety: Ernest Amory Codman. *Quality and Safety in Health Care, 11*, 104–5. Retrieved from http://www.ncbi.nlm.nih.gov/pmc/articles/PMC1743579/pdf/v011p00104.pdf

Francis Crick (1916–2004)

English co-leader of the research team that
discovered the structure of the DNA molecule

Francis Harry Compton Crick was born on June 8, 1916, in Northampton, England. Raised in comfortable middle-class surroundings, Crick studied physics at University College London, graduating in 1937. He stayed on at the school for his graduate work, but with the onset of World War II, he joined the British Admiralty Research Laboratory, developing radar and magnetic mines for naval warfare.

In 1947 Crick left the military for a research appointment at Cambridge University. In 1949 he joined Cavendish Laboratory at Cambridge, where his work increasingly focused on unraveling the mysteries of molecular biology. In 1951, the American scientist James Watson joined Crick at Cavendish. The two men soon became collaborators in an effort to uncover the structure of DNA, the primary genetic material of all cellular organisms.

In mid-1953, Crick and Watson announced their revolutionary discovery that the three-dimensional structure of the DNA molecule was a double helix, not unlike an elegant twisting ladder, capable of reproducing itself. Crick continued to study DNA and its role in genetic coding for the next several years. Working with fellow scientists like Vernon Ingram and Sydney Brenner, he made a number of additional discoveries about the chemical composition and sequencing of DNA in the late 1950s and early 1960s.

In 1962 Crick and Watson received the Nobel Prize in Physiology or Medicine with crystallographer Maurice Wilkins, whose high-resolution X-ray images of DNA fibers had laid the groundwork for the breakthrough. That same year, Crick and Brenner became co-directors of the Molecular Genetics Division of the Laboratory of Molecular Biology in Cambridge. In 1976 Crick left Cambridge for a position at the Salk Institute for Biological Studies in San Diego, California. He died on July 28, 2004, of colon cancer in La Jolla, California.

Further Reading

Edelson, E. (2000). *Francis Crick and James Watson: And the building blocks of life.* New York: Oxford University Press.

Francis Crick Papers. National Library of Medicine, Profiles in Science. Retrieved from http://profiles.nlm.nih.gov/SC/Views/Exhibit/narrative/biographical.html

Watson, J. D. (1980). *The double helix: A personal account of the discovery of the structure of DNA.* New York: Atheneum.

Dorothea Dix (1802–1887)

American advocate for persons with mental illness

Dorothea Lynde Dix was born in Hampden, Maine, on April 4, 1802, to Mary Dix and Joseph Dix, a circuit-riding preacher. She moved to Boston to live with her grandmother as an adolescent. At age 19, Dix opened a formal school on her grandmother's property, and she soon established a local reputation as a skilled teacher. When recurring health problems forced her to close the school in 1836, Dix sailed for Europe for a period of convalescence. During an extended stay in England with Quaker friends, she became acquainted with prominent social reformers like Samuel Tuke, director of the York Retreat for the Mentally Disordered, who were trumpeting more humane methods of treating people suffering from insanity and lesser forms of mental illness.

These encounters had an enormous impact on Dix, and after returning to the United States, she began investigating living conditions and treatment methods for people with mental illness in American insane asylums, almshouses, and prisons (where many people with mental illness were placed). Appalled by the filthy and miserable conditions she found, Dix resolved to lobby lawmakers for legislation that would improve conditions. This campaign took her far beyond the borders of Massachusetts into numerous other states, where she repeatedly found persons with insanity and mental illness being subjected to brutal treatment in facilities that were underfunded and almost completely unregulated by the states in which they operated. Dix documented her findings, both in testimony and in print, to state legislatures across the country in the 1840s. These efforts brought about significant changes in the way that people with mental illness were treated in many institutions and states across the United States. Moreover, Dix's crusade spurred major new investments in clinics and hospitals specifically focused on caring for indigent people suffering from severe mental illness.

In the 1850s, Dix exported her reform efforts to Europe, which made several improvements in the care and treatment of people afflicted with severe mental illness during this period. After the Civil War erupted in the United States in 1861, Dix was named Superintendent of Nurses for the Union Army. When the war ended she returned to her advocacy work on behalf of people institutionalized for mental illness. She died in Trenton, New Jersey, on July 17, 1887.

Further Reading

Gollaher, D. (1995). *Voice for the mad: The life of Dorothea Dix.* New York: Free Press.

Wilson, D. C. (1975). *Stranger and traveler: The story of Dorothea Dix, American reformer.* Boston, MA: Little, Brown.

Gerhard Domagk (1895–1964)

German researcher who discovered the antibacterial properties of sulfonamide drugs

Gerhard Johannes Paul Domagk was born on October 30, 1895, in Lagow, Germany. Domagk was studying medicine when World War I erupted across Europe. After a brief stint in the German Army (during which he was wounded), Domagk was assigned to various cholera hospitals in Russia as a member of the Sanitary Service. During this time, he repeatedly witnessed the helplessness of physicians and surgeons in the face of infectious diseases.

Domagk earned a medical degree from the University of Kiel in 1921. In 1925 he married Gertrude Strübe, with whom he eventually had four children. Two years later, he left academia to conduct research at the Bayer (Farbenindustrie) Laboratory for Experimental Pathology and Bacteriology in Wuppertal.

For the next several years, Domagk spent countless hours laboring to find a chemical antidote to the problem of infectious disease. These efforts were greatly influenced by the earlier work of Paul Ehrlich. In 1932 Domagk accidentally discovered that dimethyl benzyl dodecyl ammonium chloride was an effective antibacterial agent for skin treatments (this chemical remains the basis for hand and instrument disinfectants today). This triumph increased the scientist's determination to solve the puzzle of taming bacterial infections inside the body. In a matter of months, his research revealed that a particular sulfonamide or "sulfa drug" that came to be known by the trade name Prontosil was effective in treating streptococcus. A short time later, a desperate Domagk put his discovery to practical use by treating his daughter, who had developed a potentially deadly streptococcal infection that did not respond to traditional treatments, with Prontosil. Her rapid recovery convinced Domagk that a new age of medicine was at hand.

Domagk unveiled his discovery in 1935, and as Bayer launched commercial production of Prontosil, the death rate from post-surgical infections and scourges like meningitis and pneumonia plummeted. In 1939

Domagk was awarded the Nobel Prize in Physiology or Medicine, but he did not receive the official certificate until after World War II because of the anti-Nobel stance of Adolf Hitler's Nazi regime.

Domagk received numerous honors and awards from the scientific and medical communities in the 1940s and 1950s, during which time he continued to conduct research on antibiotics and chemotherapy treatments for cancer and tuberculosis. He died on April 24, 1964.

Further Reading

Hager, T. (2006). *The demon under the microscope.* New York: Harmony.

Paul Ehrlich (1854–1915)

German discoverer of the first effective treatment for syphilis and early pioneer in immunology and chemotherapy

Paul Ehrlich was born on March 14, 1854, in Strehlen, Upper Silesia, in the German kingdom of Prussia (the city is now known as Strzelin, in modern Poland). After receiving his medical degree from the University of Leipzig in 1878, Ehrlich took a position at Charité Hospital in Berlin, where he developed a new staining technique to identify the tuberculosis bacillus, a form of bacteria that had first been discovered by the German scientist Robert Koch. In 1883 he married Hedwig Pinkus, with whom he had two daughters.

Ehrlich's career was temporarily derailed by his own struggle with tuberculosis, but in 1890 he established his own small research laboratory at Steglitz, outside Berlin. Within a year, Koch recruited Ehrlich to join him at the Institute for Infectious Diseases. Ehrlich spent the next six years working side-by-side with Koch on treatments for cholera and tuberculosis. In 1896 he took the directorship of the new Institute for Serum Research and Serum Investigation at Steglitz, and three years later, he took a similar position at the Institute of Experimental Therapy in Frankfurt, where he conducted important studies on immunology as it related to diseases like syphilis and African sleeping sickness. Ehrlich also worked intensively during these years with such scientists as Emil von Behring on serum therapy—the treatment of humans afflicted with tetanus and diphtheria with blood serum from immune animals. It was during this period that Ehrlich developed his famous "side-chain" theory of immunology. In 1908 Ehrlich received the Nobel Prize for Physiology or Medicine for his contributions to immunological studies.

As Ehrlich's research continued into the 20th century, he increasingly moved away from serum therapy, which was proving inadequate for combating many infectious disorders. He increasingly focused on identifying chemical compounds—including those not necessarily found in nature—that could kill infections without hurting the person undergoing treatment. This turn in Ehrlich's research marked the beginnings of chemotherapy as a tool in modern medicine.

Ehrlich's quest for chemical "magic bullets" capable of combating infection without causing collateral damage to the patient led him to focus on the spirochete Treponema pallidum, the causal organism of syphilis. By 1909 he had sent hundreds of different chemical compounds into battle against the disease without success. But compound 606—a drug compound that came to be known as Salvarsan or arsphenamine—effectively treated syphilis without adverse side effects. A short time later, Ehrlich and his valued assistant, Sahachiro Hata, developed a version of Salvarsan that could be manufactured in commercial quantities. By 1910 Salvarsan was being utilized in clinics and hospitals across the country, and within a few years, it was the most widely prescribed drug in the world. It remained the preferred treatment for syphilis until 1947, when it was supplanted by penicillin.

Ehrlich remained an indefatigable researcher until December 1914, when he suffered a serious stroke. He died in Germany on August 20, 1915, after suffering a second major stroke.

Further Reading

Baumler, E. (1984). *Paul Ehrlich: Scientist for life.* New York: Holmes and Meier.
Silverstein, A. M. (1989). *A history of immunology.* London: Academic.

William Farr (1807–1883)

English pioneer in the fields of epidemiology and medical statistics

William Farr was born on November 30, 1807, in Kenley, Shropshire, England. His parents were poor, but a generous local squire bequeathed him sufficient funds to study medicine in France and Switzerland. In 1831 he entered University College London to continue his medical studies.

He earned entrance to the Apothecaries' Society one year later, and in 1833 he started a London medical practice.

Long fascinated by numbers and statistics, Farr accepted a job as a compiler of medical statistics for the Registrar General's Office in 1838. Going far beyond his official responsibilities, which merely involved tracking births and deaths in England and Wales so as to ease property transfers among the landed gentry, Farr began compiling vital medical statistics data on an annual basis, including analyses of causes of death and assessments of mortality by occupation. This effort, the first national program of vital medical statistics suitable for epidemiological study, eventually became the basis for the standard International Classification of Diseases (ICD).

Farr's skill in gathering and interpreting medical statistics was evident in 1849 and 1853, when major cholera outbreaks ripped through London, claiming thousands of lives. Like most other physicians and scientists of the era, Farr subscribed to the "miasmic theory," which said that the disease was being carried by polluted air. But when physician John Snow correctly fingered London's dreadfully contaminated water supply as the culprit, Farr dutifully examined his records. He discovered that cholera deaths were much higher in neighborhoods that received their drinking water from two companies that drew their water directly from the heavily polluted Thames River. Farr still did not concur with Snow's waterborne theory, but the data he gathered ultimately proved invaluable in helping Snow make his case.

Farr remained allegiant to the miasma theory until 1866, when another cholera epidemic swept through London. At that time, however, Farr's analysis of specific water supplies and high outbreak areas led him to conclude that Snow's theory of waterborne transmission was valid. This determination, which was also informed by growing scientific acceptance of the germ theory of disease, led the esteemed epidemiologist to call for better treatment and disposal of sewage and other public health measures in London and elsewhere.

Farr retired from the Registrar General's office in 1879. He died on April 14, 1883.

Further Reading

Halliday, W. (2000). William Farr: Campaigning statistician. *Journal of Medical Biography, 8,* 220–227.

Lilienfeld, D. E. (2007). Celebration: William Farr (1807–1883)—an appreciation on the 200th anniversary of his birth. *International Journal of Epidemiology, 36*(5), 985–987.

Alexander Fleming (1881–1955)

Scottish bacteriologist who discovered penicillin

Alexander Fleming was born on August 6, 1881, in Lochfield, a rural farming community in Ayrshire, Scotland. In his mid-teens he moved to London, where an older brother had established a medical practice. After brief stints as a shipping clerk and soldier, Fleming decided to study medicine as well. He earned his medical degree from St. Mary's Medical School in 1906, then stayed on at the school to work as a bacteriologist in its Inoculation Service.

Fleming served during World War I as a medical corps captain. During this period, Fleming watched helplessly as simple infections claimed the lives of many wounded soldiers. By the time the war ended and Fleming returned to St. Mary's, he focused determinedly on finding an effective antiseptic agent capable of warding off dangerous bacteria. In 1921 Fleming's tireless research revealed the existence of a natural protein, which he called lysozyme, with important anti-bacterial properties.

Seven years later, Fleming discovered quite by accident while cleaning up his lab that a staphylococcus culture plate featured mold with a bacteria-free circle around itself. Excited by this discovery, Fleming conducted a new round of experiments on the mold culture and found that it was tremendously potent—even in diluted form—in killing staph bacteria.

Fleming gave the active ingredient in the mold the name penicillin, then announced his findings to the world in 1929. Remarkably, his discovery initially met with a muted response from the medical community. Chemists, meanwhile, began building on Fleming's research to develop an effective form of penicillin that could be produced in large quantities. In 1945 scientists Howard Florey and Ernst Chain announced that they had found a way to produce the drug in mass quantities, and within a few years, penicillin—perhaps the most important life-saving drug in history—was being used as an antibiotic in hospitals around the world. Fleming died in London of a heart attack on March 11, 1955.

Further Reading

Brown, K. (2004). *Penicillin man: Alexander Fleming and the antibiotic revolution.* Stroud, UK: Sutton.

Bud, R. (2007). *Penicillin: Triumph and tragedy.* New York: Oxford University Press.

Sigmund Freud (1856–1939)

Austrian founder of psychoanalysis

Sigismund S. Freud was born on May 6, 1856, in Freiberg, Moravia (now part of the Czech Republic). His Jewish family moved to Vienna, Austria, when he was a small child, and he lived in that city for most of his life. In 1873 Freud entered the University of Vienna medical school, where he trained in neurology, the study of the nervous system. He received his doctorate in medicine at the age of 24, but as he grew older, Freud devoted most of his energies to the study of mental disorders—and the use of hypnosis as a method for treating such problems. These studies led him to spend several months in Paris in 1885 studying with Jean Martin Charcot, who was developing theories about the possible psychological origins of some physical problems.

In 1886, Freud returned to Vienna and opened a private practice devoted to the treatment of nervous and brain disorders. One year later, he married Martha Bernays, with whom he had six children. Over the next few years, Freud gradually turned away from hypnosis as a treatment method in favor of careful analysis of the thought processes and traumatic memories of patients—what Freud called the "talking cure"—which he came to believe were principal drivers of current emotional problems. Collaborating with Joseph Breuer at times, Freud honed his theories for treating mental illness through what he came to call "psychoanalysis"—the exposition and discussion of a subject's unconscious thoughts and feelings. By the close of the 19th century, Freud was also relying on dream analysis and free association as diagnostic tools.

In 1900 Freud published *The Interpretation of Dreams,* in which he explained his beliefs about the unconscious mind and its role in mental health. One year later he published another landmark in the history of psychoanalysis, *The Psychopathology of Everyday Life.* It was in this latter work that Freud theorized that accidental slips of the tongue—what are now known as "Freudian slips"—were actually messages freighted with deep meaning from the unconscious mind. In 1905 Freud published *Three Essays on the Theory of Sexuality*, in which he explained his famous Oedipus Complex hypothesis regarding boys and their parents (he eventually developed a similar theory for girls).

Freud's controversial theories became the basis of the modern psychoanalytic movement. Psychiatrists like Carl Jung and Eugen Bleuler studied and incorporated his ideas, and he regularly hosted gatherings of colleagues at his home or faculty office at the University of Vienna, where he had accepted a teaching position in 1902. By 1910 Freud was famous across both America and Europe, as were his ever-evolving ideas and treatments.

In 1923 Freud was diagnosed with cancer of the jaw, an affliction that probably stemmed from years of heavy cigar smoking. He endured 30 operations over the next 16 years to deal with the disease. Freud spent the last few months of his life separated from Vienna, his lifelong home. When Nazi Germany took over Austria in 1938, Freud and his wife fled to England, where he died on September 23, 1939.

Further Reading

Ferris, P. (1999). *Freud: A life*. Berkeley, CA: Counterpoint Press.
Gay, P. (2006). *Freud: A life for our time*. New York: W. W. Norton.

John Graunt (1620–1674)

English inventor of the Life Table and early demographer and medical statistician

Born on April 24, 1620, in London, England, John Graunt followed in his father's footsteps and became a prosperous local haberdasher. Knowledgeable about London's political and social affairs, he became increasingly frustrated with the city's haphazard documentation of deaths from bubonic plague and other public health threats. Convinced that better recordkeeping might give authorities better insight into how to address plague and other menaces, Graunt—who never received any formal mathematical training—decided to conduct his own study. Graunt's ultimate goal was to use his analysis of the mortality rolls in London as the basis for a sort of early warning system regarding the onset and spread of plague.

In 1662 Graunt published his findings in a pamphlet called *Natural and Political Observations mentioned in a following Index, and made upon the Bills of Mortality . . . With reference to the Government, Religion, Trade, Growth,*

Ayre, diseases, and the several Changes of the said City. This work is regarded as a foundational document in the history of epidemiology and medical statistics, for it established the idea that births, deaths, and other vital demographic statistics could be utilized to create entire "life tables"—life expectancy charts—of populations. Four editions of the influential pamphlet were published over the next several years, and *Observations* exerted a huge influence on other pioneers in the fields of epidemiology and demography, such as Sir William Petty.

Graunt's remarkable work gained him entrance into the Royal Society, but his final years were difficult ones. The Great London Fire of 1666 destroyed his shop, and liver disease and other health problems beleaguered him. He died in London on April 18, 1674.

Further Reading

Hald, A. (1990). John Graunt and his *Observations Made Upon the Bills of Mortality, 1622.* In *A history of probability and statistics and their applications before 1750* (pp. 81–105). New York: Wiley Interscience.

Alice Hamilton (1869–1970)

American physician, social reformer, and founder of occupational medicine

Alice Hamilton was born on February 27, 1869, in Fort Wayne, Indiana. The second of four daughters born to a prominent merchant grocer, Hamilton earned a doctor of medicine degree from the University of Michigan Medical School in 1893, then moved on to serve internships at the Minneapolis Hospital for Women and Children and the New England Hospital for Women and Children. Hamilton studied bacteriology and pathology at universities in Munich and Leipzig from 1895 to 1897 before taking on postgraduate work at Baltimore's Johns Hopkins University Medical School. In 1897 she moved to Chicago, where she became a professor of pathology at the Woman's Medical School of Northwestern University.

It was in Chicago that Hamilton's interests in progressive social reform and industrial toxicology fully blossomed. She spent more than a decade as a resident at Hull House, the famous Chicago settlement house established and operated by Jane Addams. During this same period, Hamilton established herself as one of the country's leading investigators of occupational health and illness in industry. Her expertise on the subject, evident in numerous studies she prepared on industrial metals, chemical compounds, workplace safety policies, and their cumulative disabling impact on the health of workers, led to her 1910 appointment to the newly formed Occupational Diseases Commission of Illinois. One year later, the U.S. Department of Labor appointed her as a special investigator. Hamilton spent the next several years publishing painstakingly researched studies on occupational health for a variety of state and federal agencies. These studies documented the toll that that unregulated industrialization was taking on public health and urban environments, and they became a key tool in progressive efforts to establish municipal and statewide boards of health and other municipal and national public health and environment agencies in the early 20th century.

In 1919 Hamilton became the first woman appointed to the faculty at Harvard Medical School, serving in the new Department of Industrial Medicine, and she also became the school's first female professor of public health. From 1924 to 1930, she served as the only female member of the League of Nations Health Committee. In 1935 she retired from Harvard and became a medical consultant to the U.S. Division of Labor Standards. She died on September 22, 1970, in Hadlyme, Connecticut.

Further Reading

Hamilton, A. (1943). *Exploring the dangerous trades: The autobiography of Alice Hamilton, MD*. Boston, MA: Little, Brown.

Sicherman, B. (2003). *Alice Hamilton: A life in letters*. Champaign, IL: University of Illinois Press.

Philip S. Hench (1896–1965)

*American physician who first isolated and used
cortisone in treating arthritis*

Philip Showalter Hench was born on February 28, 1896, in Pittsburgh, Pennsylvania. A 1916 undergraduate of Lafayette College, Hench completed his medical degree at the University of Pittsburgh in 1920, then entered a residency program at Pittsburgh's St. Francis Hospital. In 1927 he married Mary Genevieve Kahler, with whom he had four children. After pursuing postgraduate study in Germany in 1928–1929, Hench obtained a Master of Science in Internal Medicine at the University of Minnesota in 1931, and a Doctor of Science degree from Lafayette College in 1940.

Hench enjoyed a long and distinguished professional career with the Mayo Clinic in Rochester, Minnesota. This association began in 1923, after

Hench served a stint during World War I in the U.S. Army Medical Corps. By 1926 Hench was director of the clinic's Department of Rheumatic Diseases, and he spent much of the subsequent two decades specializing in treatments for arthritic disease. During this time he came to recognize that certain health conditions, most notably jaundice and pregnancy, brought remissions of pain to people suffering from arthritis. Experiments based on these observations led Hench and his colleague Edward C. Kendall to isolate a steroid from the adrenal gland cortex—later named cortisone—as the source of this pain relief.

World War II interrupted their work, as Hench returned to military service as a lieutenant colonel in the Medical Corps. As the war continued, he was promoted to Chief of the Medical Service and Director of the Army's Rheumatism Center, and he left military service in 1946 with the rank of colonel. Upon returning to Rochester, Hench and Kendall successfully treated patients suffering from rheumatoid arthritis with both cortisone and adrenocorticotrophic hormone (ACTH). Their pioneering work was recognized by the Nobel Committee, which in 1950 awarded the Nobel Prize in Physiology or Medicine to Hench, Kendall, and Swiss scientist Tadeus Reichstein for "their discoveries concerning hormones of the adrenal cortex, their structure and biological effects."

In the early 1950s, Hench and other researchers concluded that cortisone was not a cure for rheumatoid arthritis, and that it had limited long-term applications. But the breakthrough made by Hench and Kendall was still momentous, for cortisone became the cornerstone of pain-reduction therapies for myriad different conditions. Hench, who after World War II also became one of the world's leading authorities on the history of yellow fever, died in Jamaica on March 30, 1965.

Further Reading

Kendall, E. C. (1971). *Cortisone: Memoirs of a hormone hunter.* New York: Scribner's.
Philip S. Hench. Nobel Prize.org. Retrieved from http://nobelprize.org/nobel_prizes/medicine/laureates/1950/hench-bio.html

Hippocrates (ca. 460 BCE–ca. 377 BCE)

Greek physician known as the "father" of modern medicine

Hippocrates was born on the Aegean (Greek) island of Cos (Kos) around 460 BCE. Ancient biographers have stated that Hippocrates came from a family line of physicians and that he benefited from a classical education in medicine and other subjects. He worked as a physician all his life and taught medicine as well at several different points in his career.

Hippocrates' legacy as a pioneering figure in shaping modern medical thought and practice is undeniable, but historians acknowledge that many of the writings that have been attributed to him on such subjects as anatomy, prognosis and treatment of disease, surgery, and medical ethics were probably written by other physicians influenced by his insights and philosophies of medical treatment. Nonetheless, the so-called Hippocratic Corpus of more than sixty medical treatises is the basis for Hippocrates' stature as the "father" of modern medicine.

Hippocrates' central importance lay in his rejection of superstition or divine forces as the basis for human health. He believed instead that illness, disease, and disability were directly related to climate and other environmental factors, personal habits and practices, and hereditary factors—and that all of these elements could be better understood through objective scientific observation. In addition, Hippocrates devoted a great deal of time to explicating ethical and professional standards for physicians in their interactions with patients. These teachings (supplemented by others who traded on his name and reputation) became the basis for the Hippocratic Oath, a code of ethics that is still integral to modern medical practice. Hippocrates' insights thus brought about pivotal changes in the way that physicians practiced medicine and helped chart new and more effective courses of treatment.

Historians believe that Hippocrates probably died in Larissa, Greece. He died in or around the year 377 BCE, but historical accounts about the timing of his death differ.

Further Reading

Jouanna, J. (1999). *Hippocrates.* Baltimore, MD: Johns Hopkins University Press.
Levine, E. B. (1971). *Hippocrates.* New York: Twayne.

Edward Jenner (1749–1823)

English physician who developed the process of smallpox vaccination

The youngest of six children born to a Church of England clergyman, Edward Jenner was born on May 17, 1749, in Berkeley, Gloucestershire.

Jenner received his early medical training through a surgical apprenticeship in London, then studied under the famous Scottish surgeon John Hunter at St. George's Hospital. After completing his studies, Jenner returned to his hometown of Berkeley in 1773 and established his own medical practice.

Jenner spent the next two decades in comfortable obscurity, tending to his work as a surgeon and general practitioner. In the early 1790s, however, Jenner focused on devising a new treatment option for smallpox, the most feared disease in the world at the time. For many years, the chief preventive measure taken against smallpox was a type of inoculation known as variolation, in which uninfected persons were purposely exposed to material drawn from smallpox lesions in order to induce a mild form of the disease that would provide immunity from further outbreaks. Jenner, however, observed that milkmaids around Berkeley who had been exposed to a mild skin disease of cattle known as cowpox seemed to be immune to smallpox. Determined to test his hypothesis, Jenner in 1796 inoculated an area boy with cowpox, then inoculated the child with the related disease of smallpox several weeks later. When the boy showed no ill-effects from Jenner's "vaccination," as he called it in a play on the Latin word "vacca" (cow), the physician carried out the test on a number of other subjects with similar success.

In 1798 Jenner published *An Inquiry into the Causes and Effects of the Variolae Vaccinae*, which recounted his research work. Vaccination campaigns took place across Europe over the next several months, producing notable downturns in both the frequency and severity of smallpox outbreaks. Vaccination also was exported to the United States in fairly short order, and in 1809 Massachusetts enacted the nation's first mandatory vaccination law. Within another decade or so, compulsory vaccination was widely recognized as the medical community's single most effective tool for combating smallpox outbreaks.

Jenner received a number of honors and financial grants in recognition of his pioneering work in vaccination, and for many years afterward he conducted research and provided advice on the safest ways to produce, transport, and use his cowpox vaccine. Around this same time, however, he also became known as a dedicated student of fossils and archaeology, and in 1809 he was elected to the prestigious Geographic Society. His public profile diminished considerably after the death of his wife in 1815, however, and Jenner himself died in his hometown of Berkeley on January 26, 1823.

Further Reading

Basin, H. (2000). *The eradication of small pox: Edward Jenner and the first and only erad- ication of a human infectious disease.* San Diego, CA: Academic Press.

Henderson, D. A. (2009). *Smallpox: The death of a disease.* Amherst, NY: Prometheus Books.

Leo Kanner (1894–1981)

Austrian-born American child psychiatrist and researcher on autism

Leo Kanner was born Chaskel Leib Kanner in Klekotow (now Klekotiv), Austria-Hungary (now Ukraine), on June 13, 1894. He received his medical degree from the University of Berlin in 1921, then emigrated to the United States three years later to take a position at a state hospital in Yankton, South Dakota. In 1928 he joined the prestigious Johns Hopkins Hospital, where in 1930 he established the first child psychiatric clinic in a pediatric hospital (Johns Hopkins Hospital's Harriet Lane Home for Invalid Children).

Kanner's passion for child and adolescent psychiatry led him to write *Child Psychiatry* (1935), the first English-language textbook devoted to the subject of psychiatric problems in children. In 1943 he published a ground-breaking study on early infantile autism (which came to be known as Kanner Syndrome). The paper, titled "Autistic Disturbances of Affective Contact," identified autism as a distinct syndrome and established the word autism (from the Greek word "auto," meaning self) in the child psychiatry lexicon.

Kanner's paper, which came in the midst of a two-year stint as chairman of the child psychiatry section of the American Psychiatric Association, fur-ther established the author as one of the world's foremost experts in the fast-developing field of study. Over the next two decades, he published dozens of articles on autism—many of which sensitively emphasized the importance of humane treatment—as well as numerous books, articles, and studies on child psychiatry, family dynamics, history, and folklore. He was named a full professor of child psychiatry at Johns Hopkins in 1957 and became professor emeritus at the university in 1959. From 1971 to 1974 he served as editor of the *Journal of Autism and Childhood Schizophrenia.*

Kanner, who died on April 3, 1981, is remembered today as one of the seminal figures in the development of child psychiatry as an important field of medical research. Moreover, the research he conducted on autism from the 1930s through the 1950s is regarded, along with the work of fellow Austrian Hans Asperger, as foundational to the modern study of autism.

Further Reading

Eisenberg, L. (1981). In memoriam: Leo Kanner, M.D., 1894–1981. *American Journal of Psychiatry, 138*(8), 1122–1125.

Grinker, R. R. (2007). *Unstrange minds: Remapping the world of autism.* New York: Basic Books.

Sidney Katz (1924–)

American gerontologist and creator of the
Activities of Daily Living (ADL) scale

A native of Cleveland, Ohio, Sidney Katz earned both his bachelor's degree in general science (in 1944) and his medical degree (1948) from Case Western Reserve University. He interrupted his fledgling medical career by enlisting in the U.S. Army during the Korean War. He spent much of that conflict serving in a Mobile Army Surgical Hospital (MASH), and he received a Bronze Star for his role in reducing mortality from deadly outbreaks of hemorrhagic fever.

After the war, Katz enrolled in Walter Reed Army Medical Service graduate school in Washington, D.C., where he conducted additional research on hemorrhagic fever. During the 1950s, however, he gradually switched his research emphasis to gerontology, which he found much more satisfying. This change in direction was inspired in large measure by his return to Case Western Reserve University, which enjoyed a close relationship with Cleveland's Benjamin Rose Hospital for the Aged. The latter hospital was directed by Austin Chinn, a dedicated proponent of delivering high-quality services to chronically ill and disabled elderly individuals. Charged by Chinn with creating innovative programs of geriatric care and rehabilitation, Katz responded with a pioneering system for assessing the daily "functionality" of elderly people and individuals with disabilities, which could in turn be used to determine their need for various services/forms of assistance.

Katz's "Activities of Daily Living" assessment, which he first unveiled in 1957 but steadily modified and expanded in subsequent years, scored patients' ability to live independently. It did so by listing "basic activities of daily living" (BADL) necessary for fundamental aspects of self-care, such as eating, bathing, and dressing. But Katz also developed a program for measuring "instrumental activities of daily living" (IADL) necessary for independent living in a community, such as the abilities to prepare food, shop, do laundry, access transportation, and manage money.

During the 1960s and 1970s, Katz remained a leading figure in the expanding field of geriatric care, and he played an important role during this time in making "quality of life" issues a top priority for medical practitioners and policymakers involved in the fields of disability and geriatric care. In 1984 Katz earned a master's degree in medical science from Brown University, and two years later he founded Brown's Center for Gerontology and Health Care, which trains clinicians and non-clinicians in health services research with an emphasis on geriatrics, gerontology, and chronic disease management. During the mid-1980s, as chair of the Institute of Medicine's Committee on Nursing Home Regulation, Katz was instrumental in the U.S. Congress's adoption of sweeping nursing-home reforms contained in the Omnibus Budget Reconciliation Act of 1987. Katz suffered a stroke in 1993, but he remains an active voice in the field of gerontology, and he has received numerous prestigious honors and awards over the past four decades.

Further Reading

Beal, E. (2004). Interview with Dr. Sidney Katz. Benjamin Rose Institute on Aging. Retrieved from http://www.benrose.org/MythBusters/mb_sidneykatz.cfm

Hawes, C. (2009). Katz, Sidney. In R. Mullner (Ed.), *Encyclopedia of health services research*. Thousand Oaks, CA: Sage.

Robert Koch (1834–1910)

German bacteriologist who discovered the cause of tuberculosis

Born on December 11, 1843, in Clausthal, Germany, Heinrich Hermann Robert Koch was one of 13 children. The son of a local mining engineer, Koch graduated from the University of Göttingen in 1866 with a degree in medicine. He promptly opened a general practice, but his career was interrupted in 1870 by enlistment in the Franco-Prussian War, where he served as a medical officer. In 1872 he took a position as a medical officer in the German Empire district of Wollstein, in modern-day Poland.

In short order, Koch immersed himself in scientific research on anthrax, which was taking a heavy toll on local livestock. Working in isolation from the wider scientific community—and with exceedingly limited resources—Koch engaged in research that decisively proved not only that anthrax bacteria could be transmitted by blood from infected animals, but also that the bacilli could spread via hardy spores capable of living, albeit in a dormant state, for extended periods of time in practically any environment. These spores could then trigger new outbreaks of anthrax when more hospitable conditions arose.

Koch's investigation became a foundational event in the field of bacteriology, and by the late 1870s (during which time he published important studies on bacteria's role in wound infections), he had become one of Europe's most famous scientists. In 1880 Koch took a job in Berlin with the German Health Office, where he further refined the bacteriological methods he had developed in Wollstein. In 1882 he discovered the bacteria responsible for tuberculosis, as well as a system for growing it in pure culture. When he published his findings about the tubercle bacillus and its role as an infectious agent later that year, he took his place alongside Louis Pasteur in the elite pantheon of 19th-century bacteriologists.

In 1885 Koch accepted a professor of hygiene position at the University of Berlin, which also named him director of its newly established Institute of Hygiene. In 1890 he was appointed surgeon general for the city of Berlin. During these years, Koch turned his attention to cholera, traveling to Egypt and India to study outbreaks of the disease. His pioneering proposals for preventing and mitigating cholera epidemics were formally accepted by the German government in 1893. Other noteworthy scientific achievements made by Koch during these incredibly productive years included "Koch's Postulates," which established the basis for study of all types of infectious disease; the "plate" and "slide" techniques of isolating bacteria on a culture plate; and development of vital new sterilization and disinfection techniques, both in the laboratory and in public health contexts.

In the late 1890s, Koch's reputation was clouded by exaggerated claims he made about the efficacy of a tuberculosis "cure" he had developed in his laboratory. But he recovered from this blow, in part through extensive and important work in India and Africa on malaria, typhus, and livestock diseases such as rinderpest. In addition, his 1901 announcement that human and bovine tuberculosis were caused by different bacilli was an important advance in scientific understanding of the disease. In 1905 Koch was awarded the Nobel Prize for Physiology or Medicine "for his investigations and discoveries in relation to tuberculosis." Koch died on May 27, 1910, in Baden-Baden, Germany.

Further Reading

Brock, T. (1988). *Robert Koch: A life in medicine and bacteriology*. Madison, WI: Science Tech.

Robert Koch and tuberculosis. (2003). Nobelprize.org. Retrieved from http://nobelprize.org/educational/medicine/tuberculosis/readmore.html

Frank H. Krusen (1898–1973)

American physician and founder of the field
of physical medicine and rehabilitation

The famed American physiatrist Frank Hammond Krusen was born on June 26, 1898. After graduating from Philadelphia's Jefferson Medical College in 1921, Krusen intended to pursue a career in surgery. In 1924, however, he contracted pulmonary tuberculosis and was forced to undergo extended convalescence in a local sanitarium. During his recovery, Krusen experienced an epiphany about the deleterious effects of physical "deconditioning" and excessive dependence on institutional care on the minds and bodies of patients. By the time he resumed his medical career in 1926 as associate dean of Philadelphia's Temple Medical School, his passion for what came to be known as physical medicine and rehabilitation was in full flower.

In 1929, Krusen established the nation's first academic department of physical medicine at Temple. Six years later, he accepted an offer from the famed Mayo Clinic in Rochester, Minnesota, to found a department of physical medicine at that institution. In short order, he developed the country's first three-year residency program in physical medicine and established a school of physical therapy. He also helped found the American Society of Physical Therapy Physicians, a professional society for practitioners in the field of rehabilitation medicine, in 1938. Krusen served a two-year stint as president of the society, which eventually became the American Academy of Physical Medicine and Rehabilitation, in 1941 and 1942. In 1941 Krusen published the first textbook of physical medicine, titled *Physical Medicine: The Employment of Physical Agents for Diagnosis and Therapy*.

During World War II, Krusen joined other noted practitioners in the burgeoning field of physical medicine on the Baruch Committee, which produced far-reaching rehabilitation programs that were implemented by America's armed services to treat and care for soldiers and sailors suffering from disabling injuries. After the war, he played an important role in establishing a section on physical medicine and rehabilitation within the American Medical Association (AMA). This board, the American Board of Physical Medicine, was officially recognized by the AMA in 1947. In the mid-1950s Krusen went to Washington, D.C., where he played a pivotal role in bolstering the medical elements of Office of Vocational Rehabilitation programs. He also effectively promoted greater study of vocational rehabilitation process in medical schools across the country. Krusen died on September 16, 1973.

Further Reading

Krusen F. H. (1969). Historical development in physical medicine and rehabilitation during the last forty years. *Archives of Physical Medicine and Rehabilitation, 50*, 1–5.

Lanska, D. J. (2009). The historical origins of stroke rehabilitation. In J. Stein, R. L. Harvey, R. F. Macko, C. J. Winstein, & R. D. Zorowitz (Eds.). *Stroke recovery and rehabilitation.* New York: Demos Medical Publishing.

James Lind (1716–1794)

Scottish physician who developed treatments for scurvy and invented the first modern clinical medical trial

James Lind was born on October 4, 1716, in Edinburgh, Scotland. The son of a successful merchant, he was apprenticed to a prominent Edinburgh physician in 1731. In 1739 he became a surgeon's mate in the British navy, and over the next several years, his military service took him to exotic locales in the West Indies and the Mediterranean.

Lind made his mark in medical history in 1747, when, as surgeon on the *HMS Salisbury*, he carried out pioneering experiments to discover the cause of scurvy, which at that time was the scourge of the English fleet. His experiments, regarded today as the first clinical medical trial, involved treating 12 sailors suffering from scurvy with an assortment of materials, including cider, vinegar, oranges, lemons, and concoctions of garlic, horseradish, and mustard. Lind then watched in fascination as the patients who had taken the citrus fruits made rapid improvement. This trial confirmed that citrus fruits (including limes, which already had been used by mariners for health purposes for many years) were extremely effective in warding off scurvy.

Lind returned to Scotland in 1748, receiving his medical degree from the University of Edinburgh later that same year. He established a successful medical practice, and in 1754 he published his landmark *A Treatise of the Scurvy*. Three years later, he published a second tome, *On the Most Effectual Means of Preserving the Health of Seamen*. Lind used both of these works to emphasize the health benefits of citrus fruits and juices (rich sources of vitamin C) in combating scurvy on naval and merchant vessels. Unfortunately, the British Crown was slow to recognize the value of Lind's research, and scurvy remained a menace for the next several decades.

In 1758 Lind was named the chief physician of the Royal Naval Hospital at Gosport, England. He served in that capacity for the next quarter-century. When Lind retired in 1783, his son succeeded him. James Lind died on July 13, 1794, in Gosport. The following year, the British Navy finally implemented his dietary recommendations, and scurvy promptly disappeared from the ranks.

Further Reading

Bown, S. (2003). *Scurvy: How a surgeon, a mariner, and a gentleman solved the greatest medical mystery of the age of sail*. Toronto, Canada: Thomas Allen.
Watts, G. (2001, February). Twelve scurvy men. *New Scientist, 24*, 46–47.

Joseph Lister (1827–1912)

English surgeon and founder of modern antiseptic surgery

Joseph Lister was born on April 5, 1827, in Upton, Essex, England, to Joseph Jackson Lister, a prominent wine merchant and a fellow of the Royal Society. In 1844 Lister enrolled at London's University College, where he studied medicine. After graduating in 1852, he relocated to Edinburgh, Scotland, and quickly established himself as one of the city's most accomplished and learned surgeons. In 1860 he became chair of clinical surgery at the University of Glasgow, which had a close association with the Royal Infirmary.

Lister focused much of his energies over the next several years at the Infirmary, experimenting with new techniques for preventing the onset of infection when treating fractures or in the aftermath of surgical procedures. Drawing on Louis Pasteur's pioneering germ theory of disease, Lister developed a successful method of applying purified carbolic acid to wounds. Cognizant of the damage that carbolic acid could itself do to the human body, Lister then developed antiseptic wound dressings that minimized the contact of carbolic acid with human tissue. These antiseptic procedures—coupled with other Lister innovations including gauze dressings, drainage tubes, and sterilized surgical instruments and suturing materials—revolutionized the practice of surgery during the final decades of the 19th century. As infection rates plummeted, the scope of surgical procedures expanded rapidly.

Lister returned to the University of Edinburgh in 1869, and in 1877 he was appointed professor of surgery at King's College in London. By the time of his retirement in 1893, most of the skeptics in medicine and academia who had initially doubted his findings had been converted or silenced, and Lister received numerous prestigious awards and honors in these later years. He also served as president of the Royal Society from 1895 to 1900, and in 1896 he served a one-year stint as president of the British Association for the Advancement of Science. He died at his home in Walmer, Kent, on February 10, 1912.

Further Reading

Dormandy, T. (2003). *Moments of truth: Four creators of modern medicine.* Hoboken, NJ: Wiley.

Farmer, L. (1962). *Master surgeon: A biography of Joseph Lister.* New York: Harper.

Gregor Mendel (1822–1884)

German monk who undertook pioneering research in the study of genetics

Gregor Johann Mendel was born into a poor peasant farming family on July 22, 1822, in Heinzendorf (now known as Hyncice), a town in Morovia (now part of the Czech Republic). He took up studies at the St. Thomas Monastery of the Augustinian Order in Brünn in 1843 and was ordained into the priesthood four years later. Mendel's zeal for teaching subsequently led him to enroll in 1851 at the University of Vienna, where he took challenging courses in mathematics, chemistry, and the natural sciences—and acquired valuable empirical skills—that became foundations of his later genetic research.

In 1854 Mandel returned to Brünn. When not engaged in monastery duties, Mandel devoted increasing amounts of his time to the study of genetic differences among species. In 1856 he began an eight-year course of careful study of successive generations of pea plants (chosen because they could be easily pollinated and hybridized), cataloguing how traits like color and shape were passed on in the plants over time. His painstaking research revealed that hereditary characteristics were passed on to subsequent generations in accordance with two major principles: the law of segregation (which included insights into dominant and recessive genes) and the law of independent assortment (which asserted that individual traits of an organism are passed on to future generations independently of one another).

Mendel presented his findings on plant hybridization in lectures and papers in the mid-1860s. But despite his best efforts to explain and publicize his groundbreaking research, the monk's findings went largely ignored by the wider scientific community until the early 1900s, when several botanists independently verified his findings and subsequently returned to his research. From that point forward, Mendel has been known as the "father of modern genetics."

In March 1868 Mendel was elected abbot of St. Thomas Monastery. His many and varied duties as abbot forced him to curtail his genetic research, but he continued his experimentation when he could find the time. In the early 1870s, he clashed with state authorities over a new tax that was being imposed on monasteries. His defiance made him a controversial figure in his final years. Mendel died in Brünn on January 6, 1884.

Further Reading

Henig, R. M. (2000). *The monk in the garden*. Boston, MA: Houghton Mifflin.

Orel, V. (1996). *Gregor Mendel: The first geneticist*. New York: Oxford University Press.

Luc Montagnier (1932–)

French virologist who discovered the human immunodeficiency virus (HIV)

Luc Montagnier was born on August 18, 1932, in Chabris (near Tours), France, the only child of Antoine Montagnier and Marianne Rousselet. Interested in science and medicine from an early age, Montagnier attended the Collège de Châtellerault, and then the University of Poitiers, where he received an undergraduate degree in natural sciences in 1953. Two years later, he earned an advanced degree in science at the University of Paris, and in 1960 he qualified for his doctorate in medicine at the Sorbonne in Paris.

Montagnier's career as a medical researcher and virologist began at the United Kingdom's Medical Research Council in Carshalton, but in 1963 he moved on to the Institute of Virology in Glasgow, Scotland, where he conducted advanced cancer research. In 1965 Montagnier began a seven-year stint as laboratory director of the Institut de Radium (later called Institut Curie) at Orsay. In 1972 Montagnier—whose main research thrust at the time was investigating retroviruses as a potential cause of cancer—accepted the directorship of the viral oncology unit of the Pasteur Institute in Paris. By the close of the 1970s, Montagnier's research on retroviruses had firmly established him as one of the world's preeminent virologists. Montagnier greatly advanced the scientific community's understanding of the ways in which viruses can alter the genetic information of host organisms, and his research (with Edward De Maeyer and Jacquiline De Maeyer-Guignard) into the virus-fighting protein interferon helped unlock effective new treatments for viral diseases.

In 1982 a clinician from Paris's Bichat Hospital named Willy Rozenbaum approached Montagnier and the Pasteur Institute in hopes that they could help him determine whether a retrovirus was responsible for mysterious—and deadly—outbreaks of what is now known as AIDS (acquired immunodeficiency syndrome). In January 1983 Rozenbaum sent a lymph node biopsy from one of his patients to the Pasteur Institute, where Montagnier, his colleague Françoise Barré-Sinoussi, and other members of Montagnier's team subjected the biopsy to an exhaustive battery of tests and analysis. They not only confirmed Rozenbaum's hypothesis, but actually identified the retrovirus—which they initially called lymphadenopathy-associated virus (LAV)—responsible for AIDS. This discovery soon resulted in the development of a blood test that could accurately detect the presence of the virus in patients.

One year later, the pioneering work of Montagnier and his team became shadowed by controversy when American virologist Robert C. Gallo of the National Cancer Institute—who had received LAV samples from Montagnier in the fall of 1983—announced that he had discovered that AIDS was caused by a human retrovirus he called human T-cell lymphotropic virus 3 or HTLV-3. He also stated that a blood test to screen patients and the nation's blood supply for the virus would soon be commercially available. This blood test quickly received patent approval from the U.S. government, and it remains the primary means employed by medical professionals for detecting the virus. In the meantime, a blood test patent application, which had been filed by the Pasteur Institute several months earlier, was denied. Montagnier and his supporters reacted angrily to this development, especially after subsequent studies showed that Gallo's AIDS virus was in fact LAV.

The controversy quickly metastasized into an ugly war of words that did not end until 1987, when Jonas Salk helped mediate an international agreement signed by the scientists and official representatives of their respective countries. Under this agreement, Montagnier and Gallo agreed to be recognized as co-discoverers of the virus and France and the United States agreed to funnel most of the revenue from testing into AIDS research. In 1986, meanwhile, the virus names initially adopted by Montagnier and Gallo were replaced with the term human immunodeficiency virus or HIV. In 2008 Montagnier and Barré-Sinoussi—but not Gallo—received the Nobel Prize in Physiology or Medicine "for their discovery of human immunodeficiency virus."

Further Reading

Kelleher, C. (1993). Beyond HIV: Assembling the AIDS puzzle. *Omni, 15*(8), 52–57.

Montagnier, L. (1999). *Virus: The co-discoverer of HIV tracks its rampage and charts the future.* New York: W. W. Norton.

William T. G. Morton (1819–1868)

American dentist credited with first demonstrating the surgical uses of anesthesia

William Thomas Green Morton was born on August 9, 1819, in Charlton, Massachusetts. The son of a local farmer, Morton entered the Baltimore College of Dental Surgery in 1840. He left the school and city without graduating, however, partly because of legal trouble stemming from his penchant for engaging in small-time bit fraud and swindling. After brief stints in St. Louis and Cincinnati—in which he continued to showcase a proclivity for purchasing goods on credit, then disappearing without making payment—Morton landed in Hartford, Connecticut, where he studied dentistry under local dentist Horace Wells. In 1843 Morton married Elizabeth Whitman. Under pressure from Whitman's parents, he enrolled at Harvard Medical School in Boston, where he took courses under the physician-chemist Charles T. Jackson. But Morton soon abandoned his studies at Harvard and opened a dental practice in Boston.

Morton rocketed from obscurity to fame in September 1846, when he announced that he had used ether as an anesthetic on dental patients, thus enabling painless tooth extraction and other dental procedures. Morton's declaration caused an immediate stir in medical circles, and on October 16, 1846, Morton used his ether treatment on a patient at Massachusetts General Hospital so that a neck tumor could be removed. When the procedure was completed and the performing surgeon offered heartfelt praise for Morton's anesthesia treatment, the dentist's fame was assured. Physicians and surgeons around the world recognized that with a safe general anesthesia available, a new age of medical treatment was at hand.

Morton's efforts to profit financially from these developments floundered, however. Jackson came forward and claimed that *he* had told Morton about the possibility of using ether as a general anesthetic several years back, when the dentist had studied under him at Harvard. Wells issued a similar claim, asserting that he had first unlocked ether's potential as a general anesthetic and that the opportunistic Morton had in effect stolen the idea from him.

As these charges roiled around him, Morton's various efforts to parlay ether's utility as an anesthetic into personal riches came to naught. These efforts range from patents on concoctions that blended ether with inert ingredients like oil of orange to repeated petitions to the U.S. government for financial recompense. Thwarted at every turn, Morton was forced to content himself with the occasional honorary degree and his unofficial title as the "father of anesthesia." In 1862 Morton joined the Army of the Potomac as a volunteer surgeon, and he treated victims of some of the Civil War's bloodiest battles. He died on July 15, 1868, in New York City.

Further Reading

Fenster, J. M. (2002). *Ether day: The strange tale of America's greatest medical discovery and the haunted men who made it.* New York: Harper Collins.

Wolfe, R. J. (2001). *Tarnished idol: William Thomas Green Morton and the introduction of surgical anesthesia: A chronicle of the ether controversy.* San Anselmo, CA: Norman.

Joseph E. Murray (1919–)

American surgeon who performed the first successful kidney transplant operation

Joseph Edward Murray was born on April 1, 1919, in Milford, Massachusetts. He received his bachelor's degree from Holy Cross College in 1940 and his medical degree from Harvard Medical School in 1943.

He completed his surgical residency at the Harvard-affiliated Peter Bent Brigham Hospital (later Brigham and Women's Hospital), and in 1944 he began a three-year stint in the Army Medical Corps at Valley Forge General Hospital, where he performed hundreds of reconstructive surgeries of eyes and hands.

After returning to Brigham in 1947, Murray became interested in the work of Harvard researchers John Merrill and David Hume, who were researching kidney transplantation as a treatment for end-stage renal disease. Over the next few years, Murray used the work of Merrill and Hume as a springboard for his own surgical research, and he eventually developed a surgical technique for kidney transplants wherein blood vessels of donor kidneys could be connected to those in the abdomen of the recipient, and donor ureters could be implanted directly into the urinary bladder.

Murray then sought identical twins willing to volunteer for his experimental surgery, because if the donor and recipient did not share the same genetic makeup, the recipient's immune system would reject the donated organ (years later, researchers developed ways to "trick" immune systems into accepting other organs). He finally located willing twins in Ronald and Richard Herrick, the latter of whom was dying of kidney disease. The kidney transplant operation took place on December 23, 1954, and lasted for five and a half hours. The procedure went flawlessly, and Richard Herrick lived another seven years with his brother's donated kidney before dying of heart failure.

Murray performed additional successful transplant operations on identical twins over the next several years. For many years, Murray and other scientists and physicians were thwarted in their efforts to circumvent the immune reaction problem that limited such operations to identical twins. But in the early 1960s, scientific advances that suppressed the rejection response of immune systems enabled Murray to begin conducting organ and tissue transplants from non-related donors. In 1962 Murray successfully completed the first organ transplant from a cadaver.

Murray's surgical exploits in the realm of kidney transplants assured him a prominent and enduring place in the history of medicine. But he also did notable work in the realm of plastic surgery, especially for children suffering from facial birth defects. In fact, he headed the plastic surgery divisions of both Brigham (1951–1986) and Boston Children's Hospital Medical Center (1972–1985). In 1990 he was named a co-recipient of the Nobel Prize in Physiology or Medicine with E. Donnall Thomas, who conducted pioneering research into bone marrow transplants.

Further Reading

Murray, J. E. (2001). *Surgery of the soul: Reflections on a curious career.* Sagamore Beach, MA: Science History Publications.

Tilney, N. L. (2003). *Transplant: From myth to reality.* New Haven, CT: Yale University Press.

Florence Nightingale (1820–1910)

English hospital reformer and founder of modern nursing

Florence Nightingale was born in the Italian city of Florence (the inspiration for her first name) on May 12, 1820. Born into a wealthy English family, she received an extensive private education in mathematics and other subjects. Her parents initially resisted her entreaties that she be allowed to study nursing, but they eventually relented, and in 1850 Nightingale began nursing training at the Institute of St. Vincent de Paul in Alexandria, Egypt. A year later she relocated to Kaiserwerth, Germany, to study nursing at the Institute of Protestant Deaconesses and a hospital in France. In 1853 she returned to London, where she took an unpaid position as resident lady superintendent of a hospital for invalid women.

A few months later, the Crimean War broke out. As British and French troops poured into Turkey to help that nation beat back the invasion from Russia that had precipitated the conflict, outbreaks of cholera, malaria, typhus, and dysentery took a heavy toll on the British and French forces. Nightingale and other women nurses were initially rebuffed when they volunteered their help, but adverse publicity convinced the British government to reverse itself. British authorities asked Nightingale to supervise the introduction of nurses to military hospitals. Nightingale accepted the offer, thus acquiring the official title of Superintendent of the Female Nursing Establishment of the English General Hospitals in Turkey. On November 4, 1854, she arrived at an army hospital in Scutari, Turkey, with a group of carefully selected nurses in tow.

Nightingale was shocked at the primitive and unhygienic conditions that prevailed at the hospital, and she immediately set about improving the situation. She and the nurses under her charge embarked on a yeoman crusade to clean up the filthy facilities, and the male physicians became increasingly reliant on the nurses for patient care and treatment as well. Meanwhile, Nightingale established effective new sanitary methods in virtually all aspects of Scutari's operations, while simultaneously systematizing the hospital's record-keeping practices. Nightingale was thus able to use her mathematical knowledge to quantify the enormous beneficial impact of her reforms on the hospital's mortality rate.

Positive reports concerning the performance of Nightingale and her nurses flowed back to England from physicians, patients, and journalists alike. Nightingale in particular took on iconic status as "the lady with the lamp," selflessly ministering to sick and wounded soldiers without regard for her own needs. She thus returned to England as a national heroine after Russia's defeat in late 1855. Nightingale was somewhat taken aback by her sudden celebrity, but she quickly decided to use it by embarking on a campaign to reform all British military hospitals. Publication of her *Notes on Matters Affecting the Health, Efficiency and Hospital Administration of the British Army* (1857) and *Notes on Hospitals* (1859) were seminal events in changing threadbare notions about hygiene and treatment of patients in English hospitals, and she proved adept at lobbying and cajoling public officials as well. Over the next several years, many of the practices she had first introduced in Scutari were incorporated into the operations of both civilian and military hospitals across Britain and even other parts of Europe. She also remained a dedicated champion of the nursing profession, and in 1860 she and several wealthy friends established the famous Nightingale School and Home for Nurses at St. Thomas's Hospital in London.

In later life Nightingale published numerous papers and pamphlets on public health issues, but her health deteriorated badly in the 1890s. She spent her last years as an invalid before dying in London on August 13, 1910.

Further Reading

Bostridge, M. (2008). *Florence Nightingale: The making of an icon.* New York: Farrar, Straus, and Giroux.

Cook, E. T. (1913). *The life of Florence Nightingale.* London: Macmillan.

Gill, G. (2004). *Nightingales: The extraordinary upbringing and curious life of Miss Florence Nightingale.* New York: Ballantine.

Louis Pasteur (1822–1895)

French chemist who invented the pasteurization process and proved the germ theory of disease

Louis Pasteur was born on December 27, 1822, in Dôle, France. A gifted and inquisitive student, Pasteur earned degrees in mathematics and letters in the early 1840s before earning a master's degree in science (in 1845) and a doctorate in philosophy (in 1847) from the elite École Normale Supérieure in Paris. He spent the next several years teaching at Dijon Lycée secondary school and the University of Strasbourg, and in 1849 he married Marie Laurent. Three of their five children died of typhoid before reaching adulthood. These personal blows played a major role in charting the direction of Pasteur's scientific research over the years.

In 1854 Pasteur accepted a position as dean of the University of Lille's new science college. He made his mark quickly, establishing evening classes for industrial workers and launching important studies into the process of fermentation. In 1857 he began a ten-year stint as director of scientific studies at the École Normale Supérieure. It was here that he documented through careful scientific experimentation how milk could be preserved or soured, depending on the introduction and treatment of foreign bacteria. These advances in scientific understanding became the cornerstone of the process known as pasteurization.

Pasteur's reputation as one of Europe's preeminent scientists and chemists was further burnished in the mid-1860s, when his research efforts enabled France to ward off a silkworm outbreak that threatened to destroy the economically vital crop. His identification of two bacilli responsible for silkworm disease—and his documentation of methods for preventing outbreaks and detecting diseased stock—made him a national hero.

In 1867 Pasteur resigned his directorship, but he remained at the École Normale Supérieure in a private research laboratory that was supported by Emperor Napoleon III himself. It was at this time that Pasteur began to test the theory of spontaneous generation—the idea that bacterial life arises spontaneously. During the 1870s, Pasteur engaged in intensive, revolutionary field research into the bacteria that cause human and animal diseases, as well as the mechanisms of infection and immunity. He emerged from these efforts, which thoroughly eviscerated the notion of spontaneous generation, as the world's foremost champion of the germ theory of disease, which transformed the worlds of science and medicine in the late 19th century. Other triumphs followed for Pasteur as well, including his development of effective vaccines against chicken cholera, anthrax, swine erysipelas, and rabies—the latter of which had long been a particularly fearsome scourge across Europe. Pasteur's innovative research thus was pivotal in inaugurating a new era of vaccination against diseases that had terrorized the world for centuries.

In 1888 the Pasteur Institute opened in Paris under the directorship of its namesake. The research facility was headed by Pasteur until his death on September 28, 1895.

Further Reading

Debré, P. (1998). *Louis Pasteur*. Baltimore, MD: Johns Hopkins University Press.
Geison, G. L. (1995). *The private science of Louis Pasteur*. Princeton, NJ: Princeton University Press.

Philippe Pinel (1745–1826)

*French psychiatrist who championed the "humane"
treatment of people with mental illness*

Philippe Pinel was born on April 20, 1745, in the small town of Roques, France. Pinel initially pursued a life in the priesthood, enrolling in the College of Theology at Toulouse in 1767. His interests gradually drifted toward medicine, however, and in 1770 he switched his studies accordingly. He earned his medical degree from Toulouse in 1773, then continued his studies at the prestigious University of Montpellier.

In 1778 Pinel moved to Paris, where he immersed himself in further study of medicine, science, and mathematics. However, his efforts to establish a medical practice were rebuffed by Paris's medical community, which asserted that schooling from provincial universities such as Toulouse was hopelessly inferior. Pinel thus was forced to support himself throughout the 1780s and early 1790s as a writer, editor, and translator.

During this time, however, Pinel also developed a keen interest in mental illness and the treatment thereof. This interest led to several years of work at a private insane asylum in Paris. His experiences there have been cited as pivotal in the development of Pinel's psychiatric theories.

In 1793 the convulsive events of the French Revolution opened new opportunities for Pinel. Friends helped him secure an appointment as chief physician at Hospice de Bicêtre, one of the most notorious mental institutions in Paris. Upon taking his new position, Pinel and hospital governor Jean-Baptiste Pussin worked together to make sweeping changes to institutional operations. "Patients" who had previously been subjected to beatings, filthy cells, and bondage in chains were released from their restraints, given better dietary and sanitary conditions, and generally treated in a much more humane and compassionate manner.

During this same period, Pinel began to compile detailed case studies of individual patients in order to craft personalized courses of treatment. The patients' almost uniformly positive response to these reforms led the University of Paris to offer Pinel a faculty position as professor of hygiene and pathology. He maintained his association with the University of Paris for the rest of his life (he was briefly suspended from the faculty by the government in 1822 for lingering suspicions about his past associations with people involved in the Revolution, but was later reinstated as an honorary professor).

In May 1795 Pinel accepted an offer to become chief physician of Hospice de la Salpêtrière in Paris. Pinel brought his reforms and psychiatric treatments to the new facility, and over the ensuing years, the institution—which housed more than 5,000 mostly female patients—became a trailblazer in implementing modern psychiatric practices. Pinel personally explained his philosophies of treatment and care for people suffering from mental illness in *Nosographie philosophique ou méthode de l'analyse appliquée à la medicine* (1798) and *Traité médico-philosophique sur l'aliénation mentale; ou la manie* (1801). The latter work was translated into English as *Treatise on Insanity* in 1806, and its explication of "moral treatment" of people with mental illness was enormously influential on psychiatric practice in both Europe and the United States in the 19th century. Pinel remained with the Hospice de la Salpêtrière until his death on October 25, 1826.

Further Reading

Riese, W. (1969). *The legacy of Philippe Pinel: An inquiry into thought on mental alienation.* New York: Springer.

Waller, J. (2004). *Leaps in the dark: The making of scientific reputations.* New York: Oxford University Press.

Wilhelm Conrad Roentgen (1845–1923)

German physicist who discovered x-rays

Wilhelm Conrad Roentgen (an alternative German spelling is Röntgen) was born on March 27, 1845, in Lennep, Prussia. He studied physics briefly at the University of Utretcht before enrolling at the University of Zurich, where he earned a doctorate degree in 1869. His chief mentor at Zurich was the physicist August Kundt, and Roentgen served as an assistant to Kundt at various academic stops throughout the early 1870s. In 1872 he married Anna Bertha Ludwig, with whom he adopted a daughter.

In 1874 Roentgen emerged from Kundt's shadow, securing a lecturer position at France's Strasbourg University. One year later he gained a professorship at the Academy of Agriculture at Hohenheim in Württemberg, but in 1876 he returned to Strasbourg as a professor of physics. He stayed at Strasbourg for another three years, whereupon he claimed the chair of the physics department at the University of Giessen. His final academic stops were at the University of Würzburg (where he was physics chair from 1888 to 1900) and the University of Munich (where he served as chair of physics from 1900 to 1920).

Roentgen's highly successful career in academia, however, was overshadowed by his research in the field of physics. He made significant contributions in many fields of physics, including thermology and electricity, and in November 1895 he discovered "x-rays," a form of electromagnetic radiation capable of taking images inside solid objects, from metal to flesh (Roentgen also made the first radiographic images of human anatomy—his wife's hand). Roentgen's discovery of these short-wave rays, also known as Roentgen rays, revolutionized the diagnostic capabilities of medical practitioners. His achievement was formally recognized with numerous honorary doctorates and awards, including the first-ever Nobel Prize in Physics in 1901.

Unassuming and reticent, Roentgen refused to patent his discovery, accept engagements to speak about his research, or otherwise parlay the event into personal financial gain. Instead, he donated his Nobel Prize money to charity and continued to divide his time between physics research and mountaineering, which was an enduring passion. He spent his last years quietly and died in Munich on February 10, 1923.

Further Reading

Friedman, M., & Friedland, G. W. (1998). Wilhelm Roentgen and the x-ray beam. In *Medicine's ten greatest discoveries* (pp. 115–132). New Haven, CT: Yale University Press.

Shamos, M. H. (1987). William K. Roentgen (1845–1923): X-rays. In *Great experiments in physics: Firsthand accounts from Galileo to Einstein.* Mineola, NY: Dover.

Ronald Ross (1857–1932)

English entomologist and epidemiologist who discovered how the Anopheles *mosquito transmits malaria*

Ronald Ross was born on May 13, 1857, in Almora, India. He was the oldest son of Campbell C. G. Ross, a general in the English Army, and Matilda Charlotte Elderton. At the age of eight, he left British India to attend schools in England. He earned a medical degree from London's St. Bartholomew's Hospital in 1880, and one year later entered the Indian Medical Service.

A man of wide-ranging interests, Ross wrote numerous plays, poems, and works of fiction that were published in the late 19th and early 20th centuries. He even published several books on mathematics during this period. But it was in the worlds of entomology and epidemiology that Ross made his greatest contributions. In 1889 Ross returned to England, where he earned a diploma in public health and studied bacteriology. He took a particular interest in studying malaria, which he had repeatedly confronted in his various postings in British India. It was during this time that he made the acquaintance of Sir Patrick Manson, a Scottish physician who suggested to Ross that mosquitoes might be the vectors of malaria outbreaks in India and other tropical locales.

This theory, which was also being propagated by French scientist Alphonse Leveran, became the focus of Ross's research efforts when he returned to India in the early 1890s. His efforts to document the link between mosquitoes and malaria were temporarily derailed in 1897, when Ross himself struggled with a bout of the disease. Soon after recovering, however, Ross discovered the presence of a malarial parasite within the *Anopheles* species of mosquito. He then used infected birds to document the life cycle of the parasite, which traveled from its host to new victims via the bloodsucking activity of the mosquito.

Ross delivered his findings to Manson, who trumpeted the breakthrough to the 1898 meeting of the British Medical Association in Edinburgh, Scotland. Ross received numerous honors and awards for his groundbreaking research, including a knighthood and the 1902 Nobel Prize in Medicine.

In 1899 Ross resigned from the Indian Medical Service and joined the Liverpool School of Tropical Medicine, where he remained until 1912. He was then appointed Physician for Tropical Diseases at King's College Hospital in London, where he remained until 1917, when he took special consulting positions with the British government. Throughout this time, he played major roles in developing strategies of mosquito control and malaria mitigation, while also developing the first mathematical models of malaria epidemiology. These efforts took him to such far-flung tropical destinations as West Africa, Greece, Mauritius, Cyprus, and the Suez Canal Zone.

In 1926 Ross was named director of the newly created Ross Institute and Hospital of Tropical Diseases and Hygiene in London. He remained in that position until his death in London on September 16, 1932.

Further Reading

Carey, J. (Ed.). (1995). *The Faber book of science*. Boston: Faber and Faber.
Cook, G. C. (2007). *Tropical medicine: An illustrated history of the pioneers*. London: Academic Press.

Benjamin Rush (1745–1813)

*American physician, early sanitarian, and founder
of American psychiatry*

Benjamin Rush was born to John and Susanna Harvey Rush on December 24, 1745, on a plantation near Philadelphia, Pennsylvania. As a young man he attended the College of New Jersey (now Princeton University), where he earned a bachelor's degree in 1760. He then moved to Philadelphia, where he studied medicine for the next several years. In 1766 he relocated to Scotland, where he earned a doctorate in medicine from the prestigious University of Edinburgh in 1768.

Rush then returned to Philadelphia, where he quickly emerged as one of the city's most prominent and outspoken citizens. A fierce champion of American rights in the spiraling conflict with mother England, he joined the Continental Congress and was a signatory to the Declaration of Independence. But Rush was influential not only in the realm of politics, but also in the evolving worlds of science and medicine. In some respects, his influence was problematic; he was an outspoken proponent, for example, of bleeding, purging, and other heroic treatments that modern healers now view as barbaric.

But Rush had an enormously beneficial impact on other facets of medical practice. He helped advance William Cullen's theory that medical treatment should be organized in accordance with rational principles in a "system" that would simplify and improve the practice of medicine. As surgeon general of the Middle Department of the Continental Army in 1777, Rush issued *Directions for Preserving the Health of Soldiers*, a milestone document in the advancement of public health regulation, military hygiene, and preventive medicine.

Most importantly of all, Rush played an essential role in changing professional and popular attitudes about people suffering from severe mental illness. Throughout his long medical career, Rush advocated humane treatment for insane patients. He was one of the first to recognize that mental illness can stem from physical causes. Rush's observations, gleaned from decades of intense study of patients with mental illness, have led many medical historians to call him the father of American psychiatry. In fact, Rush's *Medical Inquiries and Observations on the Diseases of the Mind* (1812) is widely regarded as the first textbook ever published on the subject.

After the Revolutionary War drew to a close, Rush returned to his practice in Philadelphia. In 1783 he joined the staff of Pennsylvania Hospital, an association he maintained for the rest of his life. That same year, he played a leading role in the founding of Dickinson College in Carlisle, Pennsylvania. Also around this time, he became a lecturer at the University of the State of Pennsylvania, where his teachings on mental illness and other subjects influenced many early American medical practitioners. In 1786 he established the first free medical dispensary in America, and in 1803 Rush—a lifelong abolitionist—became president of the Pennsylvania Society for Promoting the Abolition of Slavery. His interest in sweeping social reform also led him to stake out vocal positions in support of women's rights and against capital punishment, and he made important contributions to American veterinary medicine as well. Rush died in Philadelphia on April 19, 1813.

Further Reading

Brodsky, A. (2004). *Benjamin Rush: Patriot and physician.* New York: Truman Talley Books/St. Martin's Press.

Farr, C. B. (1994). Benjamin Rush and American psychiatry. *American Journal of Psychiatry, 151*(6), 64–73.

Howard A. Rusk (1901–1989)

American physician who helped shape modern rehabilitation medicine and treatment

Howard Archibald Rusk was born in Brookfield, Missouri, on April 9, 1901. His parents were Michael Yost Rusk and Augusta Eastin Shipp Rusk. He received a bachelor's degree from the University of Missouri in 1923 and earned his medical degree at the University of Pennsylvania in 1925 after only two years of study instead of the usual four years. He then returned to Missouri to intern at St. Luke's Hospital in St. Louis, and in 1926 he established a private practice in internal medicine. That same year he married Gladys Houx, with whom he eventually had three children.

From 1926 to 1942, Rusk maintained his internal medicine practice while also rising to the position of associate chief of staff at St. Luke's. He also joined the medical school faculty of Washington University in St. Louis. Rusk's turn toward rehabilitation medicine began in 1942, when he left his practice to join the Army Air Corps during World War II. Assigned to head up the Army-Air Force Convalescent Training Program, Rusk immediately recognized that the wounded soldiers who were being crowded into wartime medical facilities needed psychological help as well as physical rehabilitation. Rusk promptly developed and implemented an ambitious convalescence program of retraining, reconditioning, and psychological readjustment and replenishment. When military authorities saw how effective Rusk's program was in reducing patients' convalescence time and recidivism rates, they ordered him to implement a program for the entire Army Air Corps. He earned the Distinguished Service Medal for his work and eventually retired as a Brigadier General in the U.S. Air Force Reserve.

After the war, Rusk relocated to New York City, where the directors of the New York University Medical School asked him to found the world's first comprehensive medical-training program in rehabilitation. Rusk headed the Institute of Physical Medicine and Rehabilitation (now known as the Howard A. Rusk Institute of Rehabilitation Medicine), which received important early funding from Bernard Baruch, from 1946 to 1978. Rusk's wartime exploits in the rehabilitation and care of soldiers suffering from disabilities also led to a regular weekly column in the *New York Times* from 1946 to 1969. Rusk used this column as a vehicle by which to spread his belief in the importance of "comprehensive" rehabilitation of people suffering from physical disabilities. According to Rusk, this approach entailed preparing disabled patients for re-integration into the general community. As Rusk put it, his rehabilitation strategies focused on "what happens to severely disabled people after the stitches are out and the fever is down." The goal, he said, was to "take them back into the best lives they can live with what they have left" (Rusk, 1956, p. 1099).

In 1955 Rusk founded the World Rehabilitation Fund, an institute designed to train professionals and publicize programs in advanced rehabilitation techniques. He directed the fund until 1982, when his son succeeded him. Rusk also wrote many articles and books during his long and distinguished career, from a 1972 autobiography to various works explicating his philosophy of rehabilitation and his support for increased investment in public health programs for elderly Americans. After receiving numerous prestigious honors and awards in recognition of his seminal role in the development of modern rehabilitation medicine, Rusk died on November 4, 1989.

Further Reading

Lanska, D. J. (2009). Profile of Howard Rusk (1901–1989): The father of comprehensive rehabilitation medicine. In J. Stein, R. L. Harvey, R. F. Macko, C. J. Winstein, & R. D. Zorowitz (Eds.), *Stroke recovery and rehabilitation.* New York: Demos Medical Publishing.

Rusk, H. A. (1956). Sick people in a troubled world. *Laryngoscope, 66,* 1094–1112. doi: 10.1288/00005537–195608000–00009

Rusk, H. A. (1972). *A world to care for: The autobiography of Howard A. Rusk, MD.* New York: Random House.

David Sackett (1934–)

American-born Canadian epidemiologist and founder of evidence-based medicine

David Lawrence Sackett was born in Chicago, Illinois, on November 17, 1934. He obtained his medical degree from the University of Illinois and his doctorate in science from the University of Bern before earning a master's degree in epidemiology from Harvard University. In 1967 he became founding Chair of Clinical Epidemiology and Biostatistics at a new medical school opened by McMaster University in Hamilton, Ontario. He remained at McMaster for the next 27 years while also serving stints as physician-in-chief at Chedoke-McMaster Hospitals and as head of the Division of General Internal Medicine for the Hamilton area. In 1994 Sackett moved on to the University of Oxford, where he took the position of foundation director of the National Health Service Research and Development Centre for Evidence-Based Medicine. He retired from clinical practice in 1999.

Sackett's wide-ranging career included significant scholarship on randomized clinical trials and "critical appraisal" strategies for clinicians. He also was part of the investigative team that documented the benefits of aspirin for patients at high risk of strokes or heart attacks, as well as studies showing that surgical repair of "hardened" arteries reduced strokes and increased life expectancies.

Sackett remains best known, however, as a leading developer and practitioner of evidence-based medicine (EBM), an effort to improve the quality of medical judgments. The basic principles of EBM, a term first coined by Sackett in the early 1990s, are to formulate answerable questions, collect evidence, confirm the validity of that evidence, apply the results in clinical practice, and evaluate the outcome. Sackett himself summarized EBM in a 1996 editorial in *BMJ-British Medical Journal* as the "conscientious, explicit, and judicious use of current best evidence in making decisions about the care of individual patients. The practice of evidence-based medicine means integrating individual clinical expertise with the best available external clinical evidence from systematic research" (p. 72).

Sackett's work on EBM has been cited as a key factor in the increased emphasis on sound empirical research and standard clinical approaches in the practice of medicine. In 2009 Sackett received the Gairdner Wightman Award, Canada's most prestigious international medical research prize.

Further Reading

Sackett, D. L. (1996). Evidence-based medicine: What it is and what it isn't. *BMJ*, *312*(7023), 71–72.

Sackett, D. L., Straus, S. E., Richardson W. S., Rosenberg, W., & Haynes, R. B. (1998). *Evidence-based medicine: How to practice and teach EBM*. New York: Harcourt.

Jonas Salk (1914–1995)

American medical researcher who developed
the first effective polio vaccine

Jonas Salk was born in New York City on October 28, 1914. He was the oldest of three children born to Daniel and Dora Salk, who were Russian-Jewish immigrants. Salk initially enrolled at City College of New York-CCNY for the purpose of pursuing a law career, but in 1934 he transferred to New York University to study medicine. One day after graduating in 1939, he married Donna Lindsay, with whom he had three children. Salk took an internship at New York's Mount Sinai Hospital for the next two years, then moved on to a research position with Dr. Thomas Francis Jr. at the University of Michigan in Ann Arbor.

During his time at Michigan, Salk provided invaluable help to Francis with an Army-sponsored effort to develop an effective flu vaccine. By 1943 Francis and Salk had produced an influenza vaccine effective against both type A and B flu viruses, and the following year (when Salk was promoted to research associate in epidemiology), they began clinical trials. In 1946 Salk was named an assistant professor of epidemiology at the university.

In 1947, Salk accepted an appointment to the University of Pittsburgh Medical School, where he conducted the studies that made him a national hero. Working under a grant from the National Foundation for Infantile Paralysis, Salk launched an intensive course of research into finding an effective vaccine against poliomyelitis, one of the most feared diseases in the world. By 1950 Salk had developed a vaccine treatment against all three types of polio viruses, and he began testing the vaccine in carefully controlled trials using polio samples he grew in cultures of monkey kidney tissue. Using heavy dosages of formaldehyde, Salk was able to kill all three polio virus strains, yet still induce immunity in his test subjects.

In April 1955 Salk announced to the world that human trials of his polio vaccine, which was administered via a series of injections, effectively shielded subjects from all three forms of polio. The stunning news made him a household name, and his meteoric rise to legend status was further accelerated when he announced that he had no intention of patenting the vaccine for personal gain. Shipments of Salk's polio vaccine went out all across the globe. By the end of 1957, more than 200 million doses of his vaccine had been administered through massive inoculation programs, and polio cases plummeted across the United States and in many other countries. Within a few years, Salk's vaccine was supplanted by a "live-virus" vaccine, which was developed by Albert Sabin and could be administered orally. But Salk's place as the man who defeated polio remained secure.

In 1960 Salk founded the Jonas Salk Institute for Biological Studies in La Jolla, California. This center for medical and scientific research formally opened in 1963. He spent the next two decades conducting scientific research into cancer, multiple sclerosis, and AIDS. He also wrote several books on science and its role in human development, including *Man Unfolding* (1972), *The Survival of the Wisest* (1973), and *World Population and Human Values: A New Reality* (1981). In 1977 he received the Presidential Medal of Freedom. Salk died on June 23, 1995, in La Jolla.

Further Reading

Kluger, J. (2005). *Splendid solution: Jonas Salk and the conquest of polio*. New York: Putnam.

Oshinsky, D. M. (2005). *Polio: An American story*. New York: Oxford University Press.

Margaret Sanger (1879–1966)

American birth control advocate and founder
of Planned Parenthood

Margaret Louise Higgins Sanger was born on September 14, 1879, in Corning, New York, to Michael Hennessey Higgins, a stonemason, and Anne Purcell Higgins. She was raised in impoverished circumstances, but older siblings helped her enroll at Claverack College and Hudson River Institute in 1896. In 1900 she entered the nursing program at White Plains Hospital in New York. She graduated from the program in 1902, the same year she married architect William Sanger. They eventually had three children.

In 1910 they moved to New York City, where Margaret Sanger took a job as a nurse. Her experiences treating poor pregnant women who were already struggling to provide for existing children turned her into a fierce critic of state and federal "Comstock Laws," which made it illegal for physicians and nurses to disseminate information about birth control options. Sanger's conviction that Comstock Laws forced working-class couples to make a difficult choice between refraining from sexual activity, seeking out illegal abortions, and raising numbers of children that far outstripped their financial and emotional resources turned her into a radical political activist.

In 1912 Sanger was able to parlay her associations with some of New York's leading left-wing intellectuals and activists into a regular sex-education column in the *New York Call*, a leading socialist newspaper. Two years later, she published the first issue of *The Woman Rebel*, a feminist monthly that asserted that birth control and sex education were essential to the economic and personal freedom of American working women. Authorities promptly indicted Sanger, charging her with sending obscene materials through the mail. A few weeks later, Sanger fled to England under the alias "Bertha Watson," where she received a hero's welcome from British radicals and feminists. She remained in England for nearly a year, during which time her marriage to William Sanger foundered.

In October 1915 Sanger returned to New York to face the postal obscenity charges. When prosecutors dropped the charges, Sanger launched a nationwide crusade for birth control, which she increasingly framed as essential to healthy female sexuality. Occasional arrests on obscenity grounds did not dissuade her, and in October 1916 she opened the nation's first birth control clinic in Brownsville, Brooklyn. Religious and political leaders denounced the clinic as an affront to basic tenets of morality, and after nine days police raided the facility. Sanger was arrested and eventually convicted on charges of illegally distributing birth control information and services. After serving a 30-day jail sentence she launched a new monthly magazine, *The Birth Control Review*, in early 1917. This periodical became Sanger's principal vehicle for advancing her message of unfettered sex education and reproductive freedom.

In 1921 Sanger founded the American Birth Control League (ABCL) in order to lobby legislators and increase public support for birth control measures. In ensuing years, however, Sanger and the ABCL increasingly couched their arguments for birth control in the language of the eugenics movement, which held that birth control should be encouraged among "inferior" ethnic stock.

In 1922 Sanger married James Noah H. Slee, a wealthy businessman who helped provide funding for Sanger's Birth Control Clinical Research Bureau, an important clinic and research center on contraception that opened in New York City in 1923. Around this time, however, her reputation as a radical was increasingly seen by the wider birth control movement as a hindrance to its cause, and in 1928 she was forced to resign from the presidency of the ABCL (which in 1939 merged with the Birth Control Clinical Research Bureau to create the Birth Control Federation of America, later renamed the Planned Parenthood Federation of America). Sanger's public profile faded from the public spotlight during the 1930s, but in the 1940s and 1950s she resumed her advocacy work for reproductive rights. She died in Tucson, Arizona, on September 6, 1966.

Further Reading

Chesler, E. (1992). *Woman of valor: Margaret Sanger and the birth control movement in America*. New York: Simon and Schuster.

Kennedy, D. M. (1991). *Birth control in America: The career of Margaret Sanger*. New Haven, CT: Yale University Press.

Sanger, M. (1931). *My fight for birth control*. New York: Farrar and Rinehart.

Lemuel Shattuck (1793–1859)

American public health statistician and advocate for public health regulation

Lemuel Shattuck was born on October 15, 1793, in Ashby, Massachusetts, to John and Betsey Shattuck, who supported themselves through farming. Shattuck had little formal schooling, but he nonetheless worked as a schoolteacher for several years before eventually establishing himself in Cambridge, Massachusetts, as a bookseller, publisher, and statistician in the mid-1830s. In 1825 he married Clarissa Baxter, with whom he had five children.

A firm believer in the utility of statistical analysis as a tool in public policymaking, Shattuck helped found the American Statistical Association in 1839. He also helped establish parameters of systematization for the collection of vital statistics in Massachusetts during the 1840s, and he urged increased use of census reports by policymakers, both at the municipal and federal levels.

It was as a public health statistician, however, that Shattuck had his greatest impact. In the 1840s he was selected to head a statistical study by the Massachusetts Sanitary Commission into possible links between urban pollution levels and disease outbreaks, which regularly cut a deadly swath through the state's fast-growing cities. This survey, technically called *Report of a General Plan for the Promotion of Public and Personal Health* but widely referred to by historians as the Shattuck Report, used detailed statistical analysis of morbidity and mortality rates across the state as a platform to call for sweeping new public health and sanitation laws in Boston and other metropolitan centers. Shattuck's report, which was published in 1850, provided convincing quantitative support for increased state regulation of water and sewage systems, garbage collection, and other environmental health services. It is regarded today as the first instance in which birth and death records and other demographic data were systematically used to describe the health of a population.

The valuable public health information contained in the Shattuck Report was slow to penetrate the consciousness of policymakers in Massachusetts. But the survey ultimately became an important factor in the establishment of Massachusetts' first state board of health in 1869, which in turn became a model for boards of health in numerous other states during the last three decades of the 19th century. Shattuck died in Boston on January 17, 1859.

Further Reading

Rosenkrantz, B. G. (1972). *Public health and the state: Changing views in Massachusetts, 1842–1936.* Cambridge, MA: Harvard University Press.

Schneider, D., & Lilienfeld, D. A. (2008). *Public health: The development of a discipline: From the age of Hippocrates to the Progressive Era.* Piscataway, NJ: Rutgers University Press.

John Snow (1813–1858)

*English physician, early anesthesiologist, and
founder of modern epidemiology*

John Snow was born at York, England, on March 15, 1813. The eldest son of a farmer with modest landholdings, Snow served a six-year apprenticeship as a youth to a surgeon in Newcastle-on-Tyne, then spent the next several years as a surgical assistant. In 1836 he enrolled at the Hunterian School of Medicine in London to continue his medical education. In 1838 he was admitted as a member of England's Royal College of Surgeons, and that same year he received his license from the Society of Apothecaries.

Snow opened his own medical practice in London in late 1838, but he continued to take advanced coursework in various medical specialties. He earned a doctorate of medicine from the University of London in 1844 and became a licentiate of the Royal College of Physicians in 1850.

Snow made his mark in the field of medicine in two different areas. In 1847 he developed an inhaler for use with anesthesia, an exciting new medical innovation of the day. Snow used his chloroform inhaler, which he designed based on his own scientific study of the effects of anesthesia on human physiology, on Queen Victoria during the delivery of two of her children. This widely publicized service, combined with Snow's published papers on anesthesiology in the late 1840s, made him one of England's acknowledged experts on the practice.

Snow's other major contribution to the world of medicine was to ascertain that cholera was a waterborne-disease. His scientific findings, based on London cholera epidemics of 1848–49 and 1853–54, launched the field of modern epidemiological research. It was during the first of these outbreaks that Snow first posited that cholera was caused by ingestion of tainted water rather than "miasmatic" air. When the second outbreak struck London, Snow offered convincing documentation for his theory that cholera was caused by sewage-contaminated water. Gathering data on cholera outbreak patterns in specific neighborhoods around London, Snow soon focused on a Broad Street water pump in South London. Wielding carefully compiled maps that showed that the heaviest concentrations of cholera events surrounded the Broad Street pump, he was able to convince local authorities to disable the water pump. The epidemic soon subsided, and Snow's place in medical history as the man who defeated cholera was secure. In the wake of his trailblazing epidemiological investigations, London and other population centers in Europe and the United States implemented new water protection regulations and sanitation systems that dramatically reduced cholera outbreaks.

Snow continued to practice medicine in London until the late 1850s, despite suffering from kidney disease and other health ailments. He suffered a debilitating stroke in 1858, however, and he died on June 16, 1858.

Further Reading

Johnson, S. (2006). *The ghost map: The story of London's most terrifying epidemic—and how it changed science, cities, and the modern world*. New York: Riverhead.

John Snow Archive and Research Companion. Retrieved from http://johnsnow .matrix.msu.edu/index.php

Jean-Andre Venel (1740–1791)

*Swiss founder of the world's first orthopedic institution
for the treatment of children with physical disabilities*

Jean-Andre Venel was born on May 28, 1740, in Morges, Switzerland, the son of a barber-surgeon. Venel's French Huguenot family had relocated to Switzerland in response to religious persecution in France. Venel was apprenticed to a local surgeon at the age of 16. He served in that capacity for six years before enrolling at the Royal College of Surgeons in Montpellier. Venel studied in Montpellier for a year but left before graduating, in all likelihood due to a lack of funding.

Venel moved on to the small town of Orbe, Switzerland, where he established a small medical practice. He went abroad on several occasions over the next few years to continue his medical studies, while also opening a local school for midwives. Venel's interest in orthopedics was sparked in the late 1770s, when he began caring for the son of a local minister who suffered from severe foot deformities, probably stemming from poliomyelitis. The boy spent a year under Venel's course of treatment, which included an ambitious regimen of massage, manipulation, and stretching exercises, and reportedly experienced considerable improvement in his condition.

This experience convinced Venel to make orthopedics the primary focus of his talents and energy. In 1780 he acquired a cluster of buildings in Orbe that had fallen into disrepair. After renovating the buildings he dedicated the complex, known as Canton de Vaud, to the care and treatment of children's skeletal deformities stemming from scoliosis, tuberculosis, poliomyelitis, and other maladies. It was the first such hospital in the world.

Venel's institute included a hospital, therapeutic baths, a classroom and occupational workshop for patients, as well as a department dedicated to the production of various braces, splints, and other treatment devices. His programs of therapy and rehabilitation, meanwhile, emphasized extensive use of braces and splints (individually crafted based on plaster molds of the deformities) as well as regular courses of massage and stretching. Venel also made a special effort to make the facility a pleasant environment for patients, adopting a paternal stance toward many of the children under his care.

Making extensive use of plaster molds to track physiological changes, Venel carefully recorded the progress of all patients at Canton de Vaud. These records, which included descriptions of all his therapeutic methods, further burnished his reputation as one of the pioneers of orthopedics. His institute, meanwhile, became a model for similar hospitals throughout Europe. Venel died of tuberculosis in 1791.

Further Reading

Peltier, L. F. (1993). *Orthopedics: A history and iconography.* San Francisco, CA: Norman.

Selman Waksman (1888–1973)

Ukrainian-born American bacteriologist who discovered streptomycin and many other antibiotics

Selman Abraham Waksman was born in the rural Ukrainian town of Novaya Priluka on July 22, 1888. In 1910 he earned his matriculation diploma from the Fifth Gymnasium in Odessa, Ukraine, and immigrated to the United States, following in the footsteps of a number of his relatives. He worked on a family farm in New Jersey for several years before enrolling at Rutgers College, where he earned a bachelor's degree in agriculture in 1915. One year later he earned his master's degree in science from Rutgers, devoting much of his energy to the study of soil bacteriology. In 1918 he earned a doctorate in biochemistry from the University of California, Berkeley.

After receiving his doctorate, Waksman returned to Rutgers, where he joined the university's bacteriology department. He was appointed associate professor in 1925 and professor in 1930, and in 1940 he was appointed head of Rutgers's Department of Microbiology. Throughout this period, Waksman engaged in intensive research into the antibacterial properties of soil bacteria. By the early 1940s his efforts, which were greatly aided by talented Rutgers colleagues like H. Boyd Woodruff and French biologist Rene Dubois, realized significant and tangible breakthroughs in combating deadly bacteria. Waksman and his staff developed a technique for identifying natural substances in soil with antibacterial properties, and they isolated a total of 18 "antibiotics" (a term coined by Waksman) using this system. The most momentous of these antibiotics were neomycin and streptomycin, the latter of which became the first antibiotic remedy for tuberculosis, one of the most feared of all diseases.

Waksman's discovery of streptomycin in 1944 gave him a pathway to great personal wealth, but although he patented and licensed streptomycin and other promising antibiotics that he found, he funneled much of his earnings back into Rutgers University. In 1951, in fact, Rutgers announced the establishment of a new Institute of Microbiology endowed and supported by Waksman's streptomycin patent royalties. The institute officially opened in 1954, two years after Waksman received the Nobel Prize in Physiology or Medicine for his discovery of streptomycin.

Waksman served as director of the Institute of Microbiology from 1954 to 1958, when he retired. The institute was formally renamed in his honor after his death in Woods Hole, Massachusetts, on August 16, 1973.

Further Reading

Rifkind, D., and Freeman, G. L. (2005). *The Nobel Prize winning discoveries in infectious diseases.* London and San Diego: Elsevier.

Waksman, S. A. (1954). *My life with the microbes.* New York: Simon and Schuster.

James Watson (1928–)

American co-leader of the research team that discovered the structure of the DNA molecule

James Dewey Watson was born on April 6, 1928, in Chicago, Illinois, to James D. Watson, a businessman, and Jean Mitchell. A brilliant young student, he earned a bachelor's degree in zoology from the University of Chicago at the age of 19. From there he earned a doctorate degree from Indiana University in the same subject in 1950. During this period, Watson also became involved in genetic research projects at Denmark's University of Copenhagen and Cold Spring Harbor Laboratory in New York State.

In 1951 Watson joined the staff at Cambridge University's Cavendish Laboratory, a leading center of biomolecular research. He quickly struck up a strong working relationship with fellow scientist Francis Crick, and for the next two years, the brilliant young researchers waged a campaign to unlock the mystery of the structure of DNA, the building blocks of all cellular organisms. In 1953 they solved the puzzle, documenting to the world that DNA molecules are shaped like a twisting three-dimensional double helix. This discovery, which they first trumpeted in the pages of the British science journal *Nature*, revolutionized research into genetics and opened the door to a host of new genetic modification techniques and areas of medical research.

In 1956 Watson became a professor of biology at Harvard University, a position he held for the next two decades. In 1962 Watson and Crick were awarded the Nobel Prize in Physiology or Medicine along with crystallographer Maurice Wilkins, whose X-ray images of DNA fibers proved invaluable in uncovering the double-helix structure of DNA. In the eventful year of 1968, Watson married Elizabeth Lewis, with whom he had two sons. That same year, he accepted the directorship of the Cold Spring Harbor Laboratory, which was revitalized as an international center of genetic research under his leadership.

In 1988 Watson joined the National Institute of Health's Human Genome Project, and in 1990 he was appointed director of the entire project, which sought to determine the chemical sequence of all DNA and map all genes in the human genome, or human species. This titanic international effort, completed in 2003, gave scientists the ability to study and understand the complete genetic blueprint for building a human being. Advocates say that this information will be of tremendous value to biomedical researchers seeking cures for thousands of hereditary disabilities and diseases.

Watson left the Human Genome Project in 1992 after it was up in running. In 1994 he became president of Cold Spring Harbor Laboratory, and in 2004 he was appointed chancellor of the institution. Watson retired from Cold Spring Harbor in 2007 after critical comments he made about the genetic qualities of African people sparked a firestorm of controversy.

Further Reading

Edelson, E. (2000). *Francis Crick and James Watson: And the building blocks of life.* New York: Oxford University Press.

Francis Crick Papers. National Library of Medicine, Profiles in Science. Retrieved from http://profiles.nlm.nih.gov/SC/Views/Exhibit/narrative/biographical.html

Watson, J. D. (1968). *The double helix: A personal account of the discovery of the structure of DNA.* New York: Atheneum.

Five

Annotated Data, Statistics, Tables, and Graphs

Many international, government, and private organizations collect data and compile statistics on people with disabilities, healthcare professionals, and facilities. They collect these data and statistics in order to: determine the demographic, health, economic, and social characteristics of the disabled; monitor and evaluate disability programs, regulations, and policies; and advocate for various disability groups and populations.

International Organizations

International organizations periodically collect multinational disability and healthcare data and statistics. For example, the World Health Organization (WHO), the directing and coordinating authority for health within the United Nations (UN) system, collects and disseminates disability and health statistics on its 193 member states. The Pan American Health Organization (PAHO), which works to improve the health and living standards of all of the countries of the Americas, collects health statistics on its 35 member nations. The Organisation for Economic Co-operation and Development (OECD), an international economic organization that brings together the governments of countries committed to democracy and the market economy, collects economic, healthcare, and social statistics on its 30 member nations, most of which are highly developed countries. The World Bank, which provides financial and technical assistance to 100 developing countries around the world, also collects data and statistics and publishes reports on various topics, such as disability in post-conflict countries, disability and its relationship to poverty, and disability and natural disasters.

Government Organizations

Government organizations often collect national disability and healthcare data and statistics. For example, in the United Kingdom, the National Health Service (NHS) and the Office for National Statistics (ONS) collect and publish disability and healthcare data and statistics on many topics. In Canada, the government organization Statistics Canada periodically conducts and publishes the results of large national surveys of disability, and the organization Health Canada publishes government guidelines and policies on disability.

In the United States, many federal government departments, as well as the various units within them, regularly collect various disability and healthcare data and statistics. At the cabinet level, the government departments that collect disability data and statistics include: U.S. Department of Commerce, U.S. Department of Education, U.S. Department of Health and Human Services (HHS), U.S. Department of Housing and Urban Development (HUD), U.S. Department of Justice, U.S. Department of Labor, and the U.S. Department of Veterans Affairs (VA).

Within the HHS, the nation's principal department for protecting the health of all Americans and providing essential human services, the following agencies, centers, and institutes collect disability and healthcare data and statistics: Agency for Healthcare Research and Quality (AHRQ); Centers for Disease Control and Prevention (CDC), which includes the National Center for Health Statistics (NCHS); Centers for Medicare and Medicaid Services (CMS); National Institutes of Health (NIH), which consists of 20 institutes and 7 centers; and the Substance Abuse and Mental Health Services Administration (SAMHSA).

Within the U.S. Department of Commerce, the U.S. Census Bureau annually conducts national surveys, some of which periodically measure the demographic, economic, and other characteristics of people with disability.

The Social Security Administration (SSA) is also an important source of national disability data. An independent government agency, the SSA administers the nation's Social Security programs. It provides benefits to millions of disabled workers and their family members. And each year, millions of individuals apply for benefits from the Supplemental Security Income (SSI) and Social Security Disability Insurance (SSDI) programs.

Private Organizations

Private organizations, including associations, research organizations, foundations, philanthropies, and academic institutions, also collect and disseminate a wide variety of disability and healthcare data and statistics. For example, in the United States, grouped by category, these organizations include: disease, injury, and condition associations (e.g., the Alzheimer's Association, American Cancer Society, American Heart Association); specific group and population associations (e.g., the AARP, American Association of People with Disabilities, National Rural Health Association); professional and trade associations (e.g., the American Hospital Association [AHA], American Medical Association [AMA], American Academy of Pediatrics); contract-research and policy organizations (e.g., the Brookings Institution, Mathematical Policy Research, RAND Corporation); foundations and philanthropies (e.g., the Commonwealth Fund, Henry J. Kaiser Family Foundation, and Robert Wood Johnson Foundation); survey research organizations (e.g., the Gallup Organization, Harris Interactive, National Opinion Research Organization [NORC]); and academic centers and university programs (e.g., Baylor College of Medicine's Center for Research on Women with Disabilities, University of Colorado's Coleman Institute for Cognitive Disabilities, Cornell University's Employment and Disability Institute).

Profile of People With Disability

Using data and statistics from various U.S. government and private organizations, this chapter presents a number of tables profiling the health and medical characteristics of people with disabilities, selected healthcare professionals (physicians, nurses, and others), and facilities (hospitals, and nursing homes).

Table 1 shows the estimated prevalence, or occurrence, of six types of disabilities in 2008, by age groups, for the civilian non-institutionalized population living in the United States. The statistics in the table are from the U.S. Census Bureau's 2008 American Community Survey (ACS), which is a large national sample survey designed to replace the Decennial Census long form.

The ACS defined disability based on six questions. A survey respondent was classified as having a disability if he or she or a proxy answered "yes" to one or more of the questions. Specifically, to determine hearing disability the respondent was asked: "Is this person deaf or does he/she have serious difficulty hearing?" The question to determine visual disability was: "Is this person blind or does he/she have serious difficulty seeing even when wearing glasses?" To determine cognitive disability, the question was: "Because of a physical, mental, or emotional condition, does this person have serious difficulty concentrating, remembering, or making decisions?" The question for ambulatory disability was: "Does this person have serious difficulty walking or climbing stairs?" For self-care disability, the question was worded: "Does this person have difficulty dressing or bathing?" Finally, independent living disability results were determined through the following question: "Because of a physical, mental, or emotional condition, does this person have difficulty doing errands alone such as visiting a doctor's office or shopping?"

In 2008, the overall estimated percentage of people with a disability for all ages in the United States was 12.1%. A total of 36,169,200 of the country's 299,852,800 individuals were estimated to have one or more disabilities. Among the six types of disabilities measured by the survey, the highest overall occurrence rate was for ambulatory disability (6.9%), while the lowest rate was for visual disability (2.3%).

By age group, the overall percentage of children 5 to 15 years of age with a disability in the country was 5.1% (an estimated 2,265,800 individuals). The highest occurrence rate for this age group was for cognitive disability (3.9%), while the lowest rate was for hearing and ambulatory disability (0.7% each). The percentage of people 16 to 20 years of age with a disability was 5.6% (1,233,700 individuals). The highest occurrence rate was for cognitive disability (3.8%), while the lowest rate was for hearing disability (0.7%). The percentage of people 21 to 64 years of age with a

Table 1 Number and Percentage of the Occurrence of Disability Among Non-Institutionalized People by Age Group—United States, 2008

Disability Type	Age Group									
	5–15 Years		16–20 Years		21–64 Years		65–74 Years		75 Years and Older	
	Number	Percent	Number	Percent	Number	Percent	Number	Percent	Number	Percent
Visual	342,600	0.8	213,000	1.0	3,314,200	1.9	925,200	4.6	1,939,800	11.2
Hearing	300,900	0.7	150,300	0.7	3,990,400	2.3	1,866,300	9.4	3,988,300	23.1
Ambulatory	300,900	0.7	192,600	0.9	9,498,200	5.4	3,342,000	16.8	5,870,000	33.9
Cognitive	1,729,100	3.9	850,400	3.8	7,213,700	4.1	1,121,100	5.6	2,548,600	14.7
Self-Care	395,600	0.9	143,700	0.7	3,240,900	1.8	974,300	4.9	2,441,200	14.1
Independent Living	—	—	418,200	1.9	6,289,600	3.6	1,732,000	8.7	4,655,500	26.9
Any Disability	2,265,800	5.1	1,233,700	5.6	18,312,900	10.4	5,287,300	26.6	8,913,300	51.5

Source: U.S. Census Bureau, American Community Survey (ACS), Erickson, W., Lee, C., & von Schræder, S. (2009). *2008 disability status report: United States.* Ithaca, NY: Cornell University Rehabilitation Research and Training Center on Disability Demographics and Statistics. Available at http://www.disabilitystatistics.org

disability was 10.4% (18,312,900 individuals). The highest occurrence rate was for ambulatory disability (5.4%), while the lowest rate was for self care disability (1.8%). The percentage of people 65 to 74 years of age with a disability was 26.6% (5,287,300 individuals). The highest occurrence rate was for ambulatory disability (16.8%), while the lowest rate was for visual disability (4.6%). Lastly, the percentage of people 75 years of age and older was 51.5% (8,913,300 individuals). The highest occurrence rate was for ambulatory disability (33.9%), while the lowest rate was for visual disability (11.2%).

It should be noted that an important limitation of the survey is that it excludes individuals in institutions such as nursing homes, chronic disease, mental, and veterans' hospitals, many of whom have a higher occurrence of disability than the general population.

Table 2 shows the estimated percentage of people 21 to 64 years of age with disabilities in 2008, ranked by state and the District of Columbia in the United States. The statistics in the table are also from the U.S. Census Bureau's 2008 ACS.

In 2008, the overall estimated percentage of people 21 to 64 years of age with disabilities in the United States was 10.4%. Geographically, the five states with the highest percentages of the disabled were: West Virginia (18.7%); Arkansas (16.6%); Kentucky (16.4%); Mississippi (16.3%); and Oklahoma (16.3%). In contrast, the five states with the lowest percentages were: Hawaii (7.2%); New Jersey (7.7%); Utah (7.9%); Minnesota (7.9%); and Colorado (8.3%).

Table 2   Percentage of People 21–64 Years of Age With Disabilities Ranked by State and the District of Columbia—United States, 2008

Rank	State	Percent
1	West Virginia	18.7
2	Arkansas	16.6
3	Kentucky	16.4
4	Mississippi	16.3

(Continued)

Table 2 (Continued)

Rank	State	Percent
5	Oklahoma	16.3
6	Alabama	15.1
7	Louisiana	13.8
8	Tennessee	13.6
9	Maine	13.4
10	Alaska	12.9
11	Vermont	12.8
12	South Carolina	12.7
13	Missouri	12.6
14	New Mexico	12.4
15	Montana	12.0
16	Wyoming	11.9
17	Michigan	11.8
18	North Carolina	11.7
19	Indiana	11.6
20	Ohio	11.6
21	Pennsylvania	11.3
22	Oregon	11.2
23	Idaho	10.9
24	Rhode Island	10.9
25	Delaware	10.8
26	Kansas	10.8
27	Arizona	10.7
28	Texas	10.6
29	Washington	10.6

Rank	State	Percent
30	Georgia	10.5
31	Florida	10.0
32	New Hampshire	9.7
33	Iowa	9.6
34	Massachusetts	9.3
35	New York	9.1
36	Wisconsin	9.1
37	District of Columbia	8.9
38	Virginia	8.9
39	Nevada	8.7
40	South Dakota	8.7
41	Maryland	8.6
42	North Dakota	8.6
43	California	8.5
44	Connecticut	8.5
45	Illinois	8.4
46	Nebraska	8.4
47	Colorado	8.3
48	Minnesota	7.9
49	Utah	7.9
50	New Jersey	7.7
51	Hawaii	7.2
Total	**United States**	**10.4**

Source: U.S. Census Bureau, American Community Survey (ACS), Erickson, W., Lee, C., & von Schrader, S. (2009). *2008 disability status report: United States*. Ithaca, NY: Cornell University Rehabilitation Research and Training Center on Disability Demographics and Statistics. Available at http://www.disabilitystatistics.org

Table 3 shows the estimated occurrence of the most common medical causes of disability in 2005, for the adult 18 years of age and older, civilian, non-institutionalized population living in the United States. The statistics in the table are from the U.S. Census Bureau's Survey of Income and Program Participation (SIPP), a large national longitudinal panel survey.

To identify the main medical causes of disability, the SIPP respondents were asked if they had difficulty doing a number of activities because of a physical or mental condition. If they responded "yes" to having difficulty with any of the activities, one or more selected impairments, or limitation in the ability to work around the house or at a job or business, they were considered to have a disability. The respondents were then given a list of medical conditions and asked to identify the main condition that caused their disability.

In 2005, an estimated 45,070,000 individuals—21.8% of the adult population—had a disability in the United States. The survey also found

Table 3   Main Cause of Disability Among Non-Institutionalized U.S. Adults With Self-Reported Disabilities—United States, 2005

Condition	Estimated Population	Percent of Adults
Arthritis or Rheumatism	8,552,000	19.0
Back or Spine Problems	7,589,000	16.8
Heart Trouble	2,988,000	6.6
Lung or Respiratory Problem	2,224,000	4.9
Mental or Emotional Problem	2,203,000	4.9
Diabetes	2,012,000	4.5
Deafness or Hearing Problem	1,908,000	4.2
Stiffness or Deformity of Limbs/Extremities	1,627,000	3.6
Blindness or Vision Problem	1,460,000	3.2
Stroke	1,076,000	2.4
Cancer	1,007,000	2.2

Condition	Estimated Population	Percent of Adults
Broken Bone/Fracture	969,000	2.1
High Blood Pressure	857,000	1.9
Mental Retardation	671,000	1.5
Senility/Dementia/ Alzheimer's Disease	546,000	1.2
Head or Spinal Cord Injury	516,000	1.1
Learning Disability	492,000	1.1
Kidney Problems	411,000	0.9
Stomach/Digestive Problems	358,000	0.8
Paralysis of Any Kind	257,000	0.6
Epilepsy	256,000	0.6
Hernia or Rupture	229,000	0.5
Cerebral Palsy	223,000	0.5
Missing Limbs/Extremities	209,000	0.5
Alcohol or Drug Problems	201,000	0.4
Tumor/Cyst/Growth	123,000	0.3
Thyroid Problems	110,000	0.2
AIDS or AIDS-Related Conditions	90,000	0.2
Speech Disorder	72,000	0.2
Other	5,830,000	12.9
Total	**45,070,000**	**100.0**

Source. Brault, M. W., Hootman, J., & Helmick, C. G. (2009). Prevalence and most common causes of disability among adults—United States, 2005. *Morbidity and Mortality Weekly Report (MMWR)* 58(16), 425, Table 2. Available at http://www.cdc.gov/mmwr/preview/ mmwrhtml/mm5816a2.htm

that women reported a significantly higher occurrence of disabilities (24.4%) compared to men (19.1%) at all ages. For both genders, the occurrence of disability doubled in successive age groups (18 to 44 years, 45 to 64 years, and 65 years of age or older).

The five most common reported medical causes of disability were: arthritis or rheumatism (affecting an estimated 8,552,000 adults, or 19.0% of adults); back or spine problems (7,589,000, 16.8%); heart trouble (2,988,000, 6.6%); lung or respiratory problem (2,224,000, 4.9%); and mental or emotional problem (2,203,000, 4.9%).

Table 4 shows the estimated percentage of individuals within the civilian, non-institutionalized population of the United States with an activity limitation caused by a chronic health condition in 2006. The statistics in the table are from the National Center for Health Statistics' (NCHS) National Health Interview Survey (NHIS), a large annual household survey that monitors the health of the country's population through the collection and analysis of data on a broad range of topics, including the occurrence of illnesses, injuries, and activity limitations.

To identify people with disability, the NHIS respondents were asked several questions. First, the NHIS asked if the respondent or a family member had a chronic health condition. If the respondent answered yes, the NHIS asked whether the chronic condition caused a limitation of daily

Table 4   Percentage of Non-Institutionalized Persons Reporting an Activity Limitation Caused by Chronic Conditions, by Selected Characteristics—United States, 2006

Age	Percent of Persons
Under 5 Years	3.9
5–17 Years	8.6
18–24 Years	4.1
25–44 Years	6.0
45–54 Years	12.5
55–64 Years	20.0
65–74 Years	24.8
75 Years and Over	41.6

Gender	
Male	11.6
Female	11.5
Race	
White Only	11.4
Black Only	14.1
American Indian or Alaska Native Only	18.4
Asian Only	6.6
Percent of Poverty Level	
Below 100%	22.1
100%–Less Than 200%	16.4
200% or More	8.7
Geographic Region	
Northeast	11.3
Midwest	12.5
South	11.9
West	10.5
Location of Residence	
Within an MSA	11.1
Outside an MSA	14.2

Source: National Center for Health Statistics. (2009). Health, United States, 2008, Table 58, p. 284. Available at http://www.cdc.gov/nchs/data/hus/hus08.pdf

Note: MSA = Metropolitan Statistical Area.

activities. If the respondent indicated that the condition limited daily activities, he or she was considered to have a disability.

The 2006 survey showed that the percentage of persons with activity limitations caused by a chronic health condition generally tended to increase with age. For example, 3.9% of children less than 5 years of age had an activity limitation, while 41.6% of individuals 75 years of age and over had an activity limitation. However, among school-age children

5 to 17 years of age, 8.6% had an activity limitation. For this group, speech problems, learning disabilities, and attention deficit/hyperactivity disorder (ADHD or ADD) were the most frequently reported causes of activity limitation.

In terms of gender, the percentage of activity limitations for males (11.6%) and females (11.5%) were very similar. By race, American Indians or Alaska Natives reported the highest percentage (18.4%) of activity limitations, while Asians reported the lowest percentage (6.6%).

Poverty level was inversely associated with activity limitations. Individuals living in poverty were more than twice (22.1%) as likely to report activity limitations as those with a family income above twice the poverty level (8.7%).

Geographically, the Census Bureau's Midwest Region (consisting of 12 states) of the country reported the highest percentage (12.5%) of individuals with activity limitations, while the West Region (13 states) reported the lowest percentage (10.5%). Individuals residing outside of a Metropolitan Statistical Area (MSA) had the highest percentage (14.2%) of activity limitations, while those living within a MSA—large urbanized areas with high population densities at its core and in surrounding towns and counties—had the lowest percentage (11.1%).

Table 5 shows the estimated percentage of adults among the civilian, non-institutionalized population of the United States reporting vision and hearing limitations in 2007. The statistics in the table are also from the NHIS.

To measure vision problems, the NHIS respondents were asked, "Do you have any trouble seeing, even when wearing glasses or contact lenses?" They were also asked, "Are you blind or unable to see at all?" In this table, "any trouble seeing" and blindness were combined into one category. To measure hearing problems, the respondents were asked, "Which statement best describes your hearing without a hearing aid: good, a little trouble, a lot of trouble, or deaf?" In this table, "a lot of trouble" and deaf were combined into one category.

The 2007 survey showed that vision and hearing problems varied greatly by gender. In terms of vision problems, women consistently reported higher percentages of trouble seeing than men, even with glasses or contact lenses. These findings applied to every age category (18 to 44 years, 45 to 54 years, 55 to 64 years, 65 to 74 years, 75 years and over).

Table 5 Percentage of Non-Institutionalized Adults 18 Years of Age and Older Reporting Vision and Hearing Limitations, by Selected Characteristics—United States, 2007

Characteristic	Any Trouble Seeing, Even With Glasses or Contacts	A Lot of Trouble, Hearing or Deaf
Gender		
Male	8.5	3.1
Female	11.2	1.6
Gender and Age		
Male:		
18–44 Years	5.6	0.5
45–54 Years	10.6	1.5
55–64 Years	10.0	4.7
65–74 Years	11.4	7.0
75 Years and Over	17.2	16.9
Female:		
18–44 Years	8.1	0.3
45–54 Years	13.9	1.0
55–64 Years	14.2	1.3
65–74 Years	14.2	2.8
75 Years and Over	18.4	11.1
Race		
White Only	9.9	2.4
Black Only	10.5	1.2
American Indian or Alaska Native Only	18.0	3.8
Asian Only	5.7	—

(Continued)

Table 5 (Continued)

Characteristic	Any Trouble Seeing, Even With Glasses or Contacts	A Lot of Trouble, Hearing or Deaf
Education		
No High School Diploma or GED	13.4	4.1
High School Diploma or GED	10.9	2.8
Some College or More	9.2	1.9
Percent of Poverty Level		
Below 100%	15.0	3.4
100% to Less Than 200%	13.0	2.8
200% or More	8.4	2.0
Geographic Region		
Northeast	8.1	1.7
Midwest	10.3	2.3
South	10.1	2.5
West	10.5	2.4
Location of Residence		
Within an MSA	9.6	2.1
Outside an MSA	11.4	3.3

Source: National Center for Health Statistics. (2009). *Health, United States, 2008,* Table 59, pp. 287–288. Available at http://www.cdc.gov/nchs/data/hus/hus08.pdf

Note: MSA = Metropolitan Statistical Area.

By race, American Indians/Alaska Natives reported the highest percentage (18.0%) of vision trouble, while Asians reported the lowest percentage (5.7%).

Education and poverty level were both inversely associated with vision trouble. Among adults with the lowest education level (no high school diploma or GED), 13.4% reported vision trouble. Among adults with at least some college, 9.2% reported vision trouble. Adults living in poverty had the highest percentage (15.0%) of vision trouble, while those who were living at two times or more above the poverty level had the lowest percentage (8.4%).

Geographically, adults in the West Region of the country had the highest percentage (10.5%) of vision trouble, while the Northeast Region had the lowest percentage (8.1%). Adults residing outside a MSA reported the highest percentage (11.4%) of vision trouble, while those residing within a MSA reported the lowest percentage (9.6%).

In terms of hearing problems, men across all age categories consistently reported higher percentages of trouble hearing or being deaf than women. By race, American Indians/Alaska Natives had the highest percentage (3.8%) of hearing trouble, while African Americans registered the lowest incidence of hearing trouble (1.2%).

Education and poverty level were both inversely associated with hearing trouble. Adults with the lowest education level had the highest incidence of hearing trouble (4.1%), whereas only 1.9% of adults at the highest education level reported hearing trouble. Adults living in poverty had the highest incidence (3.4%) of hearing trouble, while those living at two times or more above the poverty level had hearing trouble at a much lower rate (2.0%).

Geographically, adults in the South Region of the county had the highest percentage (2.5%) of hearing trouble, while the Northeast Region had the lowest percentage (1.7%). Adults residing outside a MSA reported the highest percentage (3.3%) of hearing trouble, while those residing within a MSA reported the lowest percentage (2.1%).

Table 6 shows the number and percentage of children and youths with disabilities who were served under the Individuals with Disabilities Education Act (IDEA) Part B in the United States in 2007. The statistics in the table are from the U.S. Department of Education, as published in the U.S. Census Bureau's *The 2010 Statistical Abstract: The National Data Book*.

The IDEA requires all of the states in the country to collect data about the number of children and youths ages 6 to 21 with disabilities receiving special education and related services.

In 2007, a total of 6,007,800 children and youths were reported to have a disability in the United States. The five most frequently reported disabilities were: specific learning disabilities (2,620,200 children and youths, 43.6%); speech or language impairments (1,154,200, 19.2%); other health impairments (631,200, 10.5%); mental retardation (498,200, 8.3%); and emotional disturbance (440,200, 7.3%).

Table 6   Number and Percentage of Children and Youths With
Disabilities Served Under the Individuals with Disabilities
Education Act (IDEA) Part B—United States, 2007

Disability	Number of Children and Youths	Percent of Children and Youths
Specific Learning Disabilities	2,620,200	43.6
Speech or Language Impairments	1,154,200	19.2
Mental Retardation	498,200	8.3
Emotional Disturbance	440,200	7.3
Multiple Disabilities	132,600	2.2
Hearing Impairments	72,200	1.2
Orthopedic Impairments	60,500	1.0
Other Health Impairments	631,200	10.5
Visual Impairments	26,400	0.4
Autism	258,300	4.3
Deaf-Blind	1,400	0.0
Traumatic Brain Injury	23,900	0.4
Developmental Delay	88,600	1.5
Total	**6,007,800**	**100.0**

Source: U.S. Department of Education, Office of Special Education. In U.S. Census Bureau (2009), *The 2010 statistical abstract: The national data book,* Table 183. Available at http://www .census.gov/compendia/statab/2010/tables/10s0183

Table 7 shows the number and percentage of Social Security Disability Insurance (SSDI) program beneficiaries by medical diagnostic group in the United States in December 2008. The statistics in the table are from the Social Security Administration Disabled Beneficiaries and Dependents Master Beneficiary Record file, as published in the Social Security Administration's *Annual Statistical Report on the Social Security Disability Insurance Program, 2008.*

Table 7 Number and Percentage of Social Security Disability Insurance (SSDI) Beneficiaries by Medical Diagnostic Group—United States, December 2008

Medical Diagnostic Group	Number	Percent
Congenital Anomalies	24,740	0.3
Endocrine, Nutritional, and Metabolic Diseases	291,050	3.4
Infectious and Parasitic Diseases	123,971	1.5
Injuries	334,666	3.9
Retardation	761,989	8.9
Other Mental Disorders	2,342,293	27.5
Neoplasms (Cancers)	228,035	2.7
Blood and Blood-Forming Organ Diseases	21,649	0.3
Circulatory System Diseases	693,339	8.1
Digestive System Diseases	121,781	1.4
Genitourinary System Diseases	130,900	1.5
Musculoskeletal-Connective Tissue Diseases	2,082,594	24.4
Nervous System and Sense Organ Diseases	805,884	9.4
Respiratory System Diseases	233,208	2.7
Skin and Subcutaneous Tissue Diseases	18,654	0.2
Other	19,188	0.2
Unknown	294,223	3.5
Total	**8,528,164**	**100.0**

Source. Social Security Administration. (2009). *Annual statistical report on the Social Security Disability Insurance program, 2008*, Table 6, p. 25. Washington, DC: Author. Available at http://www.ssa.gov/policy/docs/statcomps/di_asp/2008/di_asr08.pdf

The Social Security Administration uses a strict definition of disability. Its definition is based on an individual's inability to work. Specifically, an individual is only considered disabled if: the individual cannot do work that he or she did before; Social Security determines that the individual cannot adjust to other work because of his or her medical condition(s); and the individual's disability has lasted or is expected to last for at least one year or to result in death. No benefits are payable for partial disability or for short-term disability.

The SSDI program provides wage replacement income for workers who paid Social Security taxes who later become disabled (as defined by the SSA). SSDI benefits are paid to eligible disabled workers, disabled widow(er)s, or disabled adult children.

In December 2008, there were a total of 8,528,164 SSDI beneficiaries in the United States. The five most frequent medical diagnostic groups on which disability was based were: other mental disorders (2,342,293 beneficiaries, 27.5%); musculoskeletal-connective tissue diseases (2,082,594 beneficiaries, 24.4%); nervous system and sense organ diseases (805,884 beneficiaries, 9.4%); retardation (781,989 beneficiaries, 8.9%); and circulatory system diseases (693,339 beneficiaries, 8.1%).

Profile of Healthcare Professionals

Table 8 shows the number of active physicians and physician-to-population ratios in the United States in 2007. The statistics in the table are from the American Medical Association (AMA), as published in the U.S. Census Bureau's *The 2010 Statistical Abstract: The National Data Book*.

Active physicians include federal and non-federal physicians who: are working more than 20 hours per week; are not in graduate medical training; are residing in one of the 50 states or the District of Columbia; and report their primary specialty or combination of specialties as recognized by the American Medical Association. Physicians who are retired, semi-retired, or otherwise inactive are excluded.

Although physicians constitute a small part of the medical work force, they control the greatest amount of resources and make the critical decisions of admitting and discharging hospital patients, diagnosing illness, and conceptualizing overall medical treatment plans. Physicians play a vital role in treating people with disabilities, and they evaluate and certify the degree of physical or mental impairment(s) of individuals to determine their eligibility to receive disability benefits.

Table 8   Number of Active Physicians and Physician-to-Population Ratios (per 100,000 Residents) Ranked by State and the District of Columbia—United States, 2007

Rank	State	Number of Physicians	Physician/ Population Ratio
1	District of Columbia	4,745	807
2	Massachusetts	30,335	469
3	Maryland	23,680	421
4	New York	76,025	396
5	Connecticut	13,135	376
6	Rhode Island	3,955	376
7	Vermont	2,374	374
8	Hawaii	4,049	317
9	New Jersey	27,373	316
10	Pennsylvania	37,924	305
11	Minnesota	15,194	293
12	Illinois	35,932	280
13	Maine	3,662	278
14	New Hampshire	3,607	275
15	Oregon	10,253	274
16	Virginia	21,132	274
17	Washington	17,413	270
18	California	97,743	269
19	Ohio	30,615	267
20	Tennessee	16,206	264
21	Louisiana	11,487	263

(Continued)

Table 8 (Continued)

Rank	State	Number of Physicians	Physician/ Population Ratio
22	Colorado	12,576	260
23	Wisconsin	14,507	259
24	North Carolina	22,987	254
25	Delaware	2,163	251
26	Michigan	25,146	250
27	Florida	45,110	248
28	Missouri	14,462	246
29	Nebraska	4,342	245
30	New Mexico	4,785	244
31	North Dakota	1,559	244
32	Kentucky	9,843	232
33	West Virginia	4,201	232
34	South Carolina	10,122	230
35	Alaska	1,556	228
36	Kansas	6,181	223
37	Montana	2,110	221
38	South Dakota	1,743	219
39	Alabama	10,094	218
40	Georgia	20,708	217
41	Indiana	13,745	217
42	Texas	51,080	214
43	Arizona	13,321	210
44	Utah	5,553	208
45	Arkansas	5,758	203
46	Iowa	5,647	189
47	Nevada	4,796	188

Rank	State	Number of Physicians	Physician/ Population Ratio
48	Wyoming	965	184
49	Mississippi	5,196	178
50	Oklahoma	6,260	173
51	Idaho	2,526	169
Total	**United States**	**816,727**	**271**

Source: American Medical Association, *Physician characteristics and distribution in the U.S.* [annual]. In U.S. Census Bureau, *The 2010 statistical abstract: The national data bank,* Table 159. Available at: http://www.census.gov/compendia/statab

In 2007, there were an estimated 816,727 active physicians in the United States. The five states with the greatest number of physicians were California (97,743), New York (76,025), Texas (51,080), Florida (45,110), and Pennsylvania (37,924). In contrast, the five states with the fewest number of physicians were Wyoming (965), Alaska (1,556), North Dakota (1,559), South Dakota (1,743), and Montana (2,110).

Because states vary greatly in geographic size and population, physician-to-population ratios are often used to measure overall access to medical care. It is assumed that the greater the number of physicians to a standard unit of population (in this case 100,000 residents) the greater the access to care.

The overall physician-to-population ratio for the United States was 271 physicians per 100,000 residents. The five locations with the highest physician-to-population ratios were the District of Columbia (807), Massachusetts (469), Maryland (421), New York (396), and Connecticut (376). In contrast, the five states with the lowest ratios were Idaho (169), Oklahoma (173), Mississippi (178), Wyoming (184), and Nevada (188).

Table 9 shows the number of registered nurses (RNs) and nurse-to-population ratios in the United States in 2007. The statistics in the table are from the U.S. Bureau of Labor Statistics, as published in the U.S. Census Bureau's *The 2010 Statistical Abstract: The National Data Book.*

Registered nurses are responsible for the nature and quality of all nursing care patients receive, supervising practical nurses and other health personnel involved in providing patient care, and following the

Table 9 Number of Nurses and Nurse-to-Population Ratios (per 100,000 Residents) Ranked by State and the District of Columbia—United States, 2007

Rank	State	Number of Nurses	Nurse/Population Ratio
1	District of Columbia	8,110	1,380
2	South Dakota	9,670	1,215
3	Massachusetts	78,280	1,210
4	North Dakota	7,000	1,097
5	Maine	13,850	1,053
6	Minnesota	52,690	1,017
7	Pennsylvania	126,370	1,017
8	Nebraska	17,870	1,010
9	Rhode Island	10,600	1,007
10	Ohio	114,920	1,001
11	Connecticut	34,690	994
12	Iowa	29,550	990
13	Delaware	8,420	977
14	New Hampshire	12,730	970
15	Missouri	56,290	958
16	West Virginia	16,970	938
17	Kentucky	39,120	923
18	Alabama	42,180	912
19	Vermont	5,660	912
20	New Jersey	78,510	907
21	Wisconsin	50,690	905
22	Louisiana	39,090	894

Rank	State	Number of Nurses	Nurse/Population Ratio
23	Tennessee	54,960	894
24	North Carolina	80,090	886
25	Maryland	48,840	869
26	Mississippi	25,350	868
27	Kansas	24,070	867
28	Indiana	54,770	864
29	New York	166,990	859
30	Michigan	84,480	841
31	Florida	118,180	814
32	Illinois	104,130	812
33	Wyoming	4,250	812
34	Oregon	29,700	795
35	South Carolina	35,040	795
36	Arkansas	21,920	774
37	Washington	49,910	774
38	Colorado	36,850	761
39	Alaska	5,150	756
40	Hawaii	9,620	753
41	Virginia	57,740	750
42	Montana	7,160	748
43	Oklahoma	25,700	712
44	Texas	157,870	662
45	Georgia	62,230	653
46	Idaho	9,600	642

(Continued)

Table 9 (Continued)

Rank	State	Number of Nurses	Nurse/Population Ratio
47	California	233,200	641
48	Utah	16,670	625
49	New Mexico	11,400	580
50	Nevada	14,670	574
51	Arizona	34,580	544
Total	**United States**	**2,468,340**	**819**

Source: U.S. Bureau of Labor Statistics, Occupational Employment Statistics, Occupational Employment and Wages. *May 2007 wage and employment statistics.* In U.S. Census Bureau, *The 2010 statistical abstract: The national data book,* Table 159. Available at: http://www .census.gov/compendia/statab

instructions of physicians regarding patient care. Registered nurses are the largest single group of health workers in the United States.

In 2007, there were an estimated 2,468,340 registered nurses in the United States. The five states with the greatest number of registered nurses were California (233,000), New York (166,990), Texas (157,870), Florida (148,180), and Pennsylvania (126,370). In contrast, the five states with the fewest number of nurses were Wyoming (4,250), Alaska (5,150), Vermont (5,660), North Dakota (7,000), and Montana (7,160).

The overall nurse-to-population ratio for the United States was 819 nurses per 100,000 residents. The five locations with the highest nurse-to-population ratios were the District of Columbia (1,380), South Dakota (1,215), Massachusetts (1,210), North Dakota (1,097), and Maine (1,053). In contrast, the five states with the lowest ratios were Arizona (544), Nevada (574), New Mexico (580), Utah (625), and California (641).

Table 10 shows the estimated number of employees in selected healthcare occupations working in the United States in 2007. The occupations are divided into two major categories: healthcare practitioner and technical occupations, and healthcare support occupations. The statistics in the table are from the U.S. Bureau of Labor Statistics, as published in the National Center for Health Statistics' *Health, United States, 2008.*

Table 10   Number of Employees in Selected Healthcare
Occupations—United States, 2007

Occupation Title	Number
Healthcare Practitioner and Technical Occupations	
Audiologists	11,360
Cardiovascular Technologists and Technicians	46,980
Dental Hygienists	168,600
Diagnostic Medical Sonographers	46,770
Dietetic Technicians	24,540
Dietitians and Nutritionists	52,800
Emergency Medical Technicians and Paramedics	201,200
Licensed Practical and Licensed Vocational Nurse	719,240
Nuclear Medicine Technologists	20,410
Occupational Therapists	91,920
Opticians, Dispensing	62,420
Pharmacists	253,110
Pharmacy Technicians	301,950
Physical Therapists	161,850
Physician Assistants	67,160
Psychiatric Technicians	60,690
Radiation Therapists	14,620
Radiologic Technologists and Technicians	200,370
Recreational Therapists	23,240

(Continued)

Table 10 (Continued)

Occupation Title	Number
Registered Nurses	2,468,340
Respiratory Therapists	101,180
Respiratory Therapy Technicians	17,610
Speech-Language Pathologists	103,810
Healthcare Support Occupations	
Dental Assistants	283,680
Home Health Aides	834,580
Massage Therapies	45,920
Medical Assistants	434,540
Medical Equipment Preparers	43,790
Medical Transcriptionists	86,990
Nursing Aides, Orderlies, and Attendants	1,390,260
Occupational Therapist Aides	7,640
Occupational Therapist Assistants	25,130
Pharmacy Aides	49,630
Physical Therapist Aides	43,350
Physical Therapist Assistants	59,120
Psychiatric Aides	58,310

Source: National Center for Health Statistics. *Health United States, 2008,* Table 112, p. 398. Available at: http://www.cdc.gov/nchs/data/hus/hus08.pdf

In 2007, the five leading healthcare occupations in the United States were registered nurses (2,468,340); nursing aides, orderlies, and attendants (1,390,260); home health aides (834,580); licensed practical and licensed vocational nurses (719,240); and medical assistants (434,540). In contrast, the occupations supporting the smallest number of workers were occupational therapist aides (7,640); audiologists (11,360); radiation therapists (14,620); respiratory therapy technicians (17,610); and nuclear medicine technologists (20,410).

Profile of Healthcare Facilities

Table 11 shows the estimated number and percentage of workers employed by type of health service industry in the United States in 2008. The statistics in the table are from the U.S. Bureau of Labor Statistics, as published in the U.S. Census Bureau's *The 2010 Statistical Abstract: The National Data Book*.

In 2008, an estimated total of 15,819,000 workers were employed in health service industries in the United States. The five largest employers

Table 11   Number and Percentage of Workers Employed by Type of Health Service Industry—United States, 2008

Industry	Number	Percent
Ambulatory Healthcare Services		
Offices of Physicians	2,266,000	14.3
Offices of Dentists	819,000	5.2
Offices of Other Health Practitioners	629,000	4.0
Medical and Diagnostic Laboratories	219,000	1.4
Home Healthcare Services	958,000	6.0
Hospitals		
Community Hospitals	4,351,000	27.5
Psychiatric and Substance Abuse Hospitals	102,000	0.6
Other Hospitals	189,000	1.2

(Continued)

Table 11 (Continued)

Industry	Number	Percent
Nursing and Residential Care Facilities		
Nursing Care Facilities	1,614,000	10.2
Other	4,672,000	29.6
Total	**15,819,000**	**100.0**

Source: U.S. Bureau of Labor Statistics. Quarterly Census of Employment and Wages, 2008. In U.S. Census Bureau, *The 2010 statistical abstract: The national data book,* Table 156. Available at: http://www.census.gov/compendia/statab/2010/tables/10s0156.pdf

in the country were community hospitals (employing 4,351,000 workers, 27.5% of the industry total); offices of physicians (2,266,000 workers, 14.3%); nursing care facilities (1,614,000 workers, 10.2%); home healthcare services (958,000 workers, 6.0%); and offices of dentists (819,000 workers, 5.2%).

Table 12 shows the number of community hospital beds, ranked by state and inpatient admissions, across the United States in 2007. The statistics in the table are from the American Hospital Association's annual survey, as published in the *AHA Hospital Statistics, 2009.*

Community hospitals are defined as all nonfederal, short-term general, and other special hospitals that are open to the general public. They include academic medical centers, other teaching hospitals, and rehabilitation hospitals. Other hospitals, such as veterans' hospitals, prison hospitals, and college infirmaries, are excluded. Community hospitals are multipurpose institutions that provide inpatient and outpatient diagnostic and therapeutic medical services, conduct medical research, train healthcare practitioners, provide laboratories and other medical facilities, and sponsor health education and preventive healthcare programs. These hospitals play a vital role in providing medical care and preventive healthcare services to people with disabilities.

In 2007, there were 4,897 community hospitals equipped with 800,892 setup and staffed beds. That same year, community hospitals in the

Table 12 Number of Community Hospital Beds Ranked by State and the District of Columbia and Inpatient Admissions— United States, 2007

Rank	State	Beds	Admissions
1	California	69,325	3,276,372
2	New York	62,367	2,540,711
3	Texas	58,192	2,468,109
4	Florida	51,648	2,387,525
5	Pennsylvania	39,728	1,880,382
6	Illinois	34,560	1,606,241
7	Ohio	32,866	1,542,176
8	Georgia	25,483	963,583
9	Michigan	25,396	1,204,263
10	North Carolina	23,158	1,027,909
11	Tennessee	21,688	969,763
12	New Jersey	21,544	1,084,226
13	Missouri	18,454	833,114
14	Indiana	17,055	690,866
15	Virginia	16,895	787,319
16	Massachusetts	16,496	842,417
17	Minnesota	15,809	635,133
18	Louisiana	15,516	630,873
19	Alabama	15,682	696,131
20	Kentucky	14,423	611,689
21	Wisconsin	13,981	613,356

(Continued)

Table 12 (Continued)

Rank	State	Beds	Admissions
22	Mississippi	12,712	417,929
23	Arizona	12,157	675,216
24	South Carolina	12,032	518,994
25	Maryland	11,743	698,057
26	Washington	11,315	574,169
27	Oklahoma	10,862	453,977
28	Iowa	10,515	368,272
29	Kansas	10,079	325,255
30	Colorado	9,708	425,959
31	Arkansas	9,502	366,452
32	Connecticut	7,483	396,895
33	Nebraska	7,468	214,628
34	West Virginia	7,436	286,892
35	Oregon	6,841	347,089
36	Nevada	5,051	244,187
37	Utah	4,584	223,971
38	South Dakota	4,245	99,931
39	Montana	4,002	106,860
40	District of Columbia	3,418	136,488
41	New Mexico	3,696	170,081
42	Maine	3,509	151,877
43	North Dakota	3,488	89,010
44	Idaho	3,296	133,895

Rank	State	Beds	Admissions
45	Hawaii	2,920	110,788
46	New Hampshire	2,841	121,747
47	Rhode Island	2,449	128,519
48	Delaware	2,288	107,037
49	Wyoming	2,071	53,077
50	Alaska	1,554	56,584
51	Vermont	1,362	49,892
Total	**United States**	**800,892**	**35,345,986**

Source: American Hospital Association. *AHA hospital statistics,* 2009, Table 6, pp. 51–151.

United States reported 35,345,986 inpatient admissions. Most community hospitals in the country are nongovernment not-for-profit institutions (2,913), followed by state and local government institutions (1,111), and investor owned (for-profit) institutions (873). Hospitals vary greatly in bed size; the smallest hospitals have 6 to 24 beds (360), while the largest have 500 or more hospital beds (260). Most hospitals have an average bed size of 100 to 199 beds (1,083).

The five states with the highest number of community hospital beds were California (69,325 beds, 3,276,372 admissions); New York (62,367 beds, 2,540,711 admissions); Texas (58,192 beds, 2,468,109 admissions); Florida (51,648 beds, 2,387,525 admissions); and Pennsylvania (39,728 beds, 1,880,382 admissions). In contrast, the five states with the lowest number of hospital beds were: Vermont (1,358 beds, 49,892 admissions); Alaska (1,554 beds, 56,584 admissions); Wyoming (2,071 beds, 53,077 admissions); Delaware (2,288 beds, 107,037 admissions); and Rhode Island (2,449 beds, 128,519 admissions).

Table 13 shows the number and percentage of hospital-based physical rehabilitation inpatient and outpatient services and occupational health services across the United States in 2007. The statistics in the table are also from the American Hospital Association's annual survey, as published in the *AHA Hospital Statistics, 2009.*

Table 13   Number and Percentage of Hospital-Based Physical Rehabilitation and Occupational Health Services by State and the District of Columbia—United States, 2007

| | Physical Rehabilitation | | | | Occupational Health Services | |
| | Inpatient Care Unit | | Outpatient Services | | | |
State	Number	Percent	Number	Percent	Number	Percent
Alabama	20	18.2	74	67.3	50	45.5
Alaska	4	25.0	12	75.0	10	62.5
Arizona	27	43.5	43	69.4	37	59.7
Arkansas	34	33.0	72	69.9	50	48.5
California	87	26.2	228	68.1	213	63.6
Colorado	24	36.4	51	77.3	43	65.2
Connecticut	12	32.4	25	67.6	23	62.2
Delaware	3	37.5	6	75.0	6	75.0
District of Columbia	3	30.0	8	80.0	7	70.0
Florida	37	24.8	121	81.2	112	75.2
Georgia	34	29.3	91	78.4	83	71.6
Hawaii	2	10.5	11	57.9	16	84.2
Idaho	7	18.4	21	55.3	21	55.3
Illinois	49	29.5	143	86.1	113	68.1
Indiana	39	31.2	95	76.0	82	65.6
Iowa	28	22.4	107	85.6	90	72.0
Kansas	34	21.9	117	75.5	78	50.3
Kentucky	27	28.4	73	76.8	62	65.3
Louisiana	27	26.2	54	52.4	44	42.7
Maine	11	26.2	37	88.1	30	71.4

| | Physical Rehabilitation | | | | Occupational Health Services | |
| | Inpatient Care Unit | | Outpatient Services | | | |
State	Number	Percent	Number	Percent	Number	Percent
Maryland	16	26.7	43	71.7	45	75.0
Massachusetts	17	21.5	73	92.4	67	84.8
Michigan	55	36.2	129	84.9	118	77.6
Minnesota	19	17.6	93	86.1	79	73.1
Mississippi	47	43.1	59	54.1	33	30.3
Missouri	80	53.0	110	72.8	102	67.5
Montana	10	17.9	45	80.4	32	57.1
Nebraska	10	15.9	48	76.2	34	54.0
Nevada	8	27.6	21	72.4	21	72.4
New Hampshire	7	22.6	29	93.5	26	83.9
New Jersey	17	23.6	61	84.7	45	62.5
New Mexico	9	25.0	26	72.2	14	38.9
New York	66	41.3	134	83.8	125	78.1
North Carolina	34	27.6	103	83.7	88	71.5
North Dakota	8	25.8	28	90.3	16	51.6
Ohio	62	39.2	139	88.0	125	79.1
Oklahoma	34	25.4	74	55.2	52	38.8
Oregon	13	22.4	50	86.2	38	65.5
Pennsylvania	75	43.6	138	80.2	134	77.9
Rhode Island	4	33.3	9	75.0	10	83.3
South Carolina	54	65.1	58	69.9	52	62.7
South Dakota	10	18.2	39	70.9	30	54.5

(Continued)

Table 13 (Continued)

State	Physical Rehabilitation				Occupational Health Services	
	Inpatient Care Unit		Outpatient Services			
	Number	Percent	Number	Percent	Number	Percent
Tennessee	29	29.3	81	81.8	59	59.6
Texas	146	27.0	328	60.7	279	51.7
Utah	8	22.9	21	60.0	20	57.1
Vermont	3	20.0	13	86.7	13	86.7
Virginia	22	28.9	64	84.2	60	78.9
Washington	25	29.4	57	67.1	49	57.6
West Virginia	10	15.4	47	72.3	33	50.8
Wisconsin	67	47.2	111	78.2	90	63.4
Wyoming	6	20.0	16	53.3	17	56.7
Total	**1,480**	**30.2**	**3,636**	**74.2**	**3,076**	**62.8**

Source: American Hospital Association. *AHA hospital statistics, 2009,* Table 7, pp. 153, 164–165.

Physical rehabilitation inpatient services encompass a comprehensive array of restoration services for the disabled, as well as all support services necessary to help patients attain their maximum functional capacity. Physical rehabilitation outpatient services provide medical, health-related, therapy, social, and vocational services to help disabled persons attain or retain their maximum functional capacity. Occupational health services are designed to protect the safety of employees from various hazards in the work environment.

In 2007, a total of 1,480 hospitals in the United States reported they had a physical rehabilitation inpatient services unit, 3,636 maintained physical rehabilitation outpatient services, and 3,076 offered occupational health services.

The five states with the highest number of hospital-based inpatient physical rehabilitation inpatient services units were Texas (146), California (87), Missouri (80), Pennsylvania (75), and Wisconsin (67). In contrast, the five states with the lowest number of units were Hawaii (2), Delaware (3), District of Columbia (3), Vermont (3), and Alaska (4).

The five states with the highest number of hospital-based physical rehabilitation outpatient services were Texas (328), California (228), Illinois (143), Ohio (139), and Pennsylvania (138). The five states providing the lowest number of services were Delaware (6), District of Columbia (8), Alaska (12), Rhode Island (9), and Hawaii (11).

The five states with the highest number of community hospital-based occupational health services were Texas (279), California (213), Pennsylvania (134), New York (125), and Ohio (125). The five states offering the lowest number of services were Delaware (6), District of Columbia (7), Alaska (10), Rhode Island (10), and Vermont (13).

Lastly, Table 14 shows the number of nursing home beds and nursing home residents in the United States in 2008. The statistics in the table are from the Centers for Medicare and Medicaid Services' (CMS) Online Survey, Certification, and Reporting (OSCAR) database, as published in the National Center for Health Statistics' *Health, United States, 2008.*

Table 14   Number of Nursing Home Beds Ranked by State and the District of Columbia and Nursing Home Residents— United States, 2008

Rank	State	Beds	Residents
1	Texas	126,732	90,385
2	California	122,554	103,487
3	New York	120,336	110,940
4	Illinois	101,790	76,282
5	Ohio	93,039	81,395
6	Pennsylvania	87,878	79,710
7	Florida	82,067	71,833
8	Indiana	57,107	39,536
9	Missouri	55,028	37,510

(Continued)

Table 14 (Continued)

Rank	State	Beds	Residents
10	New Jersey	51,132	45,946
11	Massachusetts	49,323	43,684
12	Michigan	47,323	40,224
13	North Carolina	43,770	38,025
14	Georgia	39,762	35,276
15	Wisconsin	37,385	32,325
16	Tennessee	36,943	32,288
17	Louisiana	36,096	25,875
18	Minnesota	34,117	31,056
19	Iowa	33,658	26,292
20	Virginia	31,908	28,279
21	Oklahoma	29,786	19,518
22	Connecticut	29,678	26,819
23	Maryland	29,231	25,243
24	Alabama	26,824	23,205
25	Kansas	26,011	19,301
26	Kentucky	25,769	23,233
27	Arkansas	24,477	17,753
28	Washington	22,314	18,760
29	Colorado	19,956	16,464
30	South Carolina	18,798	17,004
31	Mississippi	18,346	16,246
32	Nebraska	16,198	12,899
33	Arizona	16,033	12,201
34	Oregon	12,473	8,113

Rank	State	Beds	Residents
35	West Virginia	10,895	9,710
36	Rhode Island	8,868	7,955
37	Utah	7,967	5,456
38	New Hampshire	7,718	6,953
39	Maine	7,243	6,591
40	Montana	7,081	5,137
41	New Mexico	6,780	5,695
42	South Dakota	6,591	6,528
43	North Dakota	6,395	5,847
44	Idaho	6,034	4,522
45	Nevada	5,675	4,724
46	Delaware	4,870	3,999
47	Hawaii	4,256	3,840
48	Vermont	3,268	2,992
49	Wyoming	2,993	2,431
50	District of Columbia	2,645	2,437
51	Alaska	725	616
Total	**United States**	**1,703,846**	**1,412,540**

Source: National Center for Health Statistics. Health, United States, 2008, Table 120, pp. 407–408. Available at: http://www.cdc.gov/nchs/data/hus/hus08.pdf

The OSCAR database includes both skilled nursing facilities and nursing facilities. Skilled nursing facilities are those that participate in both the Medicare and Medicaid programs, while nursing facilities are those that participate only in the Medicaid program.

Nursing homes are facilities licensed by states that primarily engage in providing residents with skilled nursing care and related medical and rehabilitation services. They provide skilled nursing care, personal care, room and board, supervision, medication, therapies, and rehabilitation on a 24-hour-a-day basis.

Nursing homes play a vital role in providing medical and social services to many people with injuries and disabilities. For example, many skilled nursing facilities have Alzheimer's and dementia units, brain injury units, hospice units, long-term care units, rehabilitation units, and ventilator and pulmonary units.

In 2008, there were an estimated 1,703,846 nursing home beds and 1,412,540 nursing home residents in the United States. The five states with the highest number of nursing home beds were Texas (126,732 beds, 90,385 residents); California (122,554 beds, 103,487 residents); New York (120,336 beds, 110,940 residents); Illinois (101,790 beds, 76,282 residents); and Ohio (93,039 beds, 81,395 residents). In contrast, the five states with the lowest number of nursing home beds were Alaska (725 beds, 616 residents); District of Columbia (2,645 beds, 2,437 residents); Wyoming (2,993 beds, 2,431 residents); Vermont (3,268 beds, 2,992 residents); and Hawaii (4,256 beds, residents 3,840).

Conclusion

A wealth of data and statistics on disability, healthcare professionals, and facilities are collected and disseminated by many international, government, and private organizations. This chapter has identified the major organizations that collect these data and statistics, as well as some of the specific databases and surveys used to collect them. These data and statistics can be very useful in identifying problem areas and trends, and evaluating policies. However, the users of these data and statistics face a number of problems including inconsistent definitions, fragmented data sets, and lack of timeliness. Therefore, disability data and statistics should be viewed as informative, yet a very rough sketch of the true picture.

Six

Annotated List of Organizations and Associations

This chapter identifies some of the major organizations and associations involved in the health and medical aspects of disability. The various organizations and associations are grouped into twelve categories: (1) Governmental and Nongovernmental Information Centers, Clearinghouses, and Libraries; (2) Academic Centers and University Programs; (3) Disease, Injury, and Condition Associations; (4) Group/Population Associations; (5) Professional and Trade Associations; (6) Contract-Research and Policy Organizations; (7) Accrediting Organizations; (8) Foundations and Philanthropies; (9) U.S. Government Agencies, Departments, and Institutes; (10) U.S. Government Advisory Commissions; (11) Healthcare Systems, Associations, and Programs of Other Nations; and (12) International Organizations.

1. Governmental and Nongovernmental Information Centers, Clearinghouses, and Libraries

AIDS.gov
U.S. Department of Health and Human Services (HHS)
200 Independence Avenue, SW
Washington, DC 20201
Telephone: None Listed
E-mail: contact@AIDS.gov
Web site: http://aids.gov
The mission of AIDS.gov is "to improve access to federal HIV/AIDS information programs serving minority and other communities most at-risk for, or living with, HIV, through a variety of new media channels, and to support the use of new media tools by federal and community partners."

American Association on Health and Disability (AAHD)
110 N. Washington Street, Suite 328-J
Rockville, MD 20850
Telephone: (301) 545-6140
Fax: (301) 545-6144
E-mail: contact@aahd.us
Web site: http://www.aahd.us
The AAHD's mission is to contribute to "efforts to prevent additional health complications in people with disabilities, and to identify effective intervention strategies to reduce the incidence of secondary conditions and the health disparities between people with disabilities and the general population."

Center for International Rehabilitation Research Information and Exchange (CIRRIE)
University of Buffalo
515 Kimball Tower
Buffalo, NY 14214-3079
Telephone: (716) 829-6743
Fax: (716) 829-3217
E-mail: ub-cirrie@buffalo.edu
Web site: http://cirrie.buffalo.edu
The CIRRIE works to facilitate the sharing of information and expertise in rehabilitation research between the United States and other countries through a wide range of programs.

Clearinghouse on Disability Information
Office of Special Education and Rehabilitation Services (OSERS)
550 12th Street, SW, Room 5133
Washington, DC 20202-2550
Telephone: (202) 245-7307
Fax: (202) 245-7636
E-mail: customerservice@inet.ed.gov
Web site: http://www.ed.gov/about/offices/list/osers/codi.html
The clearinghouse provides general information on disability, including areas of federal funding for disability-related programs.

Cochrane Collaboration
Center for Clinical Trials
Johns Hopkins Bloomberg School of Public Health
615 N. Wolfe Street
Mail RM W5010
Baltimore, MD 21205
Telephone: (410) 502-4650
Fax: (410) 502-4623
E-mail: uscc@jhsph.edu
Web site: http://cochrane.org
The Cochrane Collaboration is a worldwide organization of volunteers and centers (one of the U.S. centers is listed above) dedicated to making up-to-date information on the effects of healthcare available through the dissemination of systematic reviews of clinical trials and other medical and public health interventions.

Disability.gov
Office of Public Affairs
U.S. Department of Labor
Frances Perkins Building
200 Constitution Avenue, NW
Washington, DC 20210
Telephone: (202) 693-4667
E-mail: gamble.bennett@dol.gov
Web site: http://www.disability.gov
This Web site, which is maintained by the U.S. Department of Labor, contains "disability-related resources on programs, services, laws, and regulations to help people with disabilities lead full, independent lives."

Education Resources Information Center (ERIC)
c/o Computer Sciences Corporation
655 15th Street, NW, Suite 500
Washington, DC 20005
Telephone: (800) 538-3742
Web site: http://www.eric.ed.gov
*The ERIC, which is sponsored by the Institute of Education Sciences (IES) of the U.S.
Department of Education, is the world's largest digital library of education literature.*

National Center for the Dissemination of Disability Research (NCDDR)
4700 Mueller Boulevard
Austin, TX 78723
Telephone: (800) 266-1832
Fax: (512) 476-2286
E-mail: NCDRR@sedl.org
Web site: http://www.ncddr.org
*The NCDDR, which is funded by the National Institute on Disability and Rehabilitation
Research (NIDRR), works to increase the use of NIDRR-sponsored research "in shaping
new technologies, improving service delivery, and expanding decision-making options for
people with disabilities and their families."*

National Diabetes Information Clearinghouse (NDIC)
1 Information Way
Bethesda, MD 20892-3560
Telephone: (800) 860-8747
Fax: (703) 738-4929
E-mail: ndic@info.niddk.nih.gov
Web site: http://www.diabetes.niddk.nih.gov
*The NDIC is a service of the National Institute of Diabetes and Digestive and Kidney
Diseases (NIDDK); it works "to increase knowledge and understanding about diabetes
among patients, health care professionals, and the general public."*

National Digestive Diseases Information Clearinghouse (NDDIC)
2 Information Way
Bethesda, MD 20892-3570
Telephone: (800) 891-5389
Fax: (703) 738-4929
E-mail: niddic@info.niddk.nih.gov
Web site: www.digestive.niddk.nih.gov
*The NDDIC is a service of the National Institute of Diabetes and Digestive and Kidney
Diseases (NIDDK); it works "to increase knowledge and understanding about digestive*

diseases among people with these conditions and their families, health care providers, and the general public."

National Guideline Clearinghouse (NGC)
Center for Outcomes and Evidence
Agency for Healthcare Research and Quality (AHRQ)
540 Gaither Road, Suite 2000
Rockville, MD 20850
Telephone: (301) 427-1364
E-mail: info@guideline.gov
Web site: http://www.guideline.gov
Sponsored by the U.S. Agency for Healthcare Research and Quality (AHRQ), the clearinghouse provides public access to evidence-based clinical practice guidelines.

National Health Information Center
P.O. Box 1133
Washington, DC 20013-1133
Telephone: (800) 336-4797
Fax: (301) 984-4256
E-mail: info@nhic.org
Web site: http://www.health.gov/nhic
The NHIC, a service of the federal Office of Disease Prevention and Health Promotion, is a health information referral service linking health professionals and consumers who have health questions to the appropriate organizations.

National Institute of Arthritis and Musculoskeletal and Skin Diseases (NIAMS) Information Clearinghouse
National Institutes of Health
1 AMS Circle
Bethesda, MD 20892-3675
Telephone: (877) 226-4267
Fax: (301) 718-6366
E-mail: NIAMSinfo@mail.nih.gov
Web site: http://www.niams.nih.gov
The NIAMS clearinghouse "provides information on locating other sources, creating health information materials, and participating in a national federal database on health information."

National Kidney and Urologic Diseases Information Clearinghouse (NKUDIC)
3 Information Way
Bethesda, MD 20892-3580

Telephone: (800) 891-5390
Fax: (703) 738-4929
E-mail: nkudic@info.niddk.nih.gov
Web site: www.kidney.niddk.nih.gov
The NKUDIC is a service of the National Institute of Diabetes and Digestive and Kidney Diseases (NIDDK); it works "to increase knowledge and understanding about diseases of the kidneys and urologic system among people with these conditions and their families, health care professionals, and the general public."

National Library of Medicine (NLM)
8600 Rockville Pike
Bethesda, MD 20894
Telephone: (888) 346-3656
Fax: (301) 402-1384
Web site: http://www.nlm.nih.gov
One of the National Institutes of Health (NIH), the NLM is the world's largest medical library.

National Library Service for the Blind and Physically Handicapped (NLS)
The Library of Congress
1291 Taylor Street, NW
Washington, DC 20011
Telephone: (888) 657-7323
Fax: (202) 707-0712
E-mail: nls@loc.gov
Web site: http://www.loc.gov/nls/
Utilizing a national network of cooperating libraries, NLS administers a free library program of Braille and audio materials circulated to eligible borrowers in the United States by postage-free mail.

National Mental Health Consumers' Self-Help Clearinghouse
1211 Chestnut Street, Suite 1207
Philadelphia, PA 19107
Telephone: (800) 553-4539
Fax: (215) 636-6312
E-mail: info@mhselfhelp.org
Web site: http://mhselfhelp.org
The clearinghouse helps connect individuals by providing a directory of services, electronic and printed publications, and mental health consultants.

2. Academic Centers and University Programs

Association of University Centers on Disabilities (AUCD)
1010 Wayne Avenue, Suite 920
Silver Spring, MD 20910
Telephone: (301) 588-8252
Fax: (301) 588-2842
E-mail: aucdinfo@aucd.org
Web site: http://www.aucd.org
The AUCD is a membership association that supports and provides a national network of university-based interdisciplinary disability programs.

Beach Center on Disability
University of Kansas
Haworth Hall, Room 3136
1200 Sunnyside Avenue
Lawrence, KS 660045-7534
Telephone: (785) 864-7600
Fax: (785) 864-7605
Web site: http://www.beachcenter.org
The Beach Center conducts research, carries out training and technical assistance, and provides services to make a significant and sustainable difference in the quality of life of families and individuals with disabilities.

Center for Child and Human Development (CCHD)
Georgetown University
Box 571485
Washington, DC 20057-1485
Telephone: (202) 687-5000
Fax: (202) 687-8899
E-mail: gucdc@georgetown.edu
Web site: http://gucchd.georgetown.edu
The mission of the center, a division of Georgetown University's Department of Pediatrics, is "to improve the quality of life for all children and youth, children with special needs, adults with developmental and other disabilities and their families."

Center for Excellence in Disability Education, Research, and Service
University of Montana Rural Institute
52 Corbin Hall
Missoula, MT 59812

Telephone: (406) 243-5467
Fax: (406) 243-4730
Web site: http://ruralinstitute.umt.edu
The federally funded center "is committed to increasing and supporting the independence, productivity, and inclusion of persons with disabilities into the community."

Center for Research on Women with Disabilities (CROWD)
Baylor College of Medicine
1475 West Gray, Suite 165
Houston, TX 77019
Telephone: (800) 442-7693
Fax: (713) 523-0466
Web site: http://www.bcm.edu/crowd
The center's mission is "to promote, develop, and disseminate information to improve the health and expand the life choices of women with disabilities."

Coleman Institute for Cognitive Disabilities
University of Colorado
3825 Iris Avenue, Suite 200
Boulder, CO 80301
Telephone: (303) 492-0639
Fax: (303) 735-5643
Web site: http://www.colemaninstitute.org
The institute's mission "is to catalyze and integrate advances in science, engineering and technology to promote the quality of life and independent living of people with cognitive disabilities."

Disability Statistics Center
University of California, San Francisco
Institute for Health and Aging
3333 California Street, Suite 340
San Francisco, CA 94118
Telephone: (415) 502-5214
Web site: http://dsc.ucsf.edu
The center "produces and disseminates policy-relevant statistical information on the demographics and status of people with disabilities in American society."

Employment and Disability Institute
Cornell University
School of Industrial and Labor Relations
201 Dolgen Hall

Ithaca, NY 14853-3901
Telephone: (607) 255-7727
Fax: (607) 255-2763
E-mail: DisabilityStatistics@cornell.edu
Web site: http://www.ilr.cornell.edu/edi
The institute provides online access to U.S. disability statistics from the American Community Survey, Current Population Survey, and Census 2000.

Institute on Disability (IOD)

University of New Hampshire
10 West Edge Drive, Suite 101
Durham, NH 03824
Telephone: (603) 862-4329
Fax: (603) 862-0555
Web site: http://www.iod.unh.edu
The IOD provides "a coherent university-based focus for the improvement of knowledge, policies and practices related to the lives of persons with disabilities and their families."

Institute on Disability and Human Development (IDHP)

Department of Disability and Human Development
University of Illinois at Chicago
1640 W. Roosevelt Road, MC 626
Chicago, IL 60608
Telephone: (312) 413-8833
E-mail: idhd@uic.edu
Web site: http://www.idhd.org
The IDHP is dedicated to promoting the independence, productivity, and inclusion of people with disabilities into all aspects of society; it conducts research and disseminates information about disabilities.

TRENDS: Evaluating Trends in Old-Age Disability

Center on the Demography of Aging
University of Michigan
c/o Robert Schoeni
426 Thompson Street
Ann Arbor, MI 48106
Web site: http://trends.psc.isr.umich.edu
TRENDS describes itself as "a network of researchers working to accelerate scientific understanding of old-age disability and health trends"; the researchers conduct studies, review findings from new studies, and create an open discussion of cutting-edge research.

3. Disease, Injury, and Condition Associations

Alexander Graham Bell Association for the Deaf and Hard of Hearing (AG Bell)
3417 Volta Place, NW
Washington, DC 20007
Telephone: (202) 337-5220
Fax: (202) 337-8314
E-mail: info@agbell.org
Web site: http://www.agbell.org
The AG Bell helps families, healthcare providers, and educational professionals understand childhood hearing loss and the importance of early diagnosis and intervention.

ALS Association
27001 Agoura Road, Suite 250
Calabasas Hills, CA 91301-5104
Telephone: (818) 880-9007
Fax: (818) 880-9006
Web site: http://www.alsa.org
The association's mission is to lead the fight to cure and treat Amyotrophic Lateral Sclerosis (ALS), more commonly known as Lou Gehrig's Disease.

Alzheimer's Association
225 N. Michigan Ave., Fl. 17
Chicago, IL 60601-7633
Telephone: (312) 335-8700
Fax: (866) 699-1246
Web site: http://www.alz.org/index.asp
The Alzheimer's Association works to eliminate Alzheimer's disease through research; provide care and support; and reduce the risk of dementia.

American Cancer Society (ACS)
250 Williams Street, NW
Atlanta, GA 30303
Telephone: (800) 227-2345
Web site: http://www.cancer.org
The ACS is dedicated to eliminating cancer through research, education, advocacy, and service.

American Council of the Blind (ACB)
2200 Wilson Boulevard, Suite 650
Arlington, VA 22201

Telephone: (800) 424-8666
Fax: (703) 465-5085
E-mail: mailman@acb.org
Web site: http://www.acb.org
The ACB is a national, nonprofit organization that works to expand the "possibilities for people with vision loss."

American Diabetes Association (ADA)
1701 N. Beauregard Street
Alexandria, VA 22311
Telephone: (800) 342-2383
E-mail: askada@diabetes.org
Web site: http://www.diabetes.org
The ADA is a membership association that works to prevent, cure, and manage diabetes.

American Heart Association
7272 Greenville Avenue
Dallas, TX 75231
Telephone: (800) 242-8721
Web site: http://www.americanheart.org
The American Heart Association is a voluntary organization that attempts to reduce coronary heart diseases and stroke.

Amputee Coalition of America (ACA)
900 East Hill Avenue, Suite 205
Knoxville, TN 37915-2566
Telephone: (888) 267-5669
Fax: (865) 525-7917
Web site: http://amputee-coalition.org
The ACA is a national, nonprofit, consumer educational organization representing people who have experienced amputation or are born with limb differences.

Children and Adults with Attention-Deficit/Hyperactivity Disorder (CHADD)
8181 Professional Place, Suite 150
Landover, MD 20785
Telephone: (301) 306-7070
Fax: (301) 306-7090
Web site: http://www.chadd.org
The CHADD is a national, nonprofit organization providing education, advocacy, and support for individuals with attention-deficit/hyperactivity disorder.

Families of Spinal Muscular Atrophy (FSMA)
925 Busse Road
Elk Grove Village, IL 60007
Telephone: (800) 886-1762
Fax: (847) 367-7623
E-mail: info@fsma.org
Web site: http://www.fsma.org
The FSMA is dedicated to creating a treatment and cure for spinal muscular atrophy.

National Autism Association (NAA)
1330 W. Schatz Lane
Nixa, MO 65714
Telephone: (877) 622-2884
Web site: http://www.nationalautismassociation.org
The mission of the NAA is "to educate and empower families affected by autism and other neurological disorders, while advocating on behalf of those who cannot fight for their rights."

National Spinal Cord Injury Association (NSCIA)
1 Church Street #600
Rockville, MD 20850
Telephone: (800) 962-9629
Fax: (866) 387-2196
E-mail: info@spinalcord.org
Web site: http://www.spinalcord.org
The NSCIA is dedicated to improving the quality of life of Americans living with spinal cord injury and disease and providing assistance to their families.

Obesity Society
8630 Fenton Street, Suite 814
Silver Spring, MD 20910
Telephone: (301) 563-6526
Fax: (301) 563-6595
Web site: http://www.obesity.org
The Obesity Society is a scientific society dedicated to the study of obesity; it encourages research on the causes and treatment of obesity and informs the medical community and the general public of new advances.

Spina Bifida Association of America (SBA)
4590 MacArthur Boulevard, NW, Suite 250
Washington, DC 20007-4226

Telephone: (800) 621-3141
E-mail: sbaa@sbaa.org
Web site: http://www.sbaa.org
The SBA serves adults and children who have spina bifida; it also has a national clearing-house of information on the condition.

United Cerebral Palsy Association (UCPA)
1660 L Street, NW, Suite 700
Washington, DC 20036
Telephone: (800) 872-5827
Fax: (202) 776-0414
E-mail: info@ucp.org
Web site: http://www.ucp.org
The UCPA's mission is "to advance the independence, productivity and full citizenship of people with disabilities through an affiliate network."

4. Group/Population Associations

AARP
601 E Street, NW
Washington, DC 20049
Telephone: (888) 687-2277
Web site: www.aaro.org
The AARP, the nation's largest membership organization for people 50 years of age or older, attempts to enhance the quality of life for all as they age.

American Association of People with Disabilities (AAPD)
1629 K Street NW, Suite 950
Washington, DC 20006
E-mail: pViele@aapd.com
Telephone: (800) 840-8844
Fax: (202) 457-0473
Web site: http://www.aapd.com
The AAPD is the nation's largest cross-disability membership organization; it organizes the disability community to be an active voice for economic, political, and social change.

American Association on Intellectual and Developmental Disabilities (AAIDD)
501 3rd Street, NW, Suite 200
Washington, DC 20001

Telephone: (800) 424-3688
Fax: (202) 387-2193
E-mail: anam@aaidd.org
Web site: http://www.aamr.org
The AAIDD "promotes progressive policies, sound research, effective practices and universal human rights for people with intellectual and developmental disabilities."

Children's Defense Fund (CDF)
25 E Street, NW
Washington, DC 20001
Telephone: (800) 223-1200
E-mail: cdfinfo@childrensdefense.org
Web site: http://www.childrensdefense.org
The CDF is a nonprofit organization that "advocates nationwide on behalf of children to ensure children are always a priority."

Disabled American Veterans (DAV)
3725 Alexandria Pike
Cold Spring, KY 41076
Telephone: (877) 426-2838
Web site: http://www.dav.org
Chartered by the U.S. Congress as the official voice of the nation's wartime disabled veterans, DAV describes itself as a "charity dedicated to building better lives for America's disabled veterans and their families."

Easter Seals
233 S. Wacker Drive, Suite 2400
Chicago, IL 60606
Telephone: (800) 221-6827
Fax: (312) 726-1494
Web site: http://www.easterseals.com
The Easter Seals organization provides "services, education, outreach, and advocacy so that people living with autism and other disabilities can live, learn, work, and play in our communities."

Mental Health America
2000 N. Beauregard Street, 6th Floor
Alexandria, VA 22311
Telephone: (703) 684-7722

Fax: (703) 684-5968

Web site: http://www.mentalhealthamerica.net

The primary goal of Mental Health America is to educate the general public about the realities of mental health and mental illness.

National Alliance for Caregiving (NAC)

4720 Montgomery Lane, 2nd Floor

Bethesda, MD 20814

Telephone: (301) 718-8444

Fax: (301) 652-7711

Web site: http://www.caregiving.org

Established in 1996, the NAC's mission "is to be the objective national resource on family caregiving with the goal of improving the lives of family caregivers and care recipients."

National Rural Health Association (NRHA)

521 E. 63rd Street

Kansas City, MO 64110-3329

Telephone: (816) 756-3140

Fax: (816) 756-3144

E-mail: mail@NRHArural.org

Web site: http://www.ruralhealthweb.org

The NRHA is a membership association of individuals and organizations that provides leadership on rural health issues.

Veterans of Foreign Wars (VFW)

406 W. 34th Street

Kansas City, MO 64111

Telephone: (816) 756-3390

Fax; (816) 968-1149

E-mail: vfw@vfw.org

Web site: http://www.vfw.org

The VFW is a nonprofit organization that represents U.S. military veterans; it has 2.2 million members in approximately 8,100 posts worldwide.

5. Professional and Trade Associations

American Academy of Family Physicians (AAFP)

11100 Tomahawk Creek Parkway

Leawood, KS 66211-2680

Telephone: (800) 274-2237
Fax: (913) 906-6075
E-mail: contactcenter@aafp.org
Web site: http://www.aafp.org
The AAFP is a large, individual membership organization of more than 94,600 family physicians, family medicine residents, and medical students nationwide, whose mission is to "promote the science and art of family medicine and to ensure high-quality, cost-effective health care for patients of all ages."

American Academy of Pediatrics (AAP)
141 Northwest Point Boulevard
Elk Grove Village, IL 60007-1098
Telephone: (847) 434-4000
Fax: (847) 434-8000
E-mail: commun@aap.org
Web site: http://www.aap.org
The AAP is an individual membership association of 60,000 pediatricians working to attain "optimal physical, mental, and social health and well-being for all infants, children, adolescents, and young adults."

American Academy of Physical Medicine and Rehabilitation (AAPM&R)
330 North Wabash Avenue, Suite 2500
Chicago, IL 60611-7617
Telephone: (312) 464-9700
Fax: (312) 464-0227
E-mail: info@aapmr.org
Web site: http://www.aapmr.org
The AAPM&R is an individual membership association of more than 7,500 physiatrists, representing 87% of all physiatrists in the nation.

American Association of Homecare (AAHomecare)
2011 Crystal Drive, Suite 725
Arlington, VA 22202
Telephone: (703) 836-6263
Fax: (703) 836-6730
E-mail: info@aahomecare.org
Web site: http://www.aahomecare.org
The AAHomecare represents 3,000 homecare providers across the United States, as well as equipment manufacturers and other organizations in the homecare community.

American Association of Homes and Services for the Aging (AAHSA)
2519 Connecticut Avenue, NW
Washington, DC 20008-1520
Telephone: (202) 783-2242
Fax: (202) 783-2255
E-mail: info@aahsa.org
Web site: http://www.aahsa.org
The AAHSA represents 5,700 nonprofit nursing homes and other long-term care service organizations.

American Association of Preferred Provider Organizations (AAPPO)
222 S. First Street, Suite 303
Louisville, KY 40202
Telephone: (502) 403-1122
Fax: (502) 403-1129
Web site: http://www.aappo.org
The AAPPO promotes, supports, and advocates for the PPO industry.

American Chiropractic Association (ACA)
1701 Clarendon Boulevard
Arlington, VA 22209
Telephone: (703) 276-8800
Fax: (703) 243-2593
E-mail: memberinfo@acatoday.org
Web site: http://www.acatoday.org
The ACA is an individual membership association of 15,000 chiropractors; it represents the profession through lobbying, public relations, and professional education activities.

American Dental Association (ADA)
211 E. Chicago Avenue
Chicago, IL 60611-2678
Telephone: (312) 440-2500
E-mail: membership@ada.org
Web site: http://www.ada.org
The ADA, the world's largest and oldest national dental association, is an individual membership association of more than 155,000 dentists; it represents and advocates for oral health.

American Health Care Association (AHCA)
1201 L Street, NW
Washington, DC 20005

Telephone: (202) 842-4444
Fax: (202) 842-3860
Web site: http://www.ahca.org
The AHCA is the nation's largest association of long-term and post-acute care providers, representing 11,000 assisted living, nursing facilities, and developmentally disabled, and sub-acute care providers.

American Hospital Association (AHA)
One North Franklin
Chicago, Il 60606-3421
Telephone: (312) 422-3000
Web site: http://www.aha.org
The AHA is an institutional and individual membership association representing nearly 5,000 of the nation's hospitals, healthcare systems, and networks and 37,000 individual members.

American Medical Association (AMA)
515 N. State Street
Chicago, IL 60654
Telephone: (800) 621-8335
Web site: http://www.ama-assn.org
The AMA is an individual membership association representing about 236,000 physicians in the nation; it publishes the Journal of the American Medical Association as well as medical books on various topics.

American Nurses Association (ANA)
8515 Georgia Ave., Suite 400
Silver Spring, MD 20910-3492
Telephone: (301) 628-5000
Fax: (301) 628-5001
Web site: http://cms.nursingworld.org
The ANA represents the interests of the nation's 2.9 million registered nurses.

American Occupational Therapy Association (AOTA)
4720 Montgomery Lane
P.O. Box 31220
Bethesda, MD 20824-1220
Telephone: (301) 652-2682
Fax: (301) 652-7711
Web site: http://www.aota.org

The AOTA is an individual membership association representing its 39,000 member occupational therapists, occupational therapy assistants, and occupational therapy students.

American Osteopathic Association (AOA)
142 E. Ontario Street
Chicago, IL 60611
Telephone: (800) 621-1773
Fax: (312) 202-8200
Web site: http://www.osteopathic.org
The AOA is an individual membership association representing its 67,000 member osteopathic physicians.

American Physical Therapy Association (APTA)
1111 North Fairfax Street
Alexandria, VA 22314-1488
Telephone: (800) 999-2782
Fax: (703) 684-7343
Web site: http://www.apta.org
The APTA is an individual membership association representing its 72,000 members; its goal is to foster advancements in physical therapy practice, research, and education.

American Public Health Association (APHA)
800 I Street, NW
Washington, DC 20001
Telephone: (202) 777-2742
Fax: (202) 777-2534
E-mail: comments@apha.org
Web site: http://www.apha.org
The APHA is an individual membership association of 50,000 public health professionals; it works to prevent disease and promote health in the nation.

America's Health Insurance Plans (AHIP)
601 Pennsylvania Avenue, NW
South Building, Suite 500
Washington, DC 20004
Telephone: (202) 778-3200
Fax: (202) 331-7487
E-mail: ahip@ahip.org
Web site: http://www.ahip.org

AHIP represents nearly 1,300 member companies providing insurance coverage to more than 200 million Americans; its members offer medical insurance, long-term care insurance, disability income insurance, and other types of insurance coverage.

Association of American Medical Colleges (AAMC)
2450 N Street, NW
Washington, DC 20037-1126
Telephone: (202) 828-0400
Fax: (202) 828-1125
E-mail: rsherrod@aamc.org
Web site: http://www.aamc.org
The AAMC represents accredited U.S. and Canadian medical schools, major teaching hospitals and health systems, and academic and scientific societies.

Care Continuum Alliance
701 Pennsylvania Avenue, NW, Suite 700
Washington, DC 20004-2694
Telephone: (202) 737-5980
Fax: (202) 478-5113
E-mail: info@carecontinuum.org
Web site: http://www.carecontinuum.org
The Care Continuum Alliance represents disease management organizations, health plans, wellness providers, employers, and other organizations.

Gerontological Society of America (GSA)
1220 L Street, NW, Suite 901
Washington, DC 20005
Telephone: (202) 842-1275
Fax: (202) 842-1150
Web site: http://www.geron.org
The GSA is the oldest and largest interdisciplinary organization devoted to research, education, and practice in the field of aging.

National Association of County and City Health Officials (NACCHO)
1100 17th Street, NW, Second Floor
Washington, DC 20036
Telephone: (202) 783-5500
Fax: (202) 783-1583
E-mail: info@naccho.org
Web site: http://www.naccho.org

The NACCHO represents local public health departments in the nation; it supports efforts to protect and improve the health of people in communities.

Pharmaceutical Research and Manufacturers of America (PhRMA)
950 F Street, NW, Suite 300
Washington, DC 20004
Telephone: (202) 835-3400
Fax: (202) 835-3414
Web site: http://www.phrma.org
The PhRMA represents pharmaceutical research and biotechnology companies, advertising and communication services, consultants, and drug discovery software firms.

6. Contract-Research and Policy Organizations

Abt Associates Inc.
55 Wheeler Street
Cambridge, MA 02138-1168
Telephone: (617) 492-7100
Fax: (617) 492-5219
Web site: http://www.abtassociates.com
Abt Associates is a large, private, for-profit, employee-owned organization that "applies scientific research, consulting, and technical assistance expertise to a wide range of issues in social, economic, and health policy; international development; clinical trials and registries."

Brookings Institution
1775 Massachusetts Ave., NW
Washington, DC 20036
Telephone: (202) 797-6000
Web site: http://www.brookings.edu
The Brookings Institution, which is the oldest public policy organization in the nation, has three broad goals: "strengthen American democracy; foster the economic and social welfare, security, and opportunity of all Americans; and secure a more open, safe, prosperous, and cooperative international system."

Center for Studying Disability Policy (CSDP)
Mathematica Policy Research, Inc.
PO Box 2393
Princeton, NJ 08543-2393
Telephone: (609) 799-3535

Fax: (609) 799-0005
E-mail: info@mathematica-mpr.com
Web site: http://www.disabilitypolicyresearch.org
Established by Mathematica Policy Research in 2007, the CSDP collects, analyzes, and reports on issues and trends in disability policy.

Center for Studying Health System Change (HSC)
600 Maryland Ave., SW #550
Washington, DC 20024
Telephone: (202) 484-5261
Fax: (202) 484-9258
E-mail. hscinfo@hschange.org
Web site: http://www.hschange.com
The HSC is a nonpartisan policy research organization whose mission "is to inform policy makers and private decision makers about how local and national changes in the financing and delivery of health care affect people."

Institute of Medicine (IOM)
500 Fifth Street, NW
Washington, DC 20001
Telephone: (202) 334-2352
Fax: (202) 334-1412
E-mail: iomwww@nas.edu
Web site: www.iom.edu
The health arm of the National Academy of Sciences, the IOM publishes influential reports on various medical and public health topics; its mission is to serve as an advisor to the nation to improve health.

RAND Corporation
1776 Main Street
Santa Monica, CA 90401-3208
Telephone: (310) 393-0411
Fax: (310) 393-4818
Web site: http://www.rand.org
The RAND Corporation is a large, independent, nonprofit organization that conducts a broad variety of research studies on social and economic policy issues in the United States and overseas, it also has a graduate school that trains researchers and policy analysts.

RTI International
P.O. Box 12194
Research Triangle Park, NC 27709

Telephone: (919) 485-2666
E-mail: listen@rti.org
Web site: http://www.rti.org
RTI International is a large research institute providing research and technical expertise in health, education, and economic and social policy to governments and businesses in more than 40 countries.

Urban Institute
2100 M Street, NW
Washington, DC 20037
Telephone: (202) 261-5687
E-mail: paffairs@urban.org
Web site: http://www.urban.org
The Urban Institute is a nonprofit, nonpartisan policy research and educational organization that "gathers data, conducts research, evaluates programs and offers technical assistance overseas, and educates Americans on social and economic issues–to foster sound public policy and effective government."

7. Accrediting Organizations

Association for the Accreditation of Human Research Protection Programs (AAHRPP)
2301 M Street, NW, Suite 500
Washington, DC 20037
Telephone: (202) 783-1112
Fax: (202) 783-1113
E-mail: accredit@aahrpp.org
Web site: http://www.aahrpp.org
The AAHRPP is an independent, nonprofit organization that accredits human medical research programs worldwide to ensure that all research participants are respected and are protected from unnecessary harm.

Commission on Accreditation of Rehabilitation Facilities (CARF)
4891 E. Grant Road
Tucson, AZ 85712
Telephone: (520) 325-1144
Fax: (520) 318-1129
E-mail: medical@carf.org
Web site: http://carf.org
The CARF accredits rehabilitation and human services providers.

Joint Commission
One Renaissance Boulevard
Oakbrook Terrace, IL 60181
Telephone: (630) 792-5000
Web site: http://jointcommission.org
The Joint Commission accredits and certifies healthcare organizations (primarily hospitals) and programs in the United States.

National Committee for Quality Assurance (NCQA)
1100 13th Street, NW, Suite 1000
Washington, DC 20005
Telephone: (202) 955-3500
Fax: (202) 955-3599
Web site: http://www.ncqa.org
The NCQA accredits and certifies healthcare plans and managed care organizations.

URAC
1220 L Street, NW, Suite 400
Washington, DC 20005
Telephone: (202) 216-9010
Fax: (202) 216-9006
Web site: http://www.urac.org
URAC accredits providers of utilization management services, such as pharmacy benefit management and drug therapy management services, in the United States.

8. Foundations and Philanthropies

American Foundation for AIDS Research (amfAR)
120 Wall Street, 13th Floor
New York, NY 10005-3908
Telephone: (212) 806-1600
Fax: (212) 806-1601
Web site: http://www.amfar.org
The amfAR is "one of the world's leading nonprofit organizations dedicated to the support of HIV/AIDS research, HIV prevention, treatment education, and the advocacy of sound AIDS-related public policy."

American Foundation for the Blind (AFB)
2 Penn Plaza, Suite 1102
New York, NY 10121

Telephone: (800) 232-5463
Fax: (212) 502-7777
E-mail: afbinfo@afb.net
Web site: http://afb.org
The AFB is a national nonprofit foundation that works to expand possibilities for people with vision loss through broadening access to technology, increasing the quality of information tools, and promoting independent living.

Amputee Resource Foundation of America (ARFA)
2324 Wildwood Trail, Suite F104
Minnetonka, MN 55305
Telephone: (612) 812-7875
E-mail: info@amputeeresource.org
Web site: http://www.amputeeresource.org
The mission of the ARFA is to "disseminate timely and useful information, to perform charitable services, and to conduct research to enhance productivity and quality of life for amputees in America."

ARDS (Acute Respiratory Distress Syndrome) Foundation
3100 Dundee Road, Suite 402
Northbrook, IL 60062
Telephone: (312) 749-7047
Web site: http://www.ardsusa.org
The foundation's mission is "to raise awareness, increase education, and assist in funding medical research while providing a forum for all of those in the ARDS Community."

Arthritis Foundation
1330 W. Peachtree Street, Suite 100
Atlanta, GA 30309
Telephone: (800) 283-7800
E-mail: arthritisfoundation@arthritis.org
Web site: http://www.arthritis.org
The Arthritis Foundation is the world's largest, private, nonprofit contributor to arthritis research; it supports research into more than 100 types of arthritis and related conditions.

Bill and Melinda Gates Foundation
P.O. Box 23350
Seattle, WA 98102
Telephone: (206) 709-3100
E-mail: info@gatesfoundation.org
Web site: http://www.gatesfoundation.org

The Gates Foundation "works to help all people lead healthy, productive lives. In developing countries, it focuses on improving people's health and giving them the chance to lift themselves out of hunger and extreme poverty. In the United States, it seeks to ensure that all people—especially those with the fewest resources—have access to the opportunities they need to succeed in school and life."

Brain Trauma Foundation (BTF)
415 Madison Avenue, 14th Floor
New York, NY 10017
Telephone: (212) 772-0608
Web site: http://www.braintrauma.org
The BTF was founded to improve the outcome of Traumatic Brain Injury (TBI) patients by developing best practice guidelines, conducting clinical research, and educating medical personnel.

Christopher and Dana Reeve Foundation
636 Morris Turnpike, Suite 34
Short Hills, NJ 07078
Telephone: (800) 225-0293
Web site: http://www.christopherreeve.org
The foundation is "dedicated to curing spinal cord injury by funding innovative research, and improving the quality of life for people with paralysis through grants, information, and advocacy"; it has a Paralysis Resource Center that provides information to patients and their families.

Commonwealth Fund
One East 75th Street
New York, NY 10021
Telephone: (212) 606-3800
Fax: (212) 606-3500
E-mail: info@cmwf.org
Web site: http://www.commonwealthfund.org
The Commonwealth Fund, a private foundation, aims to promote a high-performing healthcare system that better addresses the needs of society's most vulnerable groups.

Cystic Fibrosis Foundation
6931 Arlington Road
Bethesda, MD 20814
Telephone: (301) 951-4422
Fax: (301) 951-6378

E-mail: info@cff.org
Web site: http://www.cff.org
The mission of the foundation is "to assure the development of the means to cure and control cystic fibrosis and to improve the quality of life for those with the disease."

Diabetes Research and Wellness Foundation (DRWF)
5151 Wisconsin Avenue, NW, Suite 420
Washington, DC 20016
Telephone: (202) 298-9211
Fax: (202) 244-4999
E-mail: diabeteswellness@diabeteswellness.net
Web site: http://www.diabeteswellness.net
The DRWF was founded to help find a cure for diabetes, and "until that goal is achieved to provide the care needed to combat the detrimental and life-threatening complications of this terrible disease."

Epilepsy Foundation of America
8301 Professional Place
Landover, MD 20785
Telephone: (800) 332-1000
Web site: http://www.epilepsyfoundation.org
The foundation is a national voluntary organization "dedicated solely to the welfare of the almost 3 million people with epilepsy in the United States and their families."

Families USA Foundation
1201 New York Avenue, NW, Suite 1100
Washington, DC 20005
Telephone: (202) 628-3030
Fax: (202) 347-2417
E-mail: info@familiesusa.org
Web site: http://www.familiesusa.org
The Families USA Foundation is a national nonprofit, nonpartisan organization "dedicated to the achievement of high-quality, affordable health care for all Americans."

Foundation Center
79 Fifth Ave./16th Street
New York, NY 10003-3076
Telephone: (800) 424-9836
Fax: (212) 807-3677
Web site: http://www.foundationcenter.org

The foundation's mission is to integrate people with disabilities into all aspects of American life.

Henry J. Kaiser Family Foundation (KFF)
2400 Sand Hill Road
Menlo Park, CA 94025
Telephone: (650) 854-9400
Fax: (650) 854-4800
Web site: http://www.kff.org
The KFF is a nonprofit, private operating foundation that focuses on the major healthcare issues facing the United States, as well as the U.S. role in global health policy.

Joseph P. Kennedy, Jr. Foundation
1133 19th Street, NW, 12th Floor
Washington, DC 20036-3604
Telephone: (202) 393-1250
Fax: (202) 824-0351
Web site: http://www.jpkf.org
The foundation's goals include enhancing the quality of life of persons with intellectual disabilities, providing seed funding for projects, increasing professional and public awareness of the needs of persons with intellectual disabilities, and working to reduce the incidence of intellectual disabilities.

Juvenile Diabetes Research Foundation International (JDRF)
120 Wall Street
New York, NY 10005-4001
Telephone: (800) 533-2873
Fax: (212) 785-9595
E-mail: info@jdrf.org
Web site: http://www.jdrf.org
The mission of the JDRF is to find a cure for diabetes and its complications through support of research.

Robert Wood Johnson Foundation (RWJF)
P.O. Box 2316
Route 1 and College Road East
Princeton, NJ 08543
Telephone: (877) 843-7953
Web site: http://www.rwjf.org
The RWJF is the nation's largest philanthropy exclusively dedicated to improving the health and healthcare of all Americans.

W. K. Kellogg Foundation
One Michigan Avenue East
Battle Creek, MI 49017-4012
Telephone: (269) 968-1611
Fax: (269) 968-0413
Web site: http://www.wkkf.org
The Kellogg Foundation "supports children, families and communities as they strengthen and create conditions that propel vulnerable children to achieve success as individuals and as contributors to the larger community and society."

9. U.S. Government Agencies, Departments, and Institutes

Administration on Aging (AOA)
One Massachusetts Avenue, NW
Washington, DC 20001
Telephone: (202) 619-0724
Fax: (202) 357-3555
E-mail: aoainfo@aoa.hhs.gov
Web site: http://www.aoa.gov
The AOA, an agency within the U.S. Department of Health and Human Services (HHS), works to "help elderly individuals maintain their dignity and independence in their homes and communities through comprehensive, coordinated, and cost effective systems of long-term care, and livable communities across the nation."

Administration on Developmental Disabilities (ADD)
Administration for Children and Families
U.S. Department of Health and Human Services (HHS)
Mail Stop: HHH 465-D
370 L'Enfant Promenade, SW
Washington, DC 20447
Telephone: (202) 690-6590
Fax: (202) 690-6904
Web site: http://www.acf.hhs.gov/programs/add/index.html
The ADD, which is part of the Administration for Children and Families, is the government agency responsible for implementing the Developmental Disabilities Assistance and Bill of Rights Act of 2000, also known as the DD Act.

Agency for Healthcare Research and Quality (AHRQ)
540 Gaither Road
Rockville, MD 20850

Telephone: (301) 427-1364

Web site: http://www.ahrq.gov

The AHRQ is the health services research arm of the U.S. Department of Health and Human Services (HHS); its areas of concentration include quality improvement and patient safety, outcomes and effectiveness of healthcare, clinical practice and technology assessment, and healthcare organization and delivery systems.

Centers for Disease Control and Prevention (CDC)

1600 Clifton Road

Atlanta, GA 30333

Telephone: (800) 232-4636

Web site: http://www.cdc.gov

The CDC is a major health unit of the U.S. Department of Health and Human Services (DHHS); through its six coordinating centers and offices and the National Institute for Occupational Safety and Health (NIOSH) it monitors, investigates, and works to prevent diseases, injuries, and disabilities.

Centers for Medicare and Medicaid Services (CMS)

7500 Security Boulevard

Baltimore, MD 21244

Telephone: (410) 786-3000

Web site: http://www.cms.hhs.gov

The CMS is the federal agency that administers Medicare, Medicaid, and the Children's Health Insurance Program.

Food and Drug Administration (FDA)

10903 New Hampshire Avenue

Silver Spring, MD 20993-0002

Telephone: (888) 463-6332

Web site: http://www.fda.gov

The FDA is an agency within the U.S. Department of Health and Human Services (HHS) that regulates drugs, medical devices, vaccines, blood and biologics, animal and veterinary products, cosmetics, radiation-emitting products, and tobacco products.

Health Resources and Services Administration (HRSA)

5600 Fishers Lane

Rockville, MD 20857

Telephone: (301) 998-7373

E-mail: callcenter@hrsa.gov

Web site: http://www.hrsa.gov

The HRSA is the primary federal agency for improving access to healthcare services for people who are uninsured, in rural areas, or are medically vulnerable.

Healthy People 2010
Office of Disease Prevention and Health Promotion (ODPHP)
U.S. Department of Health and Human Services (HHS)
1101 Wootton Parkway, Suite LL100
Rockville, MD 20852
Telephone: (240) 453-8280
Fax: (240) 453-8282
Web site: http://www.healthypeople.gov
Healthy People 2010 is "a comprehensive set of disease prevention and health promotion objectives for the nation to achieve over the first decade of the new century"; the measurable objectives were created by scientists both inside and outside of the federal government.

Indian Health Service (IHS)
The Reyes Building
801 Thompson Avenue, Suite 400
Rockville, MD 20852
Telephone: (301) 443-6394
Web site: http://www.ihs.gov
The IHS, an agency of the U.S. Department of Health and Human Services (HHS), provides federal healthcare services to American Indians and Alaska natives; it serves 1.9 million American Indians and Alaska natives residing on or near reservations.

Maternal and Child Health Bureau (MCHB)
Health Resources and Services Administration
Parklawn Building, Room 18-05
5600 Fishers Lane
Rockville, MD 20857
Telephone: (301) 443-2170
Fax: (301) 443-1797
E-mail: ctibbs@hrsa.gov
Web site: http://mchb.hrsa.gov
The MCHB works to improve the delivery of services to all mothers and children, and it seeks to reduce infant mortality and improve the health of children and families.

National Cancer Institute (NCI)
NCI Public Inquires Office
6116 Executive Boulevard, Room 3036A

Bethesda, MD 20892-8322
Telephone: (800) 422-6237
Web site: http://www.cancer.gov
The NCI, one of the National Institutes of Health (NIH), "coordinates the National Cancer Program, which conducts and supports research, training, health information dissemination, and other programs with respect to the cause, diagnosis, prevention, and treatment of cancer, rehabilitation care of cancer patients and the families of cancer patients."

National Center for Health Statistics (NCHS)
3311 Toledo Road
Hyattsville, MD 20782
Telephone: (800) 232-4636
E-mail: cdcinfo@cdc.gov
Web site: http://www.cdc.gov/nchs
The NCHS, which is part of the Centers for Disease Control and Prevention (CDC), conducts a wide range of surveys on the health characteristics of the nation's civilian population.

National Eye Institute (NEI)
Information Office
31 Center Drive, MSC 2510
Bethesda, MD 20892-2510
Telephone: (301) 496-5248
E-mail: 2020@nei.nih.gov
Web site: http://www.nei.nih.gov
The mission of the NEI, one of the National Institutes of Health (NIH), is to "conduct and support research, training, health information dissemination, and other programs with respect to blinding eye diseases, visual disorders, mechanisms of visual function, preservation of sight, and the special health problems and requirements of the blind."

National Heart, Lung, and Blood Institute (NHLBI)
NHLBI Health Information Center
P.O. Box 30105
Bethesda, MD 20824-0105
Telephone: (301) 592-8573
Fax: (240) 629-3246
E-mail: nhlbiinfo@nhlbi.nih.gov
Web site: http://www.nhlbi.nih.gov
The NHLBI, one of the National Institutes of Health (NIH), "plans, conducts, and supports research related to the causes, prevention, diagnosis, and treatment of heart, blood

vessel, lung, and blood diseases, and sleep disorders; the institute also administers national health education campaigns on women and heart disease, healthy weight for children, and other topics."

National Human Genome Research Institute (NHGRI)
Communication and Public Liaison Branch
Building 31, Room 4B09
31 Center Drive, MSC 2152
9000 Rockville Pike
Bethesda, MD 20892-2152
Telephone: (301) 402-0911
Fax: (301) 402-2218
Web site: http://www.genome.gov
The NHGRI, one of the National Institutes of Health (NIH), conducts "a broad range of studies aimed at understanding the structure and function of the human genome and its role in health and disease."

National Institute of Allergy and Infectious Diseases (NIAID)
6610 Rockledge Drive, MSC 6612
Bethesda, MD 20892-6612
Telephone: (866) 284-4107
Fax: (301) 402-3573
E-mail: niaidnews@niaid.nih.gov
Web site: http://www.niaid.nih.gov/Pages/default.aspx
The NIAID, one of the National Institutes of Health (NIH), "conducts and supports basic and applied research to better understand, treat, and ultimately prevent infectious, immunologic, and allergic diseases."

National Institute of Arthritis and Musculoskeletal and Skin Diseases (NIAMS)
Building 31, Room 4C02
Bethesda, MD 20892-2350
Telephone: (301) 496-8190
Fax: (301) 480-2814
E-mail: NIAMSinfo@mail.nih.gov
Web site: http://www.niams.nih.gov
The mission of the NIAMS, one of the National Institutes of Health (NIH), is "to support research into the causes, treatment, and prevention of arthritis and musculoskeletal and skin diseases, the training of basic and clinical scientists to carry out this research, and the dissemination of information on research programs in these diseases."

National Institute of Child Health and Human Development (NICHD), Eunice Kennedy Shriver

P.O. Box 3006

Rockville, MD 20847

Telephone: (800) 370-2943

Fax: (866) 760-5947

E-mail: NICHDinformationResourcesCenter@mail.nih.gov

Web site: http://www.nichd.nih.gov

The NICHB, one of the National Institutes of Health (NIH), "conducts and supports research on all stages of human development, from preconception to adulthood, to better understand the health of children, adults, families, and communities."

National Institute of Diabetes and Digestive and Kidney Disorders (NIDDK)

Building 31, Room 9A06

31 Center Drive, MSC 2560

Bethesda, MD 20892-2560

Telephone: (301) 496-3583

Web site: http://www2.niddk.nih.gov

The NIDDK, one of the National Institutes of Health (NIH), conducts and supports research in a broad spectrum of metabolic diseases such as diabetes, obesity, inborn errors in metabolism, endocrine disorders, mineral metabolism, digestive and liver diseases, nutrition, urology and renal disease, and hematology.

National Institute of Mental Health (NIMH)

6001 Executive Boulevard

Room 8184, MSC 9663

Bethesda, MD 20892-9663

Telephone: (866) 415-8051

Fax: (301) 443-4279

E-mail: nimhinfo@nih.org

Web site: http://www.nimh.nih.gov/index.shtml

The mission of the NIMH, one of the National Institutes of Health (NIH), is "to transform the understanding and treatment of mental illnesses through basic and clinical research, paving the way for prevention, recovery, and cure."

National Institute of Neurological Disorders and Stroke (NINDS)

NIH Neurological Institute

P.O. Box 5801

Bethesda, MD 20824

Telephone: (800) 352-9424

Web site: http://www.ninds.nih.gov
The mission of the NINDS, one of the National Institutes of Health (NIH), is to "reduce the burden of neurological diseases."

National Institute on Aging (NIA)

Building 31, Room 5C27
31 Center Drive, MSC 2292
Bethesda, MD 20892
Telephone: (301) 496-1752
Fax: (301) 496-1072
E-mail: niainfo@mail.nih.gov
Web site: http://www.nia.nih.gov
The NIA, one of the National Institutes of Health (NIH), "leads a broad scientific effort to understand the nature of aging and to extend the healthy, active years of life."

National Institute on Alcohol Abuse and Alcoholism (NIAAA)

5635 Fishers Lane, MSC 9304
Bethesda, MD 20892-9304
Telephone: (301) 443-3860
Web site: http://www.niaaa.nih.gov
The NIAAA, one of the National Institutes of Health (NIH), provides leadership in the national effort to reduce alcohol-related problems by conducting research, coordinating and collaborating with other institutes and federal programs, and translating and disseminating research findings.

National Institute on Deafness and Other Communication Disorders (NIDCD)

31 Center Drive, MSC 2320
Bethesda, MD 20892-2320
Telephone: (800) 241-1044
Fax: (301) 402-0018
E-mail: nidcdinfo@nidcd.nih.gov
Web site: http://www.nidcd.nih.gov
The NIDCD, one of the National Institutes of Health (NIH), is "mandated to conduct and support biomedical and behavioral research and research training in the normal and disordered processes of hearing, balance, smell, taste, voice, speech, and language."

National Institute on Disability and Rehabilitation Research (NIDRR)

U.S. Department of Education
400 Maryland Avenue, SW, Mailstop PCP-6038
Washington, DC 20202-2572

Telephone: (202) 245-7640
Fax: (202) 245-7323
Web site: http://www.ed.gov/about/offices/list/osers/nidrr/index.html
The NIDRR "provides leadership and support for a comprehensive program of research related to the rehabilitation of individuals with disabilities."

National Institute on Drug Abuse (NIDA)
6001 Executive Boulevard, Room 5213
Bethesda, MD 20892-9561
Telephone: (301) 443-1124
E-mail: information@nida.nih.gov
Web site: http://www.nida.nih.gov
The mission of the NIDA, one of the National Institutes of Health (NIH), is to bring "the power of science to bear on drug abuse and addiction."

National Institutes of Health (NIH)
9000 Rockville Pike
Bethesda, MD 20892
Telephone: (301) 496-4000
E-mail: NIHinfo@od.nih.gov
Web site: http://www.nih.gov
The NIH, which is composed of 27 institutes and centers, is the primary federal agency for conducting and supporting medical research.

Office on Disability (OD)
U.S. Department of Health and Human Services (HHS)
200 Independence Avenue, SW
Room 637D
Washington, DC 20201
Telephone: (877) 696-6775
E-mail: ODInfo@hhs.gov
Web site: http://www.hhs.gov/od
The mission of OD is to oversee the implementation and coordination of programs and policies within the various agencies of the Department of Health and Human Services (HHS) that enhance the health and well-being of people with disabilities.

Social Security Administration (SSA)
Office of Public Inquires
Windsor Park Building
6401 Security Boulevard

Baltimore, MD 21235
Telephone: (800) 772-1213
Web site: www.socialsecurity.gov
The SSA provides benefits to retirees and people with disabilities; it has a nationwide network of over 1,400 offices.

Substance Abuse and Mental Health Services Administration (SAMHSA)
P.O. Box 2345
Rockville, MD 20847-2345
Telephone: (877) 726-4727
Fax: (240) 221-4292
E-mail: shin@samhsa.hhs.gov
Web site: http://www.samhsa.gov
The SAMHSA is a federal agency that attempts to improve the lives of people who have (or are at risk of) mental and substance abuse disorders.

U.S. Census Bureau
4600 Silver Hill Road
Washington, DC 20233
Telephone: (800) 923-8282
Web site: http://www.census.gov
The Census Bureau conducts the population and housing census of the United States (every 10 years), the economic census of the United States (every 5 years), the American Community Survey (annually), and other surveys; some of the surveys identify the characteristics of individuals with disabilities.

U.S. Department of Education (ED)
400 Maryland Avenue, SW
Washington, DC 20202
Telephone: (800) 872-5327
Web site: http://www.ed.gov
The U.S. Department of Education establishes policy for, administers, and coordinates most federal assistance to education.

U.S. Department of Health and Human Services (HHS)
200 Independence Avenue, SW
Washington, DC 20201
Telephone: (877) 696-6775
Web site: http://www.hhs.gov

The HHS, which consists of the Office of the Secretary and 11 agencies, performs a wide variety of tasks and services, including public health, food and drug safety, health insurance, and many others.

U.S. Department of Homeland Security
245 Murray Lane, SW
Washington, DC 20528
Telephone: (202) 282-8000
Web site: http://www.dhs.gov/index.shtm
The U.S. Department of Homeland Security addresses emergency preparedness and response, counterterrorism, border security, and immigration.

U.S. Department of Justice (DOJ), Civil Rights Division, Disability Rights Section
950 Pennsylvania Avenue, NW
Disability Rights Section–NYA
Washington, DC 20530
Telephone: (202) 307-1198
Web site: http://www.justice.gov/crt/drs/drshome.php
The "primary goal of the Disability Rights Section is to achieve equal opportunity for people with disabilities in the United States by implementing the Americans with Disabilities Act (ADA)."

U.S. Department of Labor (DOL)
Frances Perkins Building
200 Constitution Avenue, NW
Washington, DC 20210
Telephone: (866) 487-2365
Web site: http://www.dol.gov
The DOL fosters and promotes the welfare of the job seekers, wage earners, and retirees of the United States by improving their work conditions, advancing their opportunities for profitable employment, protecting their retirement and healthcare benefits, helping employers find workers, strengthening free collective bargaining, and tracking changes in employment, prices, and other national economic measurements.

U.S. Department of Veterans Affairs (VA)
810 Vermont Avenue, NW
Washington, DC 20420
Telephone: (800) 827-1000
Web site: http://www.va.gov

The VA provides patient care and federal benefits to veterans and their dependents; its healthcare facilities and programs provide a broad spectrum of medical, surgical, and rehabilitative care.

U.S. Government Accountability Office (GAO)
441 G Street, NW
Washington, DC 20548
Telephone: (202) 512-3000
E-mail: contact@gao.gov
Web site: http://www.gao.gov
The GAO is an independent, nonpartisan agency that works for the U.S. Congress but also serves as a "watchdog" over congressional expenditures of taxpayer dollars. The GAO's mission statement is "to support the Congress in meeting its constitutional responsibilities and to help improve the performance and ensure the accountability of the federal government for the benefit of the American people. We provide Congress with timely information that is objective, fact-based, nonpartisan, nonideological, fair, and balanced."

10. U.S. Government Advisory Commissions

Medicare Payment Advisory Commission (MedPAC)
601 New Jersey Avenue, NW, Suite 9000
Washington, DC 20001
Telephone: (202) 220-3700
Fax: (202) 220-3759
Web site: http://www.medpac.gov
The MedPAC is an independent government agency established to advise the U.S. Congress on issues affecting the Medicare program; it publishes a number of reports that are available online.

President's Committee for People with Intellectual Disabilities (PCPID)
Aerospace Center, Suite 210
370 L'Enfant Promenade, SW
Washington, DC 20447
Telephone: (202) 619-0634
Fax: (202) 205-9519
E-mail: LRoach@acf.hhs.gov
Web site: http://www.acf.hhs.gov/programs/pcpid/index.html
The PCPID, which consists of 21 citizen members and 13 federal government members, all appointed by the president of the United States, advises the president on intellectual

disability issues; it evaluates the adequacy of current practices and programs and reviews federal agency activities impacting on people with intellectual disabilities.

Social Security Advisory Board (SSAB)
400 Virginia Avenue, SW, Suite 625
Washington, DC 20024
Telephone: (202) 475-7700
Fax: (202) 475-7715
E-mail: info@ssab.gov
Web site: http://www.ssab.gov
The SSAB is an independent, bipartisan board created to advise the president, the U.S. Congress, and the Commissioner of Social Security on matters related to Social Security and Supplemental Security Income programs; it publishes a number of reports that are available online.

11. Healthcare Systems, Associations, and Programs of Other Nations

Canadian Centre on Disability Studies (CCDS)
56 The Promenade
Winnipeg, MB
R3B 3H9
Canada
Telephone: (204) 287-8411
Fax: (204) 284-5343
E-mail: ccds@disabilitystudies.ca
Web site: www.disabilitystudies.ca
The CCDS is "dedicated to research, education, and information dissemination on disability issues."

Health Canada
Address Locator 0900C1
Ottawa, Ontario
K1A 0K9
Canada
Telephone: (866) 225-0709
Fax: (613) 941-5366
Web site: http://www.hc-sc.gc.ca
Health Canada is a detailed source of information on the healthcare system of Canada; it offers reports and publications on a variety of health-related topics for individuals and organizations.

Medicare Australia
Client Liaison Unit
Information Strategy Section
Legal, Privacy, and Information Services Branch
P.O. Box 1001
Tuggeranong DC ACT 2901
Australia
Telephone: 1800 101 099
Fax: +61 2 6124 6935
E-mail: statistics@medicareaustralia.gov.au
Web site: http://www.medicareaustralia.gov.au
Medicare Australia is part of the Australian national healthcare system that provides healthcare services and payments to Australia's population.

United Kingdom's National Health Service (NHS)
Riverside House
2A Southwark Bridge Road
London SE1 94A
England
Telephone: 020 7599 4200
Web site: http://www.nhs.uk
The NHS is the world's largest publicly funded health service.

12. International Organizations

Academic Network of European Disability (ANED)
Human European Consultancy
Maliestraat 7, 3581 SH Utrecht
The Netherlands
Telephone: +31 30 634 1422
E-mail: aned@humanconsultancy.com
Web site: http://www.disability-europe.net
The aim of ANED is to "establish and maintain a pan-European academic network in the disability field that will support policy development in collaboration with the European Commission's Disability Unit."

Disabled Peoples' International (DPI)
874 Topsail Road
Mount Pearl, Newfoundland
A1N 3J9

Canada
Telephone: (709) 747-7600
Fax: (709) 747-7603
E-mail: info@dpi.org
Web site: http://www.dpi.org
The DPI describes itself as a "network of national organizations or assemblies of disabled people, established to promote human rights of disabled people through full participation, equalization of opportunity and development."

European Commission (EC)
DG Employment, Social Affairs and Equal Opportunities
B-1049 Brussels
Belgium
Telephone: 00800 6 7 8 9 10 11
Web site: http://ec.europa.eu
The European Commission (EC) is part of the European Union (EU) economic and political partnership of 27 democratic European countries; it works in numerous EU policy areas, including coordination of the social security and healthcare rights of workers and other EU citizens.

Handicap International
6930 Carroll Avenue, Suite 240
Takoma Park, MD 20912-4468
Telephone: (301) 891-2138
Fax: (301) 891-9193
E-mail: info@handicap-international.us
Web site: http://www.handicap-international.us
Handicap International "gives assistance and aid to vulnerable groups, disabled people, displaced people and refugees"; it has 240 programs in 60 countries.

International Committee of the Red Cross (ICRC)
19 Avenue de la Paix
CH 1202 Geneva
Switzerland
Telephone: ++ 41(22) 734-6001
Fax: ++ 41(22) 733-2057
Web site: http://www.icrc.org
The ICRC is an independent, politically neutral, humanitarian organization that works to ensure the protection and assistance for victims of war and other violence.

International Society of Physical and Rehabilitation Medicine (ISPRM)
Kloosterstraat 5
B-9960 Assenede
Belgium
Telephone: +32 (0)9 344 39 59
Fax: +32 (0)9 344 40 10
E-mail: Werner@medcongress.com
Web site: http://www.isprm.org
The ISPRM is an international scientific and educational society for practitioners in the field of physical and rehabilitation medicine.

Organisation for Economic Co-operation and Development (OECD)
2, rue Andre Pascal
75775 Paris Cedex 16
France
Telephone: + 33 1 45 24 82 00
Fax: + 33 1 45 24 85 00
Web site: http://www.oecd.org
The OECD collects and publishes comparable statistics on economic, social, and health characteristics of 30 democratic countries.

Pan American Health Organization (PAHO)
525 23rd Street, NW
Washington, DC 20037
Telephone: (202) 974-3000
Fax: (202) 974-3663
Web site: http://www.paho.org
The PAHO coordinates and develops health policies for the countries of North and South America; it also serves as the Regional Office for the Americas of the World Health Organization (WHO).

Rehabilitation International (RI)
25 East 21 Street, 4th Floor
New York, NY 10010
Telephone: (212) 420-1500
Fax: (212) 505-0871
E-mail: ri@riglobal.org
Web site: http://www.riglobal.org

RI describes itself as "a global network of experts, professionals and advocates working together to empower persons with disabilities and provide sustainable solutions for a more inclusive and accessible society."

United Nations (UN)
First Avenue at 46th Street
New York, NY 10017
Telephone: (212) 963-8652
Fax: (212) 963-4116
Web site: http://www.un.org
The UN is an international organization of countries around the world. The stated purpose of the UN is to maintain international peace and security, develop friendly relationships among nations, and promote social progress, better living standards, and human rights around the globe.

United Nations Children's Fund (UNICEF)
3 United Nations Plaza
New York, NY 10017
Telephone: (212) 326-7000
Fax: (212) 887-7465
Web site: http://www.unicef.org
UNICEF works with governments, national agencies, and civil societies to prevent infant mortality by providing vaccines, food supplements, insecticide-treated bed nets, and safe hygiene practices.

U.S. Agency for International Development (USAID)
Information Center
Ronald Reagan Building
Washington, DC 20523-1000
Telephone: (202) 712-4320
Fax: (202) 216-3524
E-mail: ksc@usaid.gov
Web site: http://www.usaid.gov
The USAID, an independent agency of the federal government, provides assistance to countries worldwide; it supports economic growth, global health, and democracy.

World Bank
1818 H Street, NW
Washington, DC 29433
Telephone: (202) 473-1000

Fax: (202) 477-6391

Web site: http://www.worldbank.org

The World Bank provides financial and technical assistance to developing countries; it publishes reports on various topics, including human development, poverty, health, and disability.

World Health Organization (WHO)

Avenue Appia 20

1211 Geneva 27

Switzerland

Telephone: + 41 22 791 21 11

Fax: + 41 22 791 31 11

E-mail: info@who.int

Web site: http://www.who.int

The WHO is the health organization of the United Nations (UN); it addresses global health issues, establishes health policies and sets standards, provides technical support, and monitors health trends.

World Institute on Disability (WID)

510 16th Street, Suite 100

Oakland, CA 94612

Telephone: (510) 763-4100

Fax: (510) 763-4109

E-mail: wid@wid.org

Web site: http://www.wid.org

The mission of WID in communities and nations worldwide "is to eliminate barriers to full social integration and increase employment, economic security, and health care for persons with disabilities."

Seven

Selected Print and Electronic Resources

This chapter identifies core print and electronic resources for selected topics in medicine, public health, and disability. The resources are grouped into nine categories: (1) Reference Works; (2) U.S. Government Sources; (3) Other Nations and International Sources; (4) Data Sources and Trends; (5) Diseases, Injuries, and Conditions; (6) Public Health; (7) Clinical, Allied, and Other Health Professionals and Paraprofessionals; (8) Healthcare Organizations; and (9) Problems Experienced by People with Disability.

1. Reference Works

Albrecht, G. L. (Ed.). (2006). *Encyclopedia of disability* (5 vols.). Thousand Oaks, CA: Sage.
  This five-volume encyclopedia, containing over 1,000 entries written by more than 500 world-renowned scholars, is the largest single source of information on disability.

Albrecht, G. L., Seelman, K. D., & Bury, M. (Eds.). (2001). *Handbook of disability studies*. Thousand Oaks, CA: Sage.
  This book contains 34 chapters divided into three sections: the shaping of disability studies as a field; experiencing disability; and disability in context.

Boslaugh, S. E. (Ed.). (2008). *Encyclopedia of epidemiology* (2 vols.). Thousand Oaks, CA: Sage.

Braddock, D. L., Hemp, R., & Rizzolo, M. C. (2008). *The state of the states in developmental disabilities* (7th ed.). Washington, DC: American Association on Intellectual and Developmental Disabilities.

Breslow, L. (Ed.). (2002). *Encyclopedia of public health* (4 vols.). New York: Macmillan Reference.
This encyclopedia is considered a classic work in the field of public health.

Burch, S. (Ed.). (2009). *Encyclopedia of American disability history* (3 vols.). New York: Facts on File.

Centers for Disease Control and Prevention. (2006). *Disability and health state chart book, 2006 profiles of health for adults with disabilities.* Atlanta, GA: Centers for Disease Control and Prevention. Retrieved from http://www.cdc.gov/ncbddd/chartbook/Chartbook%20Text.pdf

Field, M. J., & Jette, A. M. (Eds.). (2007). *The future of disability in America.* Washington, DC: National Academies Press. Retrieved from http://www.nap.edu/catalog/11898.html
The report makes a number of recommendations in the areas of disability monitoring; healthcare transitions, secondary conditions, and aging with disability; environmental barriers; assistive and accessible technologies; and organizing and financing disability research.

Fisher, G. L., & Roget, N. A. (Eds.). (2009). *Encyclopedia of substance abuse prevention, treatment, and recovery* (2 vols.). Thousand Oaks, CA: Sage.

Kelly, E. B. (2009). *Encyclopedia of attention deficit hyperactivity disorder.* Santa Barbara, CA: ABC-CLIO.

Mullner, R. M. (Ed.). (2009). *Encyclopedia of health services research* (2 vols.). Thousand Oaks, CA: Sage.
This two-volume encyclopedia, containing over 400 entries written by more than 500 experts, is the largest single source of information on health services research.

Reynolds, C. R., & Fletcher-Janzen, E. (Eds.). (2007). *Encyclopedia of special education: A reference for the education of children, adolescents, and adults with disabilities and other exceptional individuals* (3rd ed., 3 vols.). Hoboken, NJ: John Wiley and Sons.

2. U.S. Government Sources

Carmona, R. M. (2005). *The Surgeon General's call to action to improve the health and wellness of people with disabilities.* Rockville, MD: Office of the Surgeon General,

Public Health Service, U.S. Department of Health and Human Services. Retrieved from http://www.surgeongeneral.gov
This was the first-ever Surgeon General's Call to Action on disability. It outlined four major goals: increase understanding nationwide that people with disabilities can lead long, healthy, and productive lives; increase knowledge among healthcare professionals and provide them with tools to screen, diagnose, and treat the whole person with a disability with dignity; increase awareness among people with disabilities of the steps they can take to develop and maintain a healthy lifestyle; and increase accessible healthcare and support services to promote independence for people with disabilities.

Federal Interagency Forum on Aging-Related Statistics. (2008). *Older Americans 2008: Key indicators of well-being.* Washington, DC: U.S. Government Printing Office. Retrieved from http://www.agingstats.gov

Jans, L., Stoddard, S., & Kraus, L. (2004). *Chartbook on mental health and disability in the United States.* An InfoUse Report. Washington, DC: U.S. Department of Education, National Institute on Disability and Rehabilitation Research. Retrieved from http://www.infouse.org/disabilitydata/mentalhealth

Manderscheid, R. W., & Berry, J. T. (Eds.). (2006). *Mental health, United States, 2004.* Rockville, MD: Substance Abuse and Mental Health Services Administration. Retrieved from http://download.ncadisamhsa.gov/ken/pdf/SMA06–4195/CMHS_2004.pdf

National Center for Health Statistics. (2009). *Health, United States 2008 with chartbook.* Hyattsville, MD: Author. Retrieved from http://www.cdc.gov/nchs/data/hus/hus08.pdf

U.S. Census Bureau. (2008). *Statistical abstract of the United States: 2009: The national data book.* Washington, DC: U.S. Government Printing Office. Retrieved from http://www.census.gov/compendia/statab

U.S. Department of Health and Human Services. (2000). *Healthy people 2010* (2nd ed., 2 vols.). Washington, DC: U.S. Government Printing Office. Retrieved from http://www.health.gov/healthypeople
This publication is the U.S. Department of Health and Human Services' public health agenda for the decade.

U.S. Social Security Administration. (2009). *Annual statistical report on the Social Security Disability Insurance Program, 2008* (SSA Pub. No. 13-11826). Washington, DC: Author. Retrieved from http://www.socialsecurity.gov/policy/docs/statcomps/di_asr

3. Other Nations and International Sources

Other Nations

Australian Institute of Health and Welfare. (2004). *Disability and its relationship to health conditions and other factors* (AIHW Cat. No. DIS 37). Canberra, Australia: Author. Retrieved from http://www.aihw.gov.au/publications/dis/drhcf/drhcf.pdf

Cossette, L., & Duclos, E. (2002). *A profile of disability in Canada, 2001* (Cat. No. 89–577-XIE). Ottawa, Canada: Statistics Canada. Retrieved from http://www.statcan.gc.ca/pub/89–577-x/pdf/4228016-eng.pdf

International Sources

Braithwaite, J., & Mont, D. (2008). *Disability and poverty. A survey of World Bank poverty assessments and implications* (Social Protection and Labor Discussion Paper No. 0805). Washington, DC: World Bank. Retrieved from http://siteresource.worldbank.org/DISABILITY/Resource/280658-1172608138489/WBPovertyAssessments.pdf

Organisation for Economic Co-operation and Development. (2009, May 14–15). *Sickness, disability and work: Keeping on track in the economic downturn.* Background Paper, High-Level Forum, Stockholm, Sweden. Retrieved from http://www.oecd.org/dataoecd/42/15/42699911.pdf

United Nations. (2006). *The convention on the rights of persons with disabilities.* New York: Author. Retrieved from http://www.un.org/disabilities

World Health Organization. (2001). *International classification of functioning, disability and health.* Geneva: Author. *The WHO maintains an ICF Browser online at http://apps.who.int/classification/icfbrowser*

World Health Organization, Disability and Rehabilitation (DAR) Team. (2006). *Disability and rehabilitation WHO action plan 2006–2011.* Geneva: World Health Organization. Retrieved from http://www.who.int/disabilities/publication/dar_action_plan_2006to2011.pdf

World Health Organization, HIV/AIDS Department. (2009). *Priority interventions: HIV/AIDS prevention, treatment and care in the health sector.* Geneva: World Health Organization. Retrieved from http://www.who.int/hiv/pub/priority_interventions_web.pdf

World Health Organization and World Bank. (2011). *World report on disability*. Geneva: World Health Organization.

4. Data Sources and Trends

Data, Statistics, and Measurement

Altman, B . M., & Bernstein, A. B. (2008). *Disability and health in the United States, 2001–2005*. Hyattsville, MD: National Center for Health Statistics. Retrieved from http://www.cdc.gov/nchs/data/misc/disability2001–2005.pdf
According to this report, on average, "during 2001–2005, almost 30% of the noninstitutionalized adult U.S. population (approximately 62 million people) had basic actions difficulty, as indicated by reporting at least some difficulty with basic movement or sensory, cognitive, or emotional difficulties."

Brault, M. W. (2008). *Americans with disabilities: 2005* (Current population reports, No. 70–117). Washington, DC: U.S. Census Bureau. Retrieved from http://www.census.gov/prod/2008pubs/p70–117.pdf
According to this report, an estimated 54.4 million Americans, or about one in five U.S. residents, had some level of disability in 2005.

Bruyere, S. M., & Houtenville, A. J. (2006, Fall). Use of statistics from national data sources to inform rehabilitation program planning, evaluation, and advocacy. *Rehabilitation Counseling Bulletin, 50*(1), 46–58.
The authors describe disability data gathered by the 2000 Decennial Census Long Form, the American Community Survey, the National Health Information Survey, the National Health Information Survey on Disability, the Current Population Survey Annual Demographics Survey, the Survey of Income and Program Participation, the Health and Retirement Survey, and administrative records such as the Rehabilitation Services Administration 911 and the Social Security Administration Title 2 and Title 16 records.

Erickson, W. A., & Lee, C. G. (2008). *2007 disability status report: United States*. Ithaca, NY: Cornell University Rehabilitation Research and Training Center on Disability Demographics and Statistics. Retrieved from http://www.ilr.cornell.edu/edi/disabilitystatistics

Mont, D. (2007). *Measuring disability prevalence* (Social Protection and Labor Discussion Paper No. 0706). Washington, DC: World Bank. Retrieved from http://siteresource.worldbank.org/DISABILITY/Resource/Data/MontPrevalence.pdf

Mont, D. (2007, May 12). Measuring health and disability. *Lancet, 369*(9573), 1658–1663. Retrieved from http://siteresource.worldbank.org/DISABILITY/Resource/Data/DanLancet.pdf

Mudrick, N. R. (2002, November). The prevalence of disability among children: Paradigms and estimates. *Physical Medicine and Rehabilitation Clinics of North America, 13*(4), 775–792.

Social Security Advisory Board. (2003). *The Social Security definition of disability.* Washington, DC: Author. Retrieved from http://www.ssab.gov/documents/SocialSecurityDefinitionOfDisability.pdf

Disability and Population Trends

Bowen, M. E., & Gonzalez, H. M. (2008, October). Racial/ethnic differences in the relationship between the use of health care services and functional disability: The health and retirement study (1992–2004). *Gerontologist, 48*(5), 659–667.
The authors state: "Nationally, health care use for Blacks and Latinos was associated with more disabilities than for Whites after we accounted for predisposing, health need, and enabling factors. The findings suggest that improving health care quality for all Americans may supersede equal access to health care for reducing ethnic and racial disparities in functional health."

Ciol, M. A., Shumway-Cook, A., Hoffman, J. M., et al. (2008, March). Minority disparities in disability between Medicare beneficiaries. *Journal of the American Geriatrics Society, 56*(3), 444–453.

Freedman, V., Martin, L. G., & Schoei, R. F. (2002, December 25). Recent trends in disability and functioning among older adults in the United States: A systematic review. *Journal of the American Medical Association, 288*(24), 3137–3146.
The authors conclude: "Several measures of old age disability and limitations have shown improvements in the last decade. Research into the causes of these improvements is needed to understand the implications for the future demand for medical care."

Kroll, T. (Ed.). (2008). *Focus on disability: Trends in research and application.* New York: Nova Science.

Manton, K. G. (2008). Recent declines in chronic disability in the U.S. population: Risk factors and future dynamics. *Annual Review of Public Health, 29,* 91–113.
The author concludes: "Recent disability declines were continuations of declines in both chronic disease and disability occurring over the past century due to improved nutrition, sanitation, and education. Concerns exist about whether disability declines will continue because of recent increases in obesity prevalence."

Manton, K. G., Lamb, V. L., & Liang, X. (2007, June). Medicare cost effects of recent U.S. disability trends in the elderly: Future implications. *Journal of Aging and Health, 19*(3), 359–381.
The authors reported "Significant declines (up to 19%) in Medicare costs were found in 2004 and 2009 assuming continuation of the 1982 to 1999 disability declines and Medicare cost trends."

Morris, M., & Hartnett, J. (2009). *Disability: Future market demand and costs of long-term services and supports.* New York: Nova Science.

Pastor, P., Reuben, C. A., & Loeb, M. (2009). *Functional difficulties among school-aged children: United States, 2001–2007* (National Health Statistics Reports, No. 19). Hyattsville, MD: National Center for Health Statistics. Retrieved from http://www.cdc.gov/NCHS/data/nhsr/nhsr019.pdf
The authors found that "approximately 18% of children aged 5–17 had basic actions difficulty in one or more of the following domains of functioning: sensory, movement, cognitive, or emotional or behavioral."

Schoeni, R. F., Martin, L. G., Andreski, P. M., et al. (2005). Persistent and growing socioeconomic disparities in disability among the elderly: 1982–2002. *American Journal of Public Health, 95*(11), 2065– 2070.

Seeman, T. E., Merkin, S. S., Crimmins, E. M., et al. (2010, January). Disability trends among older Americans: National health and nutrition examination surveys, 1988–1994 and 1999–2004. *American Journal of Public Health, 100*(1), 100–107.

Social Security Administration. (2006). *Trends in the Social Security and Supplemental Security Income disability programs* (SSA Pub. No. 13–11832). Washington, DC: Author. Retrieved from http://ssaonline.us/policy/docs/chartbooks/disability_trends/index.html
According to the publication, "the Social Security Administration administers two of the largest disability programs in the United States: the Social Security Disability Insurance (DI) program and the Supplemental Security Income (SSI) disability program. In 2003, these programs combined paid more than $990 billion in cash benefits to nearly 11.2 million disabled persons."

Spillman, B. C. (2004). Changes in elderly disability rates and the implications for health care utilization and cost. *Milbank Quarterly, 82*(1), 157–194.

U.S. Department of State and National Institute on Aging. (2007). *Why population aging matters: A global perspective.* Bethesda, MD: National Institute on Aging. Retrieved from http://nia.nih.gov
This small, informative book identifies nine population trends that are transforming the world in fundamental ways: (1) an aging population; (2) increasing life expectancy; (3) rising numbers of the oldest old; (4) growing burden of non-communicable diseases; (5) aging and population decline; (6) changing family structure; (7) shifting patterns of work and retirement; (8) evolving social insurance systems; and (9) emerging economic challenges.

5. Diseases, Injuries, and Conditions
General Works

Brault, M. W., Hootman, J., Helmick, C. G., et al. (2009, May 1). Prevalence and most common causes of disability among adults—United States, 2005. *Morbidity and Mortality Weekly Report (MMWR), 58*(16), 421–426. Retrieved from http://www.cdc.gov/mmwr
Using data from the national Survey of Income and Program Participation (SIPP), the authors found that the prevalence of disability in 2005 (21.8%) remained unchanged from 1999; however, because of the aging of the nation's population, the absolute number of persons reporting a disability increased 7.7%, from 44.1 to 47.5 million. They also noted that the most common causes of disability continued to be arthritis or rheumatism (8.6 million), back or spine problems (7.6 million), and heart trouble (3.0 million).

Falvo, D. R. (2009). *Medical and psychosocial aspects of chronic illness and disability* (4th ed.). Sudbury, MA: Jones and Bartlett.

Farmer, J. E., Donders, J., & Warschausky, S. A. (Eds.). (2006). *Treating neurodevelopmental disabilities: Clinical research and practice.* New York: Guilford Press.

Judd, S. J. (Ed.). (2005). *Brain disorders sourcebook* (2nd ed.). Detroit, MI: Omnigraphics.

Judd, S. J. (Ed.). (2007). *Ear, nose, and throat disorders sourcebook* (2nd ed). Detroit, MI: Omnigraphics.

Alzheimer's Disease and Dementia

Ballenger, J. F., Whitehouse, P. J., Lyketsos, C. G., et al. (Eds.). (2009). *Treating dementia: Do we have a pill for it?* Baltimore, MD: Johns Hopkins University Press.

Grossberg, G. T., & Kamat, S. M. (2010). *Alzheimer's: The latest assessment and treatment strategies.* Sudbury, MA: Jones and Bartlett.

National Institute on Aging. (2008). *Alzheimer's disease: Unraveling the mystery.* Bethesda, MD: National Institute on Aging.
This and other publications on Alzheimer's Disease can be obtained from the National Institute on Aging's Alzheimer's Disease Education and Referral (ADEAR) Center Web site at http://www.nia.nih/Alzheimers

Shirey, L., & Summer, L. (2000, September). *Alzheimer's disease and dementia: A growing challenge.* Washington, DC: National Academy on an Aging Society. Retrieved from http://www.agingsociety.org/agingsociety/pdf/Alzheimers.pdf

Amputation

Kirkup, J. (2006). *A history of limb amputation*. New York: Springer.

Riley, R. (2005). *Living with a below-knee amputation: A unique insight from a prosthetist/ amputee*. Thorofare, NJ: SLACK.

Smith, D. G., Michael, J. W., & Bowker, J. H. (Eds.). (2004). *Atlas of amputations of limb deficiencies: Surgical, prosthetic and rehabilitation principles* (3rd ed.). Rosemont, IL: American Academy of Orthopedic Surgeons.

Amyotrophic Lateral Sclerosis (Lou Gehrig's Disease)

Cleveland, D. W. (2008). *From Charcot to Lou Gehrig: Mechanisms and treatment of ALS*. Bethesda, MD: National Institute of Health.
This streaming video (1 hour, 13 minutes in length) is available online at http:// videocast.nih.gov/launch.asp?14223.

Miller, R. G., Gelinas, D., & O'Conner, P. (Eds.). (2005). *Amyotrophic Lateral Sclerosis*. New York: Demos Medical/American Academy of Neurology.

Mitsumoto, H. (Ed.). (2009). *Amyotrophic Lateral Sclerosis: A guide for patients and families* (3rd ed.). New York: Demos Medical.

Vincent, N., & Williams, B. J. (2010). *Principles of ALS care*. Sudbury, MA: Jones and Bartlett.

Arthritis

Dziedzic, K., & Hammond, A. (Eds.). (2010). *Rheumatology: Evidence-based practice for physiotherapists and occupational therapists*. New York: Churchill Livingstone.

Lorig, K., & Fries, J. F. (2000). *The arthritis helpbook: A tested self-management program for coping with arthritis and fibromyalgia*. New York: Perseus Books.

McNeil, M. E. A. (2005). *The first year—rheumatoid arthritis: An essential guide for the newly diagnosed*. New York: Marlowe.

Attention Deficit Hyperactivity Disorder (ADHD)

Barkley, R. A. (2010). *Attention deficit hyperactivity disorder in adults: The latest assessment and treatment strategies*. Sudbury, MA: Jones and Bartlett.

National Institute of Mental Health. (2008). *Attention deficit hyperactivity disorder (ADHD)*. Bethesda, MD: Author. Retrieved from http://www.nimh.nih.gov/ health/publications/index.shtml

Stahl, S. M., Mignon, L., & Muntner, N. (2010). *Attention deficit hyperactivity disorder.* New York: Cambridge University Press.

Autism Spectrum Disorders (ASDs)

Chez, M. G. (2010). *Autism and its medical management: A guide for parents and professionals.* Philadelphia, PA: Jessica Kingsley.

Frith, U. (2003). *Autism: Explaining the enigma* (2nd ed.), Malden, MA: Blackwell.

Lawton, S. (2007). *Asperger syndrome: Natural steps toward a better life.* Westport, CT: Praeger.

Rice, C. (2009, December 18). Prevalence of autism spectrum disorders—autism and developmental disabilities monitoring network, United States, 2006. *Morbidity and Mortality Weekly Report (MMWR), 58*(SS10).

Back Pain

Goldmann, D. R., & Horowitz, D. A. (Eds.). (2000). *DK American College of Physicians home medical guide to back pain.* New York: Dorling Kindersley.

Kostuik, J. P., Jan de Beur, S. M., & Margolis, S. (2003). *Back pain and osteoporosis.* Baltimore, MD: Johns Hopkins Medical Institution.

Santagida, P. L., Gross, A., Busse, J., et al. (2009). *Evidence report on complementary and alternative medicine in back pain utilization report* (Evidence Report/ Technology Assessment No. 177, AHRQ Pub. No. 09-E006). Rockville, MD: Agency for Healthcare Research and Quality. Retrieved from http://purl .access.gpo.gov/GPO/LPS108402
The authors of the report conclude: "There are few studies evaluating the relative utilization of various CAM therapies for back pain. For those studies evaluating utilization of individual CAM therapies, the specific characteristics of the therapy, the providers, and the clinical presentation of the back pain patients were not adequately detailed; nor was the overlap with other CAM or conventional treatments."

Cancer

Bracken, J. M. (2010). *Children with cancer: A reference guide for parents.* New York: Oxford University Press.

Carroll, W., & Finlay, J. L. (Eds.). (2010). *Cancer in children and adolescents.* Sudbury, MA: Jones and Bartlett.

Geyman, J. (2009). *The cancer generation: Baby boomers facing a perfect storm.* Monroe, ME: Common Courage Press.

Tobias, J. S., Hochhauser, D., & Souhami, R. L. (2010). *Cancer and its management*. Hoboken, NJ: Wiley-Blackwell.

Cardiac Conditions

Dunn, N., Everitt, H., & Simon, C. (2007). *Cardiovascular problems*. New York: Oxford University Press.

Kokkinos, P. (2010). *Physical activity and cardiovascular disease prevention*. Sudbury, MA: Jones and Bartlett.

Swanton, R. H. (2003). *Cardiology* (5th ed.). Malden, MA: Blackwell.

Chronic Obstructive Pulmonary Disease (COPD)

Blackler, L., Jones, C., & Mooney, C. (Eds.). (2007). *Managing chronic obstructive pulmonary disease*. Hoboken, NJ: Wiley.

Eisner, M. D., Blanc, P. D., Omachi, T. A., et al. (2011, January). Socioeconomic status, race, and COPD health outcomes. *Journal of Epidemiology and Community Health, 65*(1), 26–34.

MacNee, W., & Rennard, S. I. (2009). *Fast facts: Chronic obstructive pulmonary disease* (2nd ed.). Oxford, UK: Health Press.

Diabetes

Funnell, M. (2009). *Life with diabetes* (4th ed.). Alexandria, VA: American Diabetes Association.
This book provides a complete curriculum for delivering quality diabetes self-management education.

Holt, T. A., & Kumar, S. (2010). *ABC of diabetes* (6th ed.). Hoboken, NJ: Wiley-Blackwell/BMJ.

Kagan, A. (2009). *Type 2 diabetes: Social and scientific origins, medical complications and implications for patients and others*. Jefferson, NC: McFarland.

Matthews, D. D. (Ed.). (2003). *Diabetes sourcebook* (3rd ed.). Detroit, MI: Omnigraphics.

Epilepsy

Devinsky, O. (2007). *Epilepsy: Patient and family guide* (3rd ed.). New York: Demos Health.

Fisch, B. J. (Ed.). (2010). *Epilepsy and intensive care monitoring: Principles and practice.* New York: Demos Medical.

Reuber, M., Schachter, S. C., Elger, C. E., et al. (2009). *Epilepsy explained: A book for people who want to know more.* New York: Oxford University Press.

Fibromyalgia

Jones, K. D., & Hoffman, J. H. (2009). *Fibromyalgia.* Santa Barbara, CA: Greenwood Press/ABC-CLIO.

Ostalecki, S. (2007). *Fibromyalgia: The complete guide from medical experts and patients.* Sudbury, MA: Jones and Bartlett.

Starlanyl, D. J., & Copeland, M. E. (2001). *Fibromyalgia and chronic myofascial pain: A survival manual* (2nd ed.). Oakland, CA: New Harbinger.

Hearing Disorders and Deafness

Fiedler, D., & Krause, R. (Eds.). (2009). *Deafness, hearing loss, and the auditory system.* Hauppauge, NY: Nova Science.

Miller, M. H., & Schein, J. D. (2008). *Hearing disorders handbook.* San Diego, CA: Plural.

Stephens, D., & Kramer, S. E. (2010). *Living with hearing difficulties: The process of enablement.* Hoboken, NJ: Wiley-Blackwell.

Hip Fracture

Koval, K. J., & Zuckerman, J. D. (2000). *Hip fracture: A practical guide to management.* New York: Springer.

New Zealand Guidelines Group. (2003). *Acute management and immediate rehabilitation after hip fracture amongst people aged 65 years and over.* Wellington, New Zealand: Author. Retrieved from http://www.nzgg.org.nz/guidelines/dsp_guideline_popup.cfm?guidelineCatID=32 &guidelineID=6

Onslow, L. (2005). *Prevention and management of hip fractures.* Philadelphia, PA: Whurr.

HIV/AIDS

Durham, J. D., & Lashley, F. R. (Eds.). (2010). *The person with HIV/AIDS: Nursing perspectives.* New York: Springer.

Stolley, K. S., & Glass, J. E. (2009). *HIV/AIDS.* Santa Barbara, CA: Greenwood Press.

Weeks, B. S. (2010). *AIDS: The biological basis* (5th ed.). Sudbury, MA: Jones and Bartlett.

Intellectual and Developmental Disabilities

American Association on Intellectual and Developmental Disabilities. (2010). *Intellectual disability: Definition, classification, and systems of supports* (11th ed.). Washington, DC: Author.

Dryden-Edwards, R., & Combrinck-Graham, L. (Eds.). (2010). *Developmental disabilities from childhood to adulthood: What works for psychiatrists in community and institutional settings.* Baltimore, MD: Johns Hopkins University Press.

Eklund, L. C., & Nyman, A. S. (Eds.). (2009). *Learning and memory developments and intellectual disabilities.* Hauppauge, NY: Nova Science.

Harris, J. C. (2010). *Intellectual disability: A guide for families and professionals.* New York: Oxford University Press.

Multiple Sclerosis (MS)

Coyle, P. K., & Halper, J. (2001). *Meeting the challenge of progressive multiple sclerosis.* New York: Demos Medical.

Iezzoni, L. I. (2010). *Multiple sclerosis.* Santa Barbara, CA: Greenwood Press.

O'Mahony, D., & de Bursa, A. (Eds.). (2009). *Women and multiple sclerosis.* Hauppauge, NY: Nova Science.

Muscular Dystrophy

Abramovitz, M. (2008). *Muscular dystrophy.* San Diego, CA: Lucent Books.

Burgess, V. N. (Ed.). (2005). *Trends in muscular dystrophy research.* New York: Nova Biomedical Books.

Emery, A. E. H. (Ed.). (2001). *The muscular dystrophies.* New York: Oxford University Press.

Obesity

Bouchard, C., & Katzmarzyk, P. T. (Eds.). (2010). *Physical activity and obesity* (2nd ed.). Champaign, IL: Human Kinetics.

Fairburn, C. G., & Brownell, K. D. (Eds.). (2002). *Eating disorders and obesity: A comprehensive handbook* (2nd ed.). New York: Guilford.

Gard, M., & Wright, J. (2005). *The obesity epidemic: Science, morality and ideology.* New York: Routledge.

Waters, E. (Ed.). (2010). *Preventing childhood obesity: Evidence, policy, and practice.* Hoboken, NJ: Blackwell.

Osteoporosis

Barti, R., Frisch, B., & Barti, C. (2009). *Osteoporosis: Diagnosis, prevention, therapy* (2nd ed.). Berlin, Germany: Springer.

Mattingly, B. E., & Pillare, A. C. (Eds.). (2009). *Osteoporosis: Etiology, diagnosis, and treatment.* Hauppauge, NY: Nova Science.

Parkinson's Disease

Sharma, N. (2008). *Parkinson's disease.* Westport, CT: Greenwood Press.

Solimeo, S. (2009). *With shaking hands: Aging with Parkinson's disease in America's heartland.* New Brunswick, NJ: Rutgers University Press.

Weiner, W. J., Shulman, L. M., & Lang, A. E. (2007). *Parkinson's disease: A complete guide for patients and families* (2nd ed.). Baltimore, MD: Johns Hopkins University Press.

Psychiatric Disorders

Compton, M. T. (Ed.). (2010). *Clinical manual of prevention in mental health.* Washington, DC: American Psychiatric Publishing.

Karp, D. A., & Sisson, G. E. (Eds.). (2010). *Voices from the inside: Readings on the experiences of mental illness.* New York: Oxford University Press.

Simpson, G. A., Cohen, R. A., Pastor, P. N., et al. (2008, September). *Use of mental health services in the past 12 months by children aged 4–17 years: United States, 2005–2006* (NCHS Data Brief No. 8). Retrieved from http://www.cdc.gov/nchs/data/databriefs/db08.pdf

Spinal Cord Injury

Field-Fote, E. C. (2009). *Spinal cord injury rehabilitation.* Philadelphia, PA: F. A. Davis.

Mayo Clinic. (2009). *Mayo Clinic guide to living with a spinal cord injury: Moving ahead with your life.* New York: Demos Medical.

Palmer, S., Kriegsman, K. H., & Palmer, J. B. (2008). *Spinal cord injury: A guide for living* (2nd ed.). Baltimore, MD: Johns Hopkins University Press.

Selzer, M. E., & Dobkins, B. H. (2008). *Spinal cord injury: A guide for patients and families*. New York: Demos Medical.

Stroke

Brainin, M., & Heiss, W.-D. (Eds.). (2010). *Textbook of stroke medicine*. New York: Cambridge University Press.

Moratino, C., & Cardenas, B. (Eds.). (2009). *Hypertension, heredity, and stroke*. New York: Nova Biomedical Books.

Royal College of Physicians of London (2008). *National clinical guidelines for stroke* (3rd ed.). London: Royal College of Physicians of London.

Stein, J., Harvey, R. L., Macko, R. F., et al. (Eds.). (2009). *Stroke recovery and rehabilitation*. New York: Demos Medical.

Substance Abuse

Fields, R. (2010). *Drugs in perspective* (7th ed.). Boston, MA: McGraw-Hill.

Heinemann, A. W. (1993). *Substance abuse and physical disability*. New York: Haworth Press.

Scheier, L. M. (Ed.). (2010). *Handbook of drug use etiology: Theory, methods, and empirical findings*. Washington, DC: American Psychological Association.

Traumatic Brain Injury

Ashley, M. J. (Ed.). (2010). *Traumatic brain injury: Rehabilitation, treatment, and case management* (3rd ed.). Boca Raton, FL: CRC Press.

Chan, L. (2008). *New frontiers in traumatic brain injury: Evaluation and treatment*. Bethesda, MD: National Institute of Health.
This streaming video (1 hour, 13 minutes in length) is part of NIH Clinical Center's 2008 medicine for the public lecture series. It is available online at http://videocast.nih.gov/launch.asp?14837

High, W. M., Sander, A. M., Struchen, M. A., & Hart, K. A. (Eds.). (2005). *Rehabilitation for traumatic brain injury*. New York: Oxford University Press.

Vision Impairment and Blindness

Crandell, J. M., Jr., & Robinson, L. W. (2007). *Living with low vision and blindness: Guidelines that help professionals and individuals understand vision impairment*. Springfield, IL: Charles C Thomas.

McLannahan, H. (Ed.). (2008). *Visual impairment: A global view.* New York: Oxford University Press.

Olver, F. (2007). *Dealing with vision loss.* Bloomington, IN: Author House.

6. Public Health

General Works

Aday, L. (Ed.). (2005). *Reinventing public health: Policies and practices for a healthy nation.* San Francisco, CA: Jossey-Bass.

Centers for Disease Control and Prevention. (1999, April 2). Ten great public health achievements—United States, 1900–1999. *Morbidity and Mortality Weekly Report (MMWR), 48*(12), 241–243. Retrieved from http://www.cdc .gov/mmwr/preview/mmwrhtml/00056796.htm
The article states that during the 20th century, public health efforts increased the average life span of Americans by 25 years. The most significant public health efforts included: vaccination; motor-vehicle safety; safer workplaces; control of infectious diseases; decline in deaths from coronary heart disease and stroke; safer and healthier foods; healthier mothers and babies; family planning; fluoridation of drinking water; and recognition of tobacco use as a health hazard.

Committee on Assuring the Health of the Public in the 21st Century, Board on Health Promotion and Disease Prevention. (2003). *The future of the public's health in the 21st century.* Washington, DC: National Academies Press. Retrieved from http://www.nap.edu/catalog/10548.html

Coreil, J. (Ed.). (2010). *Social and behavioral foundations of public health* (2nd ed.). Thousand Oaks, CA: Sage.

Turnock, B. J. (2009). *Public health: What it is and how it works* (4th ed.). Sudbury, MA: Jones and Bartlett.
This is the most widely used introductory textbook on public health.

Disability

Boyle, C., & Cordero, J. F. (2005, November). Birth defects and disabilities: A public health issue for the 21st century. *American Journal of Public Health, 95*(11), 1884–1886.

Drum, C. E., Krahn, G. L., & Bersani, H. (Eds.). (2009). *Disability and public health.* Washington, DC: American Public Health Association/American Association on Intellectual and Developmental Disabilities.

This edited book, which consists of 11 chapters on various public health areas related to disability, attempts to provide a common language and a framework to mount a public health response to disability.

Mont, D., & Loeb, M. (2008). *Beyond DALYs: Developing indicators to assess the impact of public health interventions on the lives of people with disabilities* (Social Protection and Labor Discussion Paper No. 0815). Washington, DC: World Bank. Retrieved from http://siteresource.worldbank.org/SOCIALPROTECTION/Resources/SP-Discussion-papers/Disability-DP/0815.pdf

Epidemiology

Fos, P. J. (2011). *Epidemiology foundations: The science of public health.* San Francisco, CA: Jossey-Bass.

Gordis, L. (2008). *Epidemiology* (4th ed.). Philadelphia, PA: Saunders.
This is one of the most widely used introductory textbooks on epidemiology.

McDermott, S., Moran, R. R., & Platt, T. (2008). *The epidemiology of common health conditions among adults with developmental disabilities in primary care.* New York: Nova Biomedical Books.

Merrill, R. M. (2010). *Introduction to epidemiology* (5th ed.). Sudbury, MA: Jones and Bartlett.

Morbidity and Mortality Weekly Report (MMWR).
This publication is available online at http://www.cdc.gov/mmwr. The MMWR is published by the Centers for Disease Control and Prevention (CDC). It contains data on specific infectious and chronic diseases, environmental hazards, natural or human-generated disasters, occupational diseases and injuries, and intentional and unintentional injuries. Also included are reports on topics of international interest and notices of events of interest to the public health community.

Health Disparities

Agency for Healthcare Research and Quality. (2009). *National healthcare disparities report, 2008.* Rockville, MD: Author. Retrieved from http://www.ahrq.gov/qual/nhdr08/nhdr08.pdf
The U.S. Congress mandates the Agency for Healthcare Research and Quality (AHRQ) to publish an annual report on national healthcare disparities. Chapter 4 of the report addresses the problems of individuals with disabilities or special care needs.

Barr, D. A. (2008). *Health disparities in the United States: Social class, race, ethnicity, and health.* Baltimore, MD: Johns Hopkins University Press.

Dunlop, D. D., Song, J., Manheim, L. M., et al. (2007, December). Racial/ethnic differences in the development of disability among older adults. *American Journal of Public Health, 97*(12), 2209–2215.

Kaiser Family Foundation (2008). *Eliminating racial/ethnic disparities in health care: What are the options?* Menlo Park, CA: Henry J. Kaiser Family Foundation. Retrieved from http://www.kff.org/minorityhealth/upload/7830.pdf

Libard, L. C. (2010). *Diabetes and health disparities: Community-based approaches for racial and ethnic populations.* New York: Springer.

Wallace, B. C. (Ed.). (2008). *Toward equity in health: A new global approach to health disparities.* New York: Springer.
This book contains papers from the first annual Health Disparities Conference, held in March 2006 at Columbia University, New York.

7. Clinical, Allied, and Other Health Professionals and Paraprofessionals

General Works

Cockerham, W. C. (2007). *Medical sociology.* Upper Saddle River, NJ: Pearson/Prentice Hall.
This popular medical sociology textbook provides a nice overview of the U.S. healthcare system.

French, S., & Swain, J. (2008). *Understanding disability: A guide for health professionals.* Philadelphia, PA: Churchill Livingstone/Elsevier.

Nuland, S. B. (2009). *The soul of medicine: Tales from the bedside.* New York: Kaplan.

Porter, R. (Ed.). (2006). *The Cambridge history of medicine.* New York: Cambridge University Press.

Straus, E., & Straus, A. (2006). *Medical marvels: The 100 greatest advances in medicine.* Amherst, NY: Prometheus Books.

Acupuncturists

Kidson, R. (2000). *Acupuncture for everyone: What it is, why it works, and how it can help you.* Rochester, VT: Inner Traditions International.

Maciocia, G. (2005). *The foundations of Chinese medicine: A comprehensive text for acupuncturists and herbalists* (2nd ed.). Philadelphia, PA: Churchill Livingstone.

Mann, F. (1973). *Acupuncture: The ancient Chinese art of healing and how it works scientifically.* New York: Vintage Books.

Chiropractors

Haldeman, S. (Ed.). (2005). *Principles and practice of chiropractic* (3rd ed.). New York: McGraw-Hill.

McDonald, W. P. (2003). *How chiropractors think and practice: The survey of North American chiropractors.* Ada, OH: Institute for Social Research, Ohio Northern University.

Wyatt, L. H. (2005). *Handbook of clinical chiropractic care* (2nd ed.). Sudbury, MA: Jones and Bartlett.

Home Health Aides and Personal and Home Care Aides

American Medical Association. (2001). *The American Medical Association guide to home caregiving.* New York: John Wiley.

Banister, K. R. (2007). *The personal care attendant guide: The art of finding, keeping, or being one.* New York: Demos Medical.

Fuzy, J., & Leahy, W. (2011). *The home health aide handbook* (3rd ed.). Albuquerque, NM: Hartman.

Marrelli, T. M. (2008). *Home health aide: Guidelines for care: Handbook for Caregiving at Home* (2nd ed.). Boca Grande, FL: Fineline Graphics.

Zucker, E. (2000). *Being a homemaker/home health aide* (4th ed.). Upper Saddle River, NJ: Prentice Hall.

Nurses

Chang, E., & Johnson, A. (Eds.). (2008). *Chronic illness and disability: Principles for nursing practice.* New York: Churchill Livingstone/Elsevier.

D'Antonio, P. (2010). *American nursing: A history of knowledge, authority, and the meaning of work.* Baltimore, MD: Johns Hopkins University Press.

Judd, D. M., Sitzman, K., & Davis, G. M. (2010). *A history of American nursing: Trends and eras.* Sudbury, MA: Jones and Bartlett.

Raghavan, R., & Patel, P. (2005). *Learning disabilities and mental health: A nursing perspective.* Malden, MA: Blackwell.

Occupational Therapists

Atchison, B. J., & Dirette, D. K. (2006). *Conditions in occupational therapy: Effect on occupational performance* (3rd ed.). Philadelphia, PA: Wolters Kluwer/Lippincott Williams and Wilkins.

Crepeau, E. B., Cohn, E. S., & Boyt-Schnell, B. A. (Eds.). (2008). *Willard and Spackman's occupational therapy* (11th ed.). Philadelphia, PA: Wolters Kluwer/ Lippincott Williams and Wilkins.

Radomski, M. V., & Trombly-Latham, C. A. (Eds.). (2008). *Occupational therapy for physical dysfunction* (6th ed.). Philadelphia, PA: Wolters Kluwer/Lippincott Williams and Wilkins.

Soderback, I. (Ed.). (2009). *International handbook of occupational therapy interventions*. New York: Springer.

Pharmacists

Kelly, W. N. (2002). *Pharmacy: What it is and how it works.* Boca Raton, FL: CRC Press.

Posey, L. M. (2009). *Pharmacy: An introduction to the profession* (2nd ed.). Washington, DC: American Pharmacists Association.

Physical Medicine and Rehabilitation

Braddom, R., & Buschbacher, R. M. (Eds.). (2007). *Physical medicine and rehabilitation*. Philadelphia, PA: Saunders/Elsevier.

Cameron, M. H. (2009). *Physical agents in rehabilitation: From research to practice* (3rd ed.). St. Louis, MO: Saunders/Elsevier.

Frontera, W. R., Silver, J. K., & Rizzo, Jr., T. D. (Eds.). (2008). *Essentials of physical medicine and rehabilitation: Musculoskeletal disorders, pain, and rehabilitation* (2nd ed.). Philadelphia, PA: Saunders/Elsevier.

Mpofu, E., & Oakland, T. (Eds.). (2010). *Rehabilitation and health assessment: Applying ICF guidelines*. New York: Springer.

O'Sullivan, S. B., & Schmitz, T. J. (2010). *Improving outcomes in physical rehabilitation*. Philadelphia, PA: F. A. Davis.

Ward, A. B., & Barnes, M. P. (2009). *Oxford handbook of clinical rehabilitation* (2nd ed.). New York: Oxford University Press.

Weiss, L., Weiss, J., & Pobre, T. (Eds.). (2010). *Oxford American handbook of physical medicine and rehabilitation*. New York: Oxford University Press.

Zaretsky, H. H., Richter III, E. F., & Eisenberg, M. G. (Eds.). (2005). *Medical aspects of disability: A handbook for the rehabilitation professional* (3rd ed.). New York: Springer.

Physical Therapists

Irion, J. M., & Irion, G. (2010). *Women's health in physical therapy*. Philadelphia, PA: Wolters Kluwer/Lippincott Williams and Wilkins.

Moffat, M., & Vickery, S. (1999). *The American physical therapy association book of body maintenance and repair*. New York: Henry Holt.

Pagliarulo, M. A. (2006). *Introduction to physical therapy* (3rd ed.). St. Louis, MO: Mosby/Elesvier.

Phillips, M. (2006). *Physical therapy the truth: For students, clinicians, and healthcare professionals*. Bloomington, IN: Author House.

Physicians

Berenyl, A. (Ed.). (2009). *Physician supply and demand*. Hauppauge, NY: Nova Science.

Bujak, J. S. (2008). *Inside the physician mind: Finding common ground with doctors*. Chicago, IL: Health Administration Press.

Fordyce, M. A. (2007). *2005 physician supply and distribution in rural areas of the United States*. Seattle: WWAMI Rural Health Research Center, University of Washington, School of Medicine, Department of Family Medicine.

Gutkind, L. (Ed.). (2010). *Becoming a doctor: From student to specialist: Doctor-writers share their experiences*. New York: W. W. Norton.

Hing, E., & Burt, C. W. (2007). *Characteristics of office-based physicians and their practices: United States, 2003–04* (Vital and Health Statistics Series 13, No. 164. DHHS Pub. No. PHS 2007–1735). Hyattsville, MD: National Center for Health Statistics. Retrieved from http://www.cdc.gov/nchs/data/series/sr_13/sr13_164.pdf

Hoff, T. (2010). *Practice under pressure: Primary care physicians and their medicine in the twenty-first century*. New Brunswick, NJ: Rutgers University Press.

Kirkcaldy, B. D., Shephard, R. J., & Siefen, R. G. (2009). *The making of a good doctor*. Hauppauge, NY: Nova Science.

Rowe, L., & Kidd, M. (2009). *First do no harm: Being a resilient doctor in the 21st century*. New York: McGraw-Hill.

8. Healthcare Organizations

General Works

Barton, P. L. (2010). *Understanding the U.S. health services system* (4th ed.). Chicago: Health Administration Press/Association of University Programs in Health Administration.

Shi, L., & Singh, D. A. (2008). *Delivering health care in America: A systems approach* (4th ed.). Sudbury, MA: Jones and Bartlett.

Hospitals

American Hospital Association. (2009). *AHA guide to the health care field 2010: United States hospitals, health care systems, networks, alliances, health organizations, agencies, providers.* Chicago: American Hospital Association/Health Forum. *This is an annual publication that lists the characteristics of individual hospitals by city and state.*

American Hospital Association. (2009). *AHA hospital statistics 2010: The comprehensive reference sources for analysis and comparison of hospital trends.* Chicago: American Hospital Association/Health Forum.

Risse, G. B. (1999). *Mending bodies, saving souls: A history of hospitals.* New York: Oxford University Press.

Rosenberg, C. E. (1995). *The care of strangers: The rise of America's hospital system.* Baltimore, MD: Johns Hopkins University Press.

Nursing Homes and Long-Term Care

Baker, B. (2007). *Old age in a new age: The promise of transformative nursing homes.* Nashville, TN: Vanderbilt University Press.

Evashwick, C. J. (2005). *The continuum of long-term care* (3rd ed.). Clifton Park, NY: Thomas Delmar Learning.

Harris, M. (Ed.). (2009). *Handbook of home care administration* (5th ed.). Sudbury, MA: Jones and Bartlett.

Houser, A., Fox-Grage, W., & Gibson, M. J. (2009). *Across the states: Profiles of long-term care and independent living* (8th ed.). Washington, DC: AARP Public Policy Institute. Retrieved from http://assets.aarp.org/rgcenter/il/d19105_2008_ats.pdf

Jones, A. L., Dwyer, L. L., Bercovitz, A. R., et al. (2009). *The national nursing home survey: 2004 overview* (Vital and Health Statistics, Series 13, No. 167. DHHS

Pub. No. PHS 2009-1738). Hyattsville, MD: National Center for Health Statistics. Retrieved from http://www.cdc.gov/nchs/data/series/sr_13/sr13_167.pdf

Kane, R., Kane, R., & Ladd, R. (1998). *The heart of long-term care.* New York: Oxford University Press.

Pratt, J. R. (2010). *Long-term care: Managing across the continuum* (3rd ed.). Sudbury, MA: Jones and Bartlett.

Wilson, K. B. (2007). Historical evolution of assisted living in the United States, 1979 to the present. *Gerontologist, 47*(Spec. No. 3), 8–22.

Zimmerman, S., Sloane, P., & Eckert, J. (Eds.). (2001). *Assisted living: Needs, practices, and policies in residential care for the elderly.* Baltimore, MD: Johns Hopkins University Press.

9. Problems Experienced by People With Disability

General Works

Hanson, K., Neuman, T., & Voris, M. (2003). *Understanding the health-care needs and experiences of people with disabilities: Findings from a 2003 survey.* Menlo Park, CA: Henry J. Kaiser Family Foundation. Retrieved from http://www.kff.org/medicare/6106.cfm

National Organization on Disability. (2004). *National Organization on Disability/Harris 2004 survey of Americans with disabilities: Final report* (Harris Study No. 20835). New York: Harris Interactive. Retrieved from http://www.nod.org/_uploads/documents/live/harris2004_rpt.pdf

Reis, J. P., Breslin, M. L., Iezzoni, L. I ., et al. (2004). *It takes more than ramps to solve the crisis of healthcare for people with disabilities.* Chicago: Rehabilitation Institute of Chicago. Retrieved from http://www.dredf.org/healthcare/RIC_whitepaperfinal.pdf

Wittenburg, D. (2004). *A health-conscious safety net? Health problems and program use Among low-income adults with disabilities.* Washington, DC: Urban Institute. Retrieved from http://www.urban.org/url.cfm?ID=311065

Access to Healthcare

Buss, T. F., & Van de Water, P. N. (Eds.). (2009). *Expanding access to health care: A management approach.* Armonk, NY: M. E. Sharpe.

Clancy, C. M., & Andresen, E. M. (2002). Meeting the health care needs of persons with disabilities. *Milbank Quarterly, 80*(2), 381–391.

Iezzoni, L. I., Killeen, M. B., & O'Day, B. L. (2006, August). Rural residents with disabilities confront substantial barriers to obtaining primary care. *Health Services Research, 41*(4 Pt. 1), 1258–1275.

Jha, A., Patrick, D. L., MacLehose, R. F., et al. (2002, October). Dissatisfaction with medical services among medicare beneficiaries with disabilities. *Archives of Physical Medicine and Rehabilitation, 83*(10), 1335–1341.

The authors conclude "Disability is a significant independent risk factor for dissatisfaction with health care in the Medicare population. Efforts should be made to identify individuals with ADL [activities of daily living] difficulties and to improve their ease and convenience of getting to a doctor, the availability of care off hours, the access to specialists, and the follow-up care received."

Kirschner, K. L., Breslin, M. L., & Iezzoni, L. I. (2007, March 14). Structural impairments that limit access to health care for patients with disabilities. *Journal of the American Medical Association, 297*(10), 1121–1125.

Communication

Chew, K. L., Iacono, T., & Tracy, J. (2009, January–February). Overcoming communication barriers: Working with patients with intellectual disabilities. *Australian Family Physician, 38*(1–2), 10–14.

Iezzoni, L. I. (2006, Fall). Make no assumptions: Communication between persons with disabilities and clinicians. *Assistive Technology, 18*(2), 212–229.

Employment and Health Insurance

Dejong, G., Palsbo, S. E., Beatty, P. W., et al. (2002). The organization and financing of health services for persons with disabilities. *Milbank Quarterly, 80*(2), 261–301.

DeNavas-Walt, C., Proctor, B. D., & Smith, J. C. (2009). *Income, poverty, and health insurance coverage in the United States: 2008.* Washington, DC: U.S. Census Bureau. Retrieved from http://www.census.gov/prod/2009pubs/p60–236.pdf

Patterson, A. C. (Ed.). (2009). *Financial incentives for Americans with disabilities.* Hauppauge, NY: Nova Science.

Prevention

Balzi, D., Lauretani, F., Barchielli, A., et al. (2010, January). Risk factors for disability in older persons over 3-year follow-up. *Age and Aging, 39*(1), 92–98.

Kass-Bartelmes, B. L. (2002, April). Preventing disability in the elderly with chronic disease. *AHRQ Research in Action,* Issue #3. Retrieved from http://www.ahrq.gov/research/elderdis.pdf

Sinclair, S. A., & Xiang, H. (2008, August). Injuries among U.S. children with different types of disabilities. *American Journal of Public Health, 98*(8), 1510–1516.

Quality of Care

Iezzoni, L. I., Davis, R. B., Soukup, J., et al. (2003, September 22). Quality dimensions that most concern people with physical and sensory disabilities. *Archives of Internal Medicine, 163*(17), 2085–2092.

Lawthers, A. G., Pransky, G. S., Peterson, L. E., et al. (2003, August). Rethinking quality in the context of persons with disability. *International Journal for Quality in Health Care, 15*(4), 287–299.

Stigma and Discrimination

Goffman, E. (1963). *Stigma: Notes on the management of a spoiled identity.* Englewood Cliffs, NJ: Prentice-Hall.
This book is considered a classic work on stigma. It conceptualizes and presents a widely used framework for the study of stigma.

Green, G. (2009). *The end of stigma? Changes in the social experience of long term illness.* New York: Routledge.

Green, S. E. (2003, October). What do you mean "What's wrong with her?" Stigma and the lives of families of children with disabilities. *Social Science and Medicine, 57*(8), 1361–1374.

Hinshaw, S. P. (2007). *The mark of shame: Stigma of mental illness and an agenda for change.* New York: Oxford University Press.

Link, B., & Phalen, J. (2001). Conceptualizing stigma. *Annual Review of Sociology, 27*, 363–385.

Mason, T., Carlisle, C., Watkins C., & Whitehead, E. (Eds.). (2001). *Stigma and social exclusion in healthcare.* New York: Routledge.

Scambler, G. (2009, April). Health-related stigma. *Sociology of health and illness, 31*(3), 441–455.

Switzer, J. V. (2003). *Disabled rights: American disability policy and the fight for equality.* Washington, DC: Georgetown University Press.

Turner, D. M., & Stagg, K. (Eds.). (2006). *Social histories of disability and deformity.* New York: Routledge.

Van Brakel, W. H. (2006, August). Measuring health-related stigma: A literature review. *Psychology, Health, and Medicine, 11*(3), 307–334.

Glossary of Key Terms

Accountable Care Organization (ACO)   An emerging model of healthcare network that helps patients better coordinate and manage their care.

ACO   *See* Accountable Care Organization

Acquired Immunodeficiency Syndrome   *See* HIV/AIDS

Activities of Daily Living (ADLs)   A term used in healthcare to describe daily self-care tasks such as feeding, bathing, dressing, and grooming; the ability to perform ADLs provides a measurement of an individual's levels of disability and functioning.

Acute Diseases   Illnesses and conditions that are generally of short duration, sometimes curable, and often self-limiting; examples include the common cold, the flu (influenza), and sore throat.

ADA   *See* Americans with Disabilities Act of 1990

ADHD   *See* Attention Deficit Hyperactivity Disorder

ADLs   *See* Activities of Daily Living

AIDS   *See* HIV/AIDS

AIMS/AIMS2   *See* Arthritis Impact Measurement Scales

Allied Health Professionals   A term that describes clinical health professionals who are not physicians, nurses, or pharmacists; examples of the more than 100 occupational titles in this category include dental hygienists, dietitians, respiratory therapists, and speech language pathologists.

ALS   *See* Amyotrophic Lateral Sclerosis

Americans with Disabilities Act of 1990 (ADA)   A federal civil rights statute that creates broad legal protection for people with disabilities; it affects access to employment, government programs and services, places of public accommodation, transportation, and telecommunications.

Amyotrophic Lateral Sclerosis (ALS)   Often referred to as Lou Gehrig's disease, this degenerative disease of the nerve cells in the brain and spinal cord is associated with a high degree of disability.

Arthritis Impact Measurement Scales (AIMS/AIMS2)   An assessment used to measure the physical, social, and emotional well-being of patients with rheumatic diseases.

ASD   *See* Autism Spectrum Disorders

Attention Deficit Hyperactivity Disorder (ADHD)   A developmental disorder characterized by chronic and impairing behavior patterns that involve diminished attention, impulsivity, hyperactivity, or their combination.

Autism Spectrum Disorders (ASD)   A set of five pervasive developmental disorders that appear in early childhood and are characterized by varying degrees of impairment in communication skills and social interactions, as well as by patterns of restricted, repetitive, and stereotyped behavior.

CAM   *See* Complementary and Alternative Medicine

CCRC   *See* Continuing Care Retirement Community

Chronic Diseases   Illnesses and conditions that are generally of long duration, progressive, and not cured once they are acquired; examples include arthritis, diabetes, and heart disease.

Chronic Obstructive Pulmonary Disease (COPD)   A group of diseases—including emphysema, chronic bronchitis, and in some cases asthma—that cause airflow blockage and breathing-related problems; COPD is a leading cause of illness, disability, and death in the United States.

CLASS   *See* Community Living Assistance Services and Supports

Clinical Health Professionals   Professionals such as physicians, nurses, and pharmacists who examine and treat individual patients or clients, including those with disabilities.

Community Living Assistance Services and Supports (CLASS)   Established under the Patient Protection and Affordable Care Act (PPACA), this voluntary national long-term care insurance program provides individuals with a cash benefit if they have functional limitations or disability.

Complementary and Alternative Medicine (CAM)   A term used to describe a group of diverse medical practitioners and healthcare systems and products—such as chiropractors and acupuncturists—that are not usually considered part of conventional medicine, as it is practiced by physicians, nurses, pharmacists, and allied health professionals.

Condition-Specific Outcome Measures   Diagnostic, physiologic, cognitive, and functional assessments and evaluations of quality of life that focus on specific health conditions and are used to inform clinical decisions and the provision of services; examples include the Arthritis Impact Measurement Scales (AIMS/AIMS2), Disabilities of the Arm, Shoulder, and Hand (DASH) Outcome Measure, and Kurtzke Expanded Disability Status Scale (EDSS).

Continuing Care Retirement Community (CCRC)   Sometimes referred to as a life-care community, this type of residential facility provides residents with access to three levels of housing and care in one location: independent living, assisted living, and skilled nursing home care.

COPD   *See* Chronic Obstructive Pulmonary Disease

DALY   *See* Disability-Adjusted Life Years

DASH   *See* Disabilities of the Arm, Shoulder, and Hand Outcome Measure

DD   *See* Developmental Disabilities

Developmental Disabilities (DD)   A diverse group of severe chronic conditions that originate at birth or during childhood and usually last throughout a person's lifetime; categories of DD include nervous system disabilities, sensory-related disabilities, metabolic disorders, and degenerative disorders.

Disabilities of the Arm, Shoulder, and Hand (DASH) Outcome Measure   A self-administered questionnaire that assesses the physical function and symptoms for several musculoskeletal disorders of the upper limbs.

Disability   An evolving concept that results from the interaction between persons with impairments and attitudinal and environmental barriers that hinder their full and effective participation in society on an equal basis with others.

Disability-Adjusted Life Years (DALY)   A summary measure created by the World Health Organization (WHO) to represent the burden of disease in terms of years of life lost due to either disability or premature death.

Donabedian Model   A framework that uses the components of structure, process, and outcome to measure the quality of healthcare.

Dual Eligibility   A term used to describe individuals who are eligible for federal healthcare coverage under both the Medicare and Medicaid programs; Medicare covers their acute care services, while Medicaid covers their Medicare premiums, cost sharing, and long-term care services.

EDSS   *See* Kurtzke Expanded Disability Status Scale

Function   The normal physiological action or activity of a body part, organ, or system.

Functional Model of Disability   A conceptual model that focuses primarily on the expression of disability, such as the inability of an individual to perform a number of functional activities; it stresses the adoption of treatment regimens, strategies, and services that improve functional capacity rather than exclusively addressing the underlying condition or impairment.

Gehrig's Disease, Lou   *See* Amyotrophic Lateral Sclerosis

HCERA   *See* Health Care and Education Reconciliation Act

Health Care and Education Reconciliation Act (HCERA)   Also known as P.L. 111-152, this 2010 legislation amended portions of the Patient Protection and Affordable Care Act (PPACA) and combined it with the Student Aid and Fiscal Responsibility Act (SAFRA).

Healthcare Organizations   Facilities such as community hospitals, rehabilitation centers, nursing homes, and home healthcare agencies that provide a wide array of services across the life span of individuals with disabilities.

Health Services Research   A multidisciplinary field that focuses on the study of the access, costs, quality, and outcomes of healthcare services.

Healthy Life Expectancy (HLE)   A summary measure of the expected number of remaining years of life spent in good health from a particular age, assuming current rates of mortality and morbidity.

HIV/AIDS   HIV (human immunodeficiency virus) is the virus that causes AIDS (acquired immunodeficiency syndrome). HIV attacks the body's immune system; AIDS is the final stage of HIV infection, when the virus has weakened a person's immune system to the point at which the body has a difficult time fighting infection.

HLE   *See* Healthy Life Expectancy

Human Immunodeficiency Virus   *See* HIV/AIDS

ICC   *See* Interagency Coordinating Council on Emergency Preparedness and Individuals with Disabilities

ICF   *See* Intermediate Care Facility; International Classification of Functioning, Disability, and Health

ICF/DD   *See* Intermediate Care Facility for the Developmentally Disabled

Impairment   Any loss, abnormality, or disturbance of psychological, physiological, or anatomical structure or function that interferes with normal activities and may be temporary or permanent.

Integrated Models of Disability   Any of a number of conceptual models that attempt to integrate various components of the medical, functional, and social models of disability.

Interagency Coordinating Council on Emergency Preparedness and Individuals with Disabilities (ICC)   Established by President George W. Bush in 2004, the ICC coordinates the activities of 23 federal departments and agencies to support the safety and security of individuals with disabilities in all types of emergency situations.

Intermediate Care Facility (ICF)   A facility that provides care for individuals who are recovering from acute medical conditions but who do not need continuous care or daily therapeutic services.

Intermediate Care Facility for the Developmentally Disabled (ICF/DD)   A type of residential facility certified by Medicare and Medicaid that provides a wide variety of services for the complex needs of intellectual and developmentally disabled individuals who also have significant physical impairments and need 24-hour nursing care.

International Classification of Functioning, Disability, and Health (ICF)   Released in 2001 by the World Health Organization (WHO), this conceptual model of disability integrates the medical and social models; it views disability and functioning as outcomes of the interactions between health conditions and contextual factors.

Kurtzke Expanded Disability Status Scale (EDSS)   A widely used outcome measure of multiple sclerosis (MS).

Lou Gehrig's Disease   *See* Amyotrophic Lateral Sclerosis

MD   *See* Muscular Dystrophy

Medicaid   Established under Title XIX of the Social Security Act, this federal-state program provides health insurance for individuals and families with low incomes and limited resources; it covers children, the elderly, blind, and/or the disabled.

Medical Model of Disability   A conceptual model that focuses on diseases, injuries, and conditions that impair the physiological or cognitive functioning of an individual; it defines disability as a condition or deficit that resides within the individual and can be cured or ameliorated, or its progression stopped, through a treatment or a particular intervention.

Medicare   Created under Title XVIII of the Social Security Act, this federal government program provides healthcare coverage for elderly Americans and individuals with certain disabilities; it consists of Part A (hospital insurance), Part B (medical insurance), Part C (managed-care plans), and Part D (prescription drug coverage).

MS   *See* Multiple Sclerosis

Multiple Sclerosis (MS)   A progressive neurodegenerative disease characterized by inflammation, destruction, and scarring of cells that protect the neurons in the central nervous system; it is one of the most common disabling neurological diseases in young people.

Muscular Dystrophy (MD)   A group of more than 30 inherited diseases that causes slow, progressive muscle weakness; the main types of MD include Duchenne, Becker, limb-girdle, faciosapulohumeral, oculopharyngeal, and myotonic dystrophy.

Paratransit   Also known as "dial-a-ride," this type of public transportation provides individualized rides without fixed routes or schedules for people whose disabilities make it unfeasible for them to use the fixed routes within the transit system.

Patient Protection and Affordable Care Act (PPACA)   Also known as P.L. 111-148, this sweeping 2010 healthcare reform legislation requires that all Americans have health insurance; bars health insurance companies from discriminating based on pre-existing medical conditions, health status, or gender; prohibits lifetime limits on coverage; prohibits rescission (dropping) of customers by insurers; creates insurance exchanges; requires employers with 50 workers or more to offer health insurance benefits or pay a fee; expands Medicaid and provides premium assistance; and creates temporary insurance pools for consumers with pre-existing conditions until insurance exchanges open in 2014.

Physiatrist   A physician who specializes in physical medicine and rehabilitation (PM&R); the primary role of the physiatrist is to manage a patient's medical issues as the patient participates in the rehabilitation process.

Physical Medicine and Rehabilitation (PM&R)   Also referred to as rehabilitation medicine, this specialty is concerned with evaluating, diagnosing, and treating patients with physical disabilities; subspecialties include hospice and palliative medicine, neuromuscular medicine, pain medicine, pediatric rehabilitation medicine, spinal cord injury medicine, and sports medicine.

PM&R   *See* Physical Medicine and Rehabilitation

PPCA   *See* Patient Protection and Affordable Care Act

Public Health Professionals   Professionals such as scientists and researchers, health educators, public policymakers, public health physicians, public health nurses, occupational health and safety professionals, social workers, sanitarians, and nutritionists who work to prevent disease and promote health within groups of people, from small communities to entire countries.

QALY   *See* Quality-Adjusted Life Years

Quality-Adjusted Life Years (QALY)   A summary measure of disease burden that includes both the quality and quantity of life.

Skilled Nursing Facility (SNF)   A facility that provides short-term nursing and rehabilitation care, generally to assist individuals during their recovery following hospitalization for acute medical conditions.

SNF   *See* Skilled Nursing Facility

Social Model of Disability   A conceptual model that focuses on the barriers an individual with disabilities faces when interacting with the environment; it defines disability as a problem that lies primarily outside the individual, in the lack of accommodations in the surrounding environment and in the negative attitudes of people without disabilities.

Social Security Disability Insurance (SSDI)   A federal government program that provides wage replacement income for individuals who have worked and paid Social Security taxes and become disabled according to Social Security criteria; its benefits are paid to disabled workers, their widows, widowers, and children, and eligible adults disabled since childhood.

SSDI   *See* Social Security Disability Insurance

SSI   *See* Supplemental Security Income

Summary Measures   A measurement that combines mortality, morbidity, and other social and personal attributes using several different methods to represent overall population health in a single number; examples include disability-adjusted life years (DALY), quality-adjusted life years (QALY), and healthy life expectancy (HLE).

Supplemental Security Income (SSI)   A federal government income supplement program that is designed to help low-income people who are elderly, blind, or disabled meet their basic needs for food, clothing, and shelter.

TBI   *See* Traumatic Brain Injury

Ticket to Work and Work Incentives Improvement Act of 1999 (TWWIIA)   A federal government program intended to help pave avenues to employment for people with disabilities; it also allows people with disabilities to maintain Medicare eligibility for four additional years.

Traumatic Brain Injury (TBI)   An injury caused by a blow or jolt to the head or a penetrating head injury that disrupts the normal function of the brain; TBI can cause a wide range of functional changes affecting thinking, sensation, language, and/or emotions.

TWWIIA   *See* Ticket to Work and Work Incentives Improvement Act of 1999

Universal Design   The concept of designing all products and environments to be usable to the greatest extent possible by everyone, regardless of their age, ability, or status in life.

Veterans Health Administration (VHA)   The component of the U.S. Department of Veterans Affairs (VA) that provides medical care and services for U.S. veterans with disabilities.

VHA   *See* Veterans Health Administration

Index

Osteoporosis, 14, 303
"Other diseases/conditions"
    category, 9
OTs (occupational therapists), 29–30,
    262–263, 309
Outcome measures, 63–70, 110

PAHO (Pan American Health
    Organization), 126, 206
Pan American Health Organization
    (PAHO), 107, 126, 206, 287
Paraprofessionals, 32–33, 307
Paratransit services, 50
Parkinson's disease, 14, 93, 303
Pasteur, Louis, 101, 103, 186–188
Patient Protection and Affordable Care
    Act (PPACA), 70–76, 151–152
Patient safety, 63
PCPID (President's Committee for
    People with Intellectual
    Disabilities), 283–284
Pellegra, 112
Penicillin, 116, 120, 124, 164–165
Personal and home care aides,
    32–33, 308
Pharmaceutical Research and
    Manufacturers of America
    (PhRMA), 265
Pharmacies/pharmacists, 28–29, 90,
    93, 129, 268, 309
Phenylketonuria (PKU), 130
Philanthropies, 268–273
PhRMA (Pharmaceutical Research and
    Manufacturers of America), 265
PHS (Public Health Service), 91–92
Physiatrists, 27, 119, 260
Physical diseases/conditions
    category, 9, 10–15
Physical medicine, 118
Physical medicine and rehabilitation
    (PM&R), 26–27
    biographies of key contributors,
        176–177
    historical highlights, 119, 121, 127
    organizations, 260, 287
    resources, 309–310

Physical rehabilitation and
    occupational health services,
    237–241
Physical therapy, 29, 30–31,
    114, 263, 310
Physicians, 24–26, 128, 224,
    259–260, 310
Physician-to-population
    ratios, 224–227
Physiotherapy, 113
Pinel, Philippe, 188–189
PKU (phenylketonuria), 130
Plagues, 84, 85
Planned Parenthood, 198–199
PM&R. *See* Physical medicine and
    rehabilitation (PM&R)
Policy organizations, 265–267
Polio
    biographies of key
        contributors, 196–197
    historical highlights, 112, 114,
        116, 120, 125, 126–127,
        129, 141, 144
Polytrauma, 37
PPACA (Patient Protection and
    Affordable Care Act),
    70–76, 151–152
Preexisting conditions, 71, 73
Preferred provider organizations
    (PPO), 261
President's Committee for People
    with Intellectual Disabilities
    (PCPID), 283–284
Prevention, 63, 313–314
Primary care physicians, 25–26
Private organizations, 208
Private transportation, 49
Process measures of healthcare, 63, 64
Professional/trade associations,
    259–265
Psychiatry
    biographies of key contributors,
        172–173, 192–193
    historical highlights, 85, 90–91,
        93, 96
    hospitals for, 35